EXERCISE PROGRESSION FOR LOW BACK DISORDERS

A PROFESSIONAL'S MANUAL

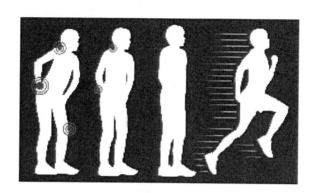

WWW.THENIHS.COM

ISBN 978-1-4276-3327-9

Preface

This book began as I was working with spinal rehabilitation clients and needing some sort of handout to give them to ensure that they would do their exercises and "homework" while away from the clinic. Little did I know how far this need would take me. As a personal trainer, massage therapist, and medical exercise specialist working with doctors and the like, I quickly learned how different the two schools of thought are on exercising with injuries and pain. I decided it was my duty to utilize my own experiences to help bridge this gap of "not enough exercise" on one side and "too much exercise" on the other. It is my goal with this manual to build a common understanding in our professional community of terms, anatomy, injury mechanisms, and exercise concepts for those with low back pain. This manual can be used by chiropractors, physical therapists, personal trainers, massage therapists, and other like-minded professionals with the common goal of improving low back pain through exercise and lifestyle changes. The level of skill necessary to implement the assessments and programs of Exercise Progression is high. It takes many years of experience, training and working with people before these concepts can be understood and applied safely. That is why The National Institute of Health Specialists (NIHS) has created a training program (see following pages) that will ensure the proper use of this manual. I applaud you for your dedication on this road to helping others and wish you the best of luck in improving the most prevalent pain disorder our society has; low back pain.

CHRIS HALLFORD

President, NIHS

Forward

There has always been a large divide between Health Care Professionals and Fitness Professionals. However both of these professions deal with a common client, that is one that has some form of Low Back complaint.

What Chris Hallford does throughout this book is cover in detail the topic of Low Back Disorders, and what exercises, slow progressions and assessments can be used when dealing with this population for the Health Care Professional to the Personal Trainer. Getting all of these professions together with the same understanding, the same terminology and the same approach to helping the client is essential and Chris does this incredibly well. From stretching protocols, the anatomy and physiology, full body assessments to the exercises and movement prescription, every component is covered to allow the professional a full understanding of what causes and what helps alleviate Low Back Pain.

I recommend this book to any professional dealing with clients with any form of mild low back issues, which today is almost everyone at some stage within their life cycle. This is the first brave step to truly integrating the different professionals within the Health and Fitness industry and I applaud Chris for creating such a thorough yet easy to follow guide in this book Exercise Progression, Low Back Disorders.

Recommend this to every Health and Fitness Professional you know.

RICHARD BOYD

Co Founder, Personal Training on the Net
Largest educational resource for fitness professionals in the world

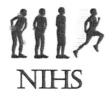

**National Institute of
Health Specialists**

About

Our focus at NIHS is to help as many people as we can reach their potential in the arenas of health, fitness, and pain relief. We do this by a) training professionals in our methods and systems, and b) seeing clients at various locations. Our methods and courses consist of three components;

    1) Pain Release Techniques - PRT   2) Exercise training   3) Health coaching.

Each of these follows a system that is laid out in their corresponding books or manuals. The combination of these three components makes for a professional that is able to help a wide variety of people. This new type of health professional is one that is capable of restoring function and self-reliance in non-acute clients and patients. Our goal is to empower and reduce the growing population that is wandering around between "specialists" with no clear direction for their ailments.
We achieve this by incorporating the following modalities.

- Cutting edge assessments that get to the root of each ailment.
- Post-rehabilitation exercise for the spine, shoulder, elbow, knee, hip, foot, and hand.
- Post-rehabilitation PRT for all injuries, aches, and pains.
- PRT for stress relief and general aches and pains.
- Corrective exercise programs for general aches and pains.
- Exercise programs for those seeking weight loss, increased energy, and improved health.
- Sports specific training for athletes of all levels.
- Health coaching for all who seek health.
- Continuing education credits (CEC's) through courses, workbooks, videos, and workshops for personal trainers and massage therapists.

Mission

To lead the way in creating a new type of health professional while giving our clients and students the highest level of care and direction available

Purpose

To help people live to their potential

Values

- Evidence
- Excellence
- Leadership
- Results

Vision

To enhance the medical community by creating a health professional that is able to significantly impact the lives of those in pain and poor health

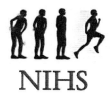

NIHS

The Programs

Injury Exercise Specialist

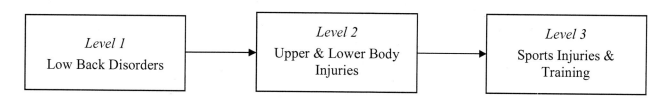

| *Level 1*
 Low Back Disorders | → | *Level 2*
 Upper & Lower Body Injuries | → | *Level 3*
 Sports Injuries & Training |

Soft Tissue Specialist

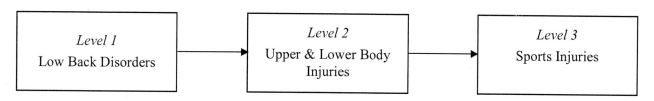

| *Level 1*
 Low Back Disorders | → | *Level 2*
 Upper & Lower Body Injuries | → | *Level 3*
 Sports Injuries |

Health Coach

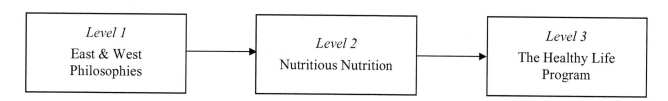

| *Level 1*
 East & West Philosophies | → | *Level 2*
 Nutritious Nutrition | → | *Level 3*
 The Healthy Life Program |

POST-GRADUATE TRAINING

Pain & Injury Specialist

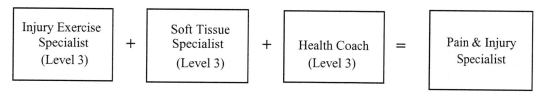

Injury Exercise Specialist (Level 3) + Soft Tissue Specialist (Level 3) + Health Coach (Level 3) = Pain & Injury Specialist

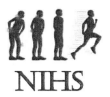

NIHS

Injury Exercise Specialist

Level 1: Low Back Disorders

A level 1 graduate is someone who is able to handle any type of low back disorder client; whether it's creating an exercise program or referring them to the appropriate specialist. This professional will be in high demand and have the ability to work with doctors and surgeons alike to ensure the proper care for every client.

While most professionals can take the pre-requisites, only those with at least five years of related experience can go on to the mentorship program and therefore graduate.

Level 1 Program

A) Pre-requisites
- Workshops &/or videos
- Workbook test

B) Mentorship Program
- Workshops
- Correspondence classes
- Case studies
- Homework assignments

C) Final Exam
- Written
- Hands-on

List of Competencies

- Identify red flags and contraindications to exercise for low back pain (LBP) clients.
- Learn clinical anatomy and pathology mechanisms of low back disorders (LBD).
- Learn how to assess and find the root cause of LBP by using clinically proven methods in ROM, posture, muscle testing, pain patterns, and more.
- Learn an exercise system that is evidence based and clinically proven to improve LBP and its recurrence.
- Learn how to design individualized exercise programs for LBP clients by utilizing 1) assessment findings, 2) contraindications guidelines, and 3) a systematized exercise program.
- Learn how to identify and design programs for nine different LBD.
- Learn how to keep clients motivated and educated with handouts.
- Learn how to stretch LBP clients safely.
- Learn how to assess CORE function.
- Learn which muscles cause specific dysfunctions and postural distortions affecting the low back.
- Learn how to improve specific dysfunctions and imbalances throughout the kinetic chain with exercises, stretches and daily activity modifications (D.A.M's).
- Learn the necessary D.A.M's associated with LBP.
- Learn the six components to every successful exercise program.
- Learn when to refer to a licensed professional.
- Learn how to establish referral-based relationships in the medical community.
- Learn the scope of practice for a level one graduate.

Dedication

To my mom,

who taught me that the best way to help myself

is through helping others, unconditionally.

Acknowledgments

Life has blessed me with the experience of my own chronic low back pain, injuries in every major joint, a 25 year sports career, working with spinal clinics and doctor's offices, amazing mentors in Toby Hansen (acupuncturist, applied kinesiology specialist, philosopher, and bodyworker), Steven Collins (sports chiropractor), Thomas Santucci (chiropractor, applied kinesiology specialist, Ph. D), many more physical therapists, personal trainers, psychologists, and chiropractors I have got to work with and ask an overwhelming amount of questions to, and of course the thousands of clients that have turned my job into my passion.

A special thanks to Mike Baxter and Charlie Provance for being at my disposal and taking thousands of pictures over many days to capture all of the images you see in this manual. Also to Primal Pictures for their amazing anatomy images that enhance the learning process.

CONTENTS

Volume I

Part I The Components

Part II The Low Back

Part III The Exercise Programs

Part IV Appendix

SPECIFIC CONTENTS

Volume I

Muscles

Boxes, Tables, & Figures

Chapter 1 Exercise Progression

Exercise Progression aims to bridge the gap between health care and fitness professionals by educating and creating a progressive and systematic exercise program that not only improves strength, power, endurance, flexibility, balance, coordination, cardiovascular health, percentage of lean body mass, and exercise knowledge, but also post-rehabilitates injuries, decreases pain, improves daily functioning, and prepares the body for whatever activity it wishes to engage in.

The diversity of Exercise Progression makes it useful for personal trainers, physical therapists, chiropractors, and doctors alike who wish to encourage active care for aches and pains or progress someone to an elite level of fitness.

This is a necessary change from the non-specific exercise routines found in most programs that build strength in one dimension only, basically training the body to sit, stand, or lay in place while lifting, pushing, pulling, bending, extending, or twisting (rarely) against resistance, oftentimes causing repetitive microtraumas and strains and encouraging poor posture.

A middle ground needs to be found that combines the all too common under-active and non-specific exercise programs prescribed in general health care and the over-active or inappropriate exercise programs utilized in the general fitness environment.

This requires an exchange of knowledge between doctors and fitness professionals regarding the treatment philosophies of certain dysfunctions. Collaboration between the different schools of thought will ensure a more complete treatment plan for each person, as well as encourage active care.

In order to reach a common ground, fitness professionals must learn new terminology, post-rehabilitation protocols, legalities, paperwork, and an entirely different training philosophy than the general fitness approach offers.

This manual was created to enhance this alliance by educating about anatomy, injury mechanisms, biomechanics, exercise contraindications, how to efficiently progress exercises, and the difference between health and fitness. A full understanding of body mechanics and a detailed assessment is essential to helping most people and hurting no one, rather than helping some and hurting some by playing the odds

with a general protocol regimen. Designing a specific program from x-rays, MRI's, and evaluations is ideal. Once the problem is found, or narrowed down, a list of do's and don'ts can be made, and then appropriate exercises from any approach may be used to progress the person towards health. ***A program is only as good as the assessment.***

In regards to low back pain (LBP), there are many treatment programs that claim to reduce LBP. This is not very impressive when considering the large studies which showed LBP (no neurological symptoms) has a natural healing course that normally resolves itself within four weeks regardless of the treatment.[147,156,157]

In other words, just about any treatment method can seem effective in the right situation. Unfortunately, these methods usually do not produce beneficial results in the long run.

Exercise Progression will utilize an exercise program that is proven to achieve long-term results for LBP sufferers, such as reduced recurrence of LBP.

Exercise Progression consists of six components that are progressed together in four different phases and can be used to post-rehabilitate or progress someone to a level of fitness suitable for almost any situation.

Success is dependent upon utilization of all six components, although two more components, manual therapy and nutrition, are often necessary to improve certain situations.

Manual therapy is not necessary for everyone and is thus not considered a main component, but it should always be considered a factor in improvement. Nutrition details are also out of the scope of this text, although a brief questionnaire on nutrition should always be part of a professional's "tool box."

Creating an exercise program without thorough evaluation can lead to debilitation instead of rehabilitation. The key to exercising is to be able to affect the way the body functions statically and dynamically in a positive manner in all aspects of health: balance, coordination, posture, flexibility, cardiovascular, strength, immune system, etc.

Many subacute and chronic pain or injury exercise programs focus on functional restoration as a means for pain relief and prevention of recurrences. In this manual, corrective exercise will be the foundation of the exercise program, post-rehabilitative or not, in order to improve the potential for functional restoration.

The word "functional" implies utilization of the neuromuscular system, but this system operates at decreased levels if postural distortions or pain exist.

Therefore, if functional activities are restored in a person that has musculoskeletal imbalances or pain, then the restoration of function will be limited, like building a new house on an uneven foundation.

An exception where functional training may proceed if major imbalances still exist is when the training can be done without compensating, or immediate restoration of function is a priority over long-term results; i.e., an athlete or worker has to immediately return to action.

The Six Components of Exercise Progression		
Assessment	Cardio	Proprioception
Strength	Flexibility	D.A.M.'s

The following descriptions are brief and are elaborated on fully in their appropriate chapters.

Assessment: Figure out which areas need the most attention, and what kind of attention they need; i.e., stretching, strengthening, etc.

Cardio: Improve cardiovascular efficiency, increase endurance, and improve overall health.

Proprioception: Improve body awareness and neuromuscular efficiency with balance and reflex training, and improve stability, strength, and movement control with PNF techniques where appropriate.

Stretching: Increase blood flow, decrease stress, and create structural and functional balance by lengthening the muscles that are too short or limited by adhesions.

Strengthening: Activate muscles that are inhibited in order to create balance surrounding a joint, build confidence in the body's ability to perform ordinary and extraordinary tasks, and achieve proper posture through specific strength training.

Daily Activity Modifications (D.A.M.'s): Teach proper body mechanics (bending, lifting, etc.) and apply them to a daily routine. Unlearn the movements that cause problems. It will be a long road to optimal functioning if someone does all the right exercises but improperly unloads the washing machine or picks up their child every day.

Corrective Exercising

The modern day lifestyle in urban areas is becoming more and more sedentary with each new invention that is made for our "convenience." This impairs the normal functioning of almost every system in the body unless corrective actions are taken.

The necessary corrections are those that move the body towards structural alignment and challenge the neuromuscular system (including the heart and cardiovascular system) in a way that promotes health.

This is done with simple movements and exercises based on assessment findings that focus on activating inhibited areas and relaxing overactive muscles. Without this organized system, common strength exercises (if performed on already tight muscles) can increase tightness and reinforce any related antagonistic inhibitions and joint dysfunctions.

Corrective exercise is the foundation of Exercise Progression and is necessary for people who want to function efficiently at any level with less or no aches and pains.

It is possible to go through life without ever exercising and lead a relatively happy life. But, it is also possible for that same person to increase their energy and ease of daily living by performing corrective exercises.

In general, corrective exercising will:

- Decrease daily or activity-related soreness.
- Improve overall energy and functioning by creating a more efficient vehicle.
- Make ordinary and extraordinary tasks easier.
- Decrease the chances of future injuries by improving joint mechanics and muscle coordination.

The hard part to keep in mind is that many people have major imbalances, and yet no pain or discomfort, and seem to live a normal life. This makes it difficult to suggest that all major imbalances are significant, but the following analogy, shared with the author from Tobe Hansen[9], can be used to shed light on why people with similar imbalances can have very different symptoms.

Imagine the body's pain and injury tolerance as an empty cup. Each negative factor that contributes to pain and injury, such as genetics, coping mechanisms, fitness routine, nutrition, daily activities, age, history of injuries, etc., is a drop of water in the cup. Certain instances, such as traumatic events, create larger drops that can fill the cup quickly.

Once the cup overflows, pain and injury occur. But by receiving manual therapy, chiropractic adjustments, or performing corrective exercises, one can remove drops from the cup and thus increase their potential to withstand cumulative trauma.

What causes the last drop is not as important as it being the last drop. Something as simple as bending over to pick up a child or sleeping crooked can be drops added every day that eventually overflow and manifest into symptoms.

Therefore, correcting as many imbalances and habits, starting with the most influential, and scooping out as many drops from the cup as possible is very relevant to preventing and correcting a variety of ailments.

It can be very difficult to convince an asymptomatic person to use corrective exercise in order to improve their lifestyle. It should be impressed upon them, however, that corrective exercise will improve the body's overall function potential and decrease the risk of future injury, aches, and pains by "emptying out their cup."

Corrective exercise is the best first option for non-serious musculoskeletal disorders when combined with the necessary manual therapy, changing of faulty habits, and education. It is a much better option than the others that are utilized, such as medication, non-specific massage and exercise, and rest, which all focus on the symptoms and ignore the cause.

A large part of the success of corrective exercise depends on the exercises being performed often and correctly, which is made easier with handouts and a home exercise program.

Based on the *Law of Facilitation*, once an impulse passes through a given set of neurons to the exclusion of others, it will tend to follow the same course on future occasions, and every time it does, the resistance will be less.

Therefore, in order to initially transform the body, good habits and exercises must outweigh the improper ones. So one hour a day will hardly make an impact on an eight-hour day of sitting. The exercises, D.A.M.'s, and Healthful Hints need to be integrated into daily movements and thoughts so that the body can slowly adapt to a new and healthier lifestyle.

The Kinetic Chain

The body is physically shaped by how it sits, stands, sleeps, eats, plays, and what it plays. Imbalances accumulate very quietly through bad habits and repetitive stress, announcing themselves only when "the cup overflows" or the tissues can no longer

tolerate the strains placed upon them; i.e., not enough rest, too much or too little activity, repetitive stress, poor nutrition, etc.

Posture is the manifestation of myofascial, neurological, and articular functioning and interaction. These three components make up the *kinetic chain*.[14,41,101,102]

Box 1-1 *Components of the Kinetic Chain*

Myofascial	Articular	Neural
• Fascia	• Bones	• Nerves
• Muscles	• Joints	• Proprioception
• Connective tissue		• Neuromuscular function

Dysfunction in one component will induce compensations in the other components and lead to decreased neuromuscular efficiency and performance along with increased chance of injury. There is no such thing as an isolated dysfunction. Once a muscle is lengthened or shortened beyond its optimum length, it will be limited in the amount of tension it can produce[14,41,61,67,101,102] and therefore force other areas to compensate.

There are predictable patterns of dysfunction created by misalignments in posture[4,11,41], some of which are upper and lower crossed syndrome and are described in more detail in chapters 12 and 13.

These dysfunctions are in response to the abnormal stresses placed on the structures and tissues throughout the kinetic chain by poor posture, repetitive stress, and unhealthy habits.

For example, when the head and shoulders are slouching forward, the lower trapezius and posterior neck muscles and ligaments have to strain to keep the head up against the increased gravitational pull on the head, not to mention all of the shortened anterior muscles and altered joint mechanics. This can lead to tension headaches, shoulder problems, low back pain, and numerous other dysfunctions.

Dysfunctional patterns are created from *five main types of neuromuscular compensation: 1) reciprocal inhibition, 2) reciprocal facilitation, 3) synergistic dominance, 4) arthrokinetic inhibition, 5) mental influences.*

Reciprocal Inhibition

There are two types of reciprocal inhibition, the first being the normal functioning of reflexes, such as when a muscle contracts, it forces its antagonist to relax.[19] The second deals with a dysfunctional pattern that occurs when a tight or dominant muscle decreases the neural drive to its antagonist.[27,41,101,102]

This latter inhibition results in a weakness in that antagonist muscle which can often be instantly strengthened by "waking it up" through stretching of the antagonist and proper activation of the agonist (inhibited muscle).

For example, a tight and facilitated psoas muscle can inhibit its antagonist, the gluteus maximus; but if the psoas is stretched and specific exercises are performed for the gluteus maximus, the inhibition will be changed into normal activation levels, which will last as long as the psoas is at a normal length.

This relationship is vital to functioning because of an antagonist's stabilization influence on a joint at the beginning of a movement[4]; if the antagonist is inhibited, then certain movements in the joint will not have the proper force couples (muscle recruitment patterns) and thus create a progression of problems, starting with altered joint mechanics and instability.

If the inhibition is a relatively new occurrence, then full strength can be regained quickly; but if it has been a chronic problem, then more time and an in-depth strengthening program are needed to restore strength.

Reciprocal Facilitation

This term has not yet been used (to this author's knowledge), but is an appropriate term for an already accepted theory and will thus be used in this manual.

Reciprocal facilitation is essentially the opposite phenomenon of reciprocal inhibition and describes the resultant tightness that occurs in a muscle (i.e. hip adductors) due to a weak antagonist (gluteus medius).

George Goodheart was the first to pioneer this theory (although he did not use the term "reciprocal facilitation") that a weakness can cause tightness in the antagonist. This concept is hard to grasp if one has always focused on treating the tightness, but it is important to understand that it is a basic concept of the body's innate protective mechanisms.

When a weak muscle contracts, it will force its antagonist (which should be inhibited by the contraction) to become more active in order to protect the joint from a ROM or position that cannot be stabilized by the weak muscle, eventually causing a shortening in the resting length of the antagonist. This results in tightness and shortening of the antagonist, which can be confusing if the muscle is classified as a stabilizer and supposed to become inhibited in response to stress; i.e., hip adductors.

See pg. 9 for classifications.

Reciprocal inhibition and reciprocal facilitation can seemingly occur at the same time in the same joint; i.e., which came first, the chicken or the egg?

Seem confusing? It is. But hopefully the following thought will help.

Regardless of the cause, weakness or tightness, the corrective actions are virtually the same. The main goal is to balance tension around the joint. It is up to the clinical wisdom of the professional to figure out whether or not more time should be spent strengthening or stretching, but either way, both need to be implemented in order to have long-lasting effects.

The only exception is an acute situation or injury that can be resolved by simply relieving the disturbance.

See the ROM and Weakness section on pg. 41 for more on balancing tension surrounding a joint.

Synergistic Dominance

This occurs when a synergist compensates for a muscle that is weak or inhibited.[41,101,102] A common example is the hamstrings and erector spinae muscles synergistically dominating hip extension because the gluteus maximus is inhibited by a tight psoas muscle.

This leads to altered joint mechanics and muscle recruitment patterns which eventually cause injury and deterioration.

Arthrokinetic Inhibition

Takes place when a joint dysfunction creates muscular inhibition surrounding the joint.[101,102] The inhibition can be a result of altered mechanics or pain in the joint.

Reciprocal inhibition, synergistic dominance, and arthrokinetic inhibition can usually be corrected with appropriate strengthening and stretching exercises, but arthrokinetic inhibition sometimes requires surgery in cases where damage is present. Manual therapy is also important for correcting the above dysfunctions.

Correcting these types of imbalances is crucial for an exercise program, because if left alone, they can cause inefficient movement patterns and increased wear and tear.

For instance, Vladimir Janda[48] showed that *tight* erector spinae muscles are activated during sit-ups, and that stretching them before the sit-ups will increase EMG activity in the abdominals and decrease it in the erectors, therefore allowing a more efficient workout of the abdominal muscles.

Mental Influences

Negative thoughts or feelings can cause dysfunctional

nerve impulses that decrease neuromuscular potential, and therefore physical functioning and well being.

Depression, anxiety, fear, anger, disgust, sadness, etc. are all emotions that produce a unique excitation, inhibition, pain, tightness, or altered muscle recruitment patterns and joint mechanics in areas that are related to the emotion.

For instance, many times when someone is injured they will store associated feelings in the area surrounding the injury as well as other places, and once the injury is healed, those feelings remain and maintain the sub-par functioning levels along with signs of pain that should already be gone. This is most obvious when an individual is not improving in pain or function levels but all signs of tissue damage and healing are improved.

It can be difficult to see mental influences on neuromuscular behavior, because during the assessment, the muscles can test strong or normal if the person's demeanor is relatively normal, but once they are in a negative state of mind, which can be triggered by specific people, thoughts, or activities, the neuromuscular system, in a way, short circuits in the areas related to the event, emotion, attitude, etc.

These short circuits can be detected by a trained examiner, i.e., through muscle testing and then brought to attention, if appropriate, and improved through positive reinforcement associations or cognitive-behavior therapy techniques.

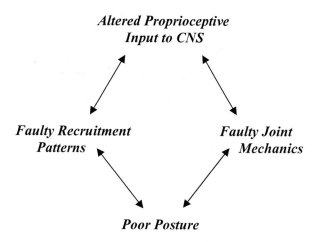

Fig. 1-1. Relationship between poor posture and the kinetic chain.

Muscular Reactions to Stress

This manual is geared for exercising, but not to the exclusion of mentioning influential factors regarding health and fitness.

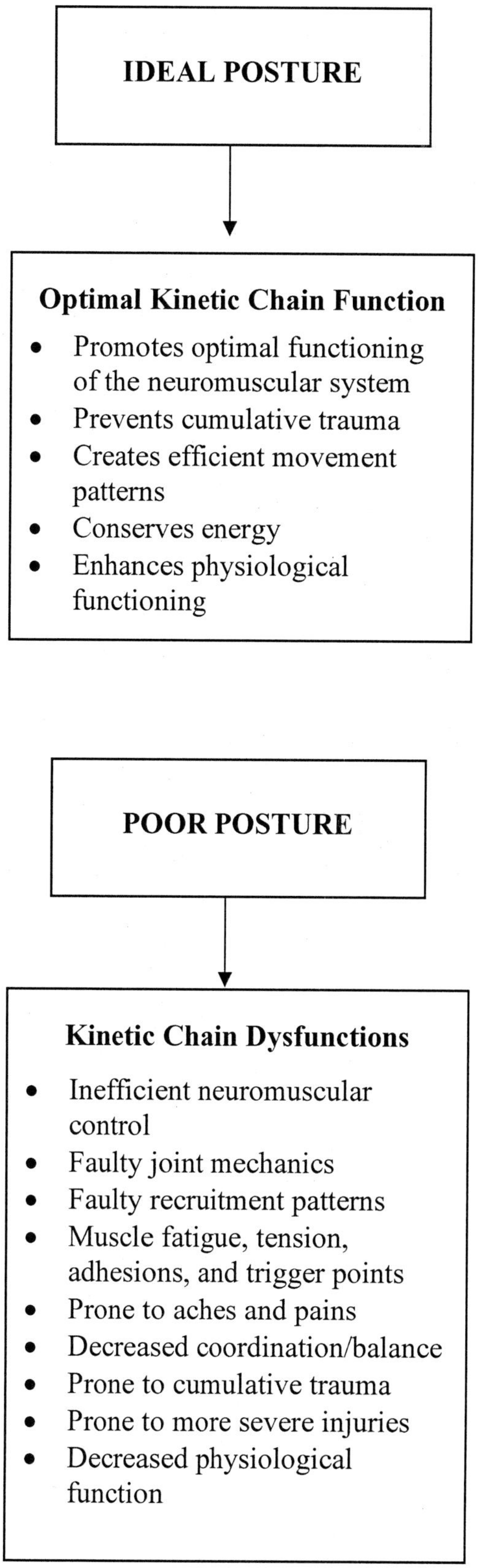

IDEAL POSTURE

↓

Optimal Kinetic Chain Function

- Promotes optimal functioning of the neuromuscular system
- Prevents cumulative trauma
- Creates efficient movement patterns
- Conserves energy
- Enhances physiological functioning

POOR POSTURE

↓

Kinetic Chain Dysfunctions

- Inefficient neuromuscular control
- Faulty joint mechanics
- Faulty recruitment patterns
- Muscle fatigue, tension, adhesions, and trigger points
- Prone to aches and pains
- Decreased coordination/balance
- Prone to cumulative trauma
- Prone to more severe injuries
- Decreased physiological function

Fig. 1-2 This above contains muscular and soft tissue reactions to dysfunctions in the body, mostly concerning the kinetic chain; many of them require manual therapy to correct their condition rather than self-stretching and corrective exercise.

It is important to learn and differentiate between the qualities of muscular dysfunction, because, according to Liebenson[41] "*Clinical decision making would be better served if muscle tension or stiffness is viewed as being related to either viscoelastic, connective tissue, and or neuromuscular factors.*"

The following terms are grouped together, as they are commonly misused or misinterpreted. Although they have similar definitions, it is imperative to differentiate between their subtleties in order to learn their causes and recognize how to correct each one.

- Trigger point/Taut band/Adhesion
- Contraction/Contracture/Spasm
- Short/Tight/Taut/Hypertonic/Facilitated
- Weak/Elongated/Inhibited

Trigger Point

The following description is based on the brilliant work of Travell and Simons[7,8] and barely scratches the surface of the knowledge and treatment of trigger points (TP's).

TP's are tender nodules in soft tissue within a palpable taut band that elicit a distinct referred pain pattern if digital pressure is applied or they are aggravated enough.

They create an environment in the muscle which makes it: 1) more susceptible to fatigue, 2) facilitated and overactive, or 3) inhibited, 4) hypersensitive to pain, 5) shortened and painful in response to stretching.

Evidence indicates that TP's can transmit their influence (facilitation, inhibition, spasm, tension, etc.) to other muscles throughout the kinetic chain by way of the CNS, especially if those areas already house TP's.

TP's are formed when stress or trauma creates a dysfunction at the motor endplate and damages the sarcoplasmic reticulum, causing it to release excessive calcium that signals the release of excessive acetylcholine in the synapses. This event cycles on and creates a sustained sarcomere shortening (contracture) which leads to an energy crisis in the muscle fiber.

The contracted muscle fibers require energy to allow the muscle to relax (ATP molecule binds to myosin head to facilitate cross-bridge detachment), and so because of the constant tension and energy usage created by a TP, that sarcomere remains in a state of contracture, which can only be relieved by improving the TP.

TP's are formed once adequate physical (cumulative or acute trauma) or physiological (nutritional deficiencies, allergies, and more) stress is placed on a muscle. They can be dormant or active,

both of which can cause referred pain, but an active TP will refer a familiar pain that the person has been experiencing recently.

Treating TP's is done with a variety of methods, such as postisometric relaxation techniques (PIR), ischemic compression, and many other manual therapy techniques that are described in great detail in the Myofascial Pain and Dysfunction manual's[7,8] and the two volumes of Clinical Applications of Neuromuscular Techniques.[4,11]

Applying each technique depends on the location of the TP, which can be towards the middle (central TP) or at the attachment of a muscle. Stretching can aggravate attachment TP's but inactivate central TP's. It is recommended to release any central TP's that are on the same taut band as an attachment TP before addressing that attachment TP.

Taut Band

A taut band is a palpable cord that consists of a group of muscle fibers, oftentimes housing a TP somewhere along its course, which ultimately ends at the muscle's attachment site, although, taut bands can be found in normal muscles.[7]

Taut bands are treated, if accompanied by a TP, by treating the TP. This should be distinguished from a taut muscle, which is not necessarily related to TP's.

Adhesion

Adhesions are formed by unorganized fibrous cross-linking, i.e., scar tissue, and can be found in ligaments, muscles, fascia, cartilage, or tendons.[40] They are formed when joint degeneration, prolonged immobilization, or trauma occurs[40], or when tissues can no longer tolerate the cumulative stresses placed upon them.

Myofascial and articular adhesions can greatly reduce ROM as well as cause pain with certain movements. Myofascial adhesions limit soft tissue pliability and can directly spread their restrictiveness along the entire kinetic chain by way of the myofascial meridians, which connect from head to toe. For more details on myofascial meridians, see the Kinetic Chain Anatomy manual.

Improving or eliminating adhesions is short lived if the process by which they are formed is not also corrected. Once the source is dealt with, adhesions can be treated with PIR techniques, manual therapy, and manipulations.

Contraction

Contracture, contraction, and spasm all involve muscle contractions, but only a contraction is voluntary and controllable. Most functional movements utilize contractions, both subconsciously (eyes blinking, breathing, postural adjustments, etc.) and consciously (sports, dancing, cooking, etc.). Contractions are the only normal occurrence listed here and are necessary for daily functioning.

Contracture

Contractures result from two different situations, both resulting in decreased ROM and strength potential. One is from soft tissue shortening due to fibrosis[7,8], which can occur from chronic adaptations to kinetic chain distortions or traumatic injuries. The other is more complicated and involves an *involuntary muscular contraction that remains in a state of constant contraction in the absence of action potentials*; the contracture seems to be maintained by a neuromuscular dysfunction at the motor endplate of the muscle fiber and is thought to be a product of TP's.[7,8]

The presence of a contracture or palpable taut band is therefore significant to exercise programming due to the probable existence of a nearby TP which is causing multiple dysfunctions, interfering with exercise and function. Treating a contracture is recommended before performing complex exercises and is done with PIR techniques and manual therapy.

Spasm

Spasms are like a contraction in that they involve action potentials that increase tension with or without muscle shortening, but they differ by their involuntary nature.[7,8] They usually act as a protective mechanism that attempts to restrict movement surrounding an injured or diseased area. This type of spasm responds well to placing the protected tissues in a resting position[4] and resolving the underlying issue.

Another form of spasm is a referred spasm induced from TP's. This referred spasm is more likely to occur in muscles that already harbor TP's or in certain susceptible muscles (lumbar paraspinals, upper trapezius, masseter, and posterior cervicals) and is independent of referred pain patterns.[7] Contractures and spasms can occur in nearby tissues.[4]

Treating a spasm should only proceed once its cause is known. Treatment for a *protective* spasm, which can look and feel just like a TP spasm, should not focus on the spasm, it should be aimed at improving the cause; otherwise the protected tissues will become

vulnerable; i.e., underlying disc herniation or hypermobile joints.

Treating a referred or TP spasm, however, is done effectively with PIR techniques[7,42] and or TP release and manual therapy, but only if it is clear that no acute underlying issues are present.

Short

Short muscles are just that, short, although figuring out why they are short can require great skill. A short muscle will feel tight if it is in a constant state of semi-contraction. Short muscles are prone to tightness, weakness, TP's, and contractures, and are accompanied by their elongated and weak antagonistic muscles. This combination creates immediate joint imbalances and more wide-spread distortions throughout the entire kinetic chain. Chronically shortened muscles eventually become weak in what Janda[115] calls *"tightness weakness"*; i.e., the psoas or quadratus lumborum.

A short muscle's length is limited by numerous influences that range from the muscular reactions mentioned in this section (contractures, spasm, etc.) to genetic deficiencies and compensating for distant or nearby kinetic chain imbalances. A short muscle's strength can appear greater than normal if it is only tested in its shortened position but will show signs of weakness if tested for endurance, coordination, or after briefly lengthening it.

How to lengthen short muscles depends on the condition of the muscle and its surroundings. It can take quite an investigation to figure out if the antagonist needs to be strengthened or if simply stretching the short muscle will improve both the short and elongated/weak muscles.

See ROM and Weakness section on pg. 41 for details about weaknesses limiting ROM.

If the short muscle is in combination with other factors, i.e., is facilitated, tight, weak, has contractures, etc., then additional strategies should follow the guidelines mentioned for each additional factor.

Tight

Muscle tightness leads to loss of flexibility and produces palpable sensations that are similar to stiffness, firmness, rigidity, and tautness. It is a general term that relates to tissue which is dysfunctional and prone to TP's and contractures and often requires a thorough examination to figure out the cause of the tightness. Tightness alone is not a good indicator for specific treatment plans, because it is present with numerous types of dysfunctions; therefore, other

7

observations are needed, along with the presence of tightness, to deduce a treatment plan.

Taut

Using the words of Kendall and McCreary[49], "*Taut* means stretched out fully, not slack."

If a muscle becomes taut before reaching its normal ROM limit, then the muscle is short. It is not unusual for a muscle to palpate as tight or rigid without being taut; i.e., the upper trapezius and erector spinae. This definition should be distinguished from "taut band."

Hypertonic

Hypertonic muscles exhibit excessive tone and tension that is visibly noticeable. Unfortunately, it is just like tightness, in that it is only a sign of dysfunction that requires further examination in order to discover the reasons for the hypertonicity.

Facilitated

Muscles that are facilitated tend to be overactive and dominate movements in which a related synergist or antagonist is weak/inhibited even if the movement is not the muscle's main duty.

Facilitation can be spread throughout the kinetic chain to various regions of related function and requires special training to correct it due to the Law of Facilitation.

Common interactions of facilitated and inhibited muscles, along with their corrective actions, will be mentioned throughout the manual.

Weak

Weakness can be due to neurological (nerve root compression or peripheral entrapment), disuse atrophy, anatomical (length/tension relationship) and or neuromuscular factors (inhibition). Weakness is related to muscle length abnormalities and will lead to joint instability and antagonistic tightness in the surrounding area, eventually spreading compensation throughout the kinetic chain. Its treatment depends on its source, which can be in distant or nearby dysfunctions.

See the Correcting Tightness and Weakness section below for details on corrective actions.

Elongated

Elongated muscles are the opposite of short muscles in regards to length but are associated with myofascial tension, as are short muscles. The difference is, a tense elongated muscle usually produces a noticeable weakness compared to a tense short muscle.

The complex interactions of the surrounding muscles and influential areas of the kinetic chain need to be understood before planning a corrective actions program for elongated muscles.

Inhibited

Inhibition here refers to decreased neural drive to a muscle and seems impossible without facilitation of the antagonist. Inhibition causes weakness in the muscle that can be quickly improved with specific exercises if the weakness is relatively new, or it can take much longer if the (Law of Facilitation) has settled in. Inhibition can also be referred from distant TP's.[7]

Correcting inhibitions is, once again, done most effectively by utilizing the interactions of the kinetic chain to find the key influences. Once it is certain that the inhibited muscle needs to be strengthened, specific activation techniques can be used to "jump start" the neuromuscular connection to the muscle. This will speed up the strengthening process and encourage proper utilization of the muscle for specific unassisted strengthening exercises.

Correcting Tightness and Weakness

Many people adhere to the principle of shortness/tightness causing weakness/elongation of a muscle, but George Goodheart, DC (the "father" of applied kinesiology), had incredible success treating muscle tension by simply strengthening the weak antagonists of tight muscles; therefore, showing that weakness can cause tightness.

It is dependent upon the belief of the professional as to which strategy should be used for correcting tight or weak muscles; either focusing on stretching tight muscles or strengthening weak muscles.

It is useful to note that both strategies seem effective if applied to the appropriate situation; in other words, sometimes weakness/elongation is a priority, and other times tightness/shortness is a priority.

Always remember however that true weakness in a muscle is not improved by stretching its antagonist.

Muscle Classifications

The exercise philosophy of this manual is largely based on the classification of muscles and can be summed up with two main principles:

1. There are three types of muscles: global and local stabilizers, and mobilizers. Each can be placed into one of two categories: 1) hypoactive, 2) hyperactive.

Classifications of Muscle Groups
"Stress Response"

Box 1-2

Hypoactive Group	Hyperactive Group
Usually stabilizers *Tend to weaken/lax* *Fatigues easily* *Prone to inhibition and delayed activation patterns* *Requires special training* *Dominated*	*Usually mobilizers* *Tend to tighten/shorten* *Predominantly used* *Prone to facilitation* *Prone to TP's first* *Increased resting tone* *Spasm in response to pain* *Dominate*
Arm extensors Deep cervical stabilizers Deep erector spinae Deep neck flexors Gluteals Infraspinatus Internal oblique Middle/Lower trapezius Multifidus Paraspinal muscles (not erector spinae) Pectoralis major (lower) Peroneals Posterior deltoid Psoas major (posterior fascicles) Rectus abdominis (lower) Rhomboids Serratus anterior Teres minor Tibialis anterior Tibialis posterior Transverse abdominis VMO	Hip adductors Arm flexors Erector spinae Gastrocnemius Hamstrings Latissimus dorsi Levator scapula Pectoralis major (upper) Pectoralis minor Piriformis Psoas Quadradtus Lumborum Rectus femoris Rectus abdominis (upper) Soleus Sternocleidomastoid Teres major Tensor Fascia Lata Upper trapezius

This box is a combination from Norris[59], Jull and Janda[60], Janda[61], and Chaitow and DeLaney.[4] Some of the muscles (scalenes, external obliques, and others) are not agreed upon and will therefore be left out. It is possible for muscles to start as one type (hyper or hypoactive), and then evolve into the other type if sufficient demands are placed on it from faulty postures; i.e., the scalenes.[4, 41]

2. These muscles must be activated and strengthened in a progressive order; otherwise the larger muscles will dominate the smaller ones and create instability altered activation patterns.

Many great minds[59,60,61,138,139,140] in the past have contributed to the evolution of classifying muscles, and to this day there is still disagreement on one classification system that fits all. There has been more confusion with the naming of the classifications than the actual functions for each group of muscles.

For instance, it is generally agreed that the hamstrings have a tendency to shorten or tighten when chronically stressed, but they are labeled as postural muscles by Janda[61], which seems confusing, due to the fact that they are electromyographically silent during quiet standing, on one or two feet [99,142]

This author combines the compatible theories into *two* similar classification systems that are helpful for figuring out the corrective actions and common tendencies for specific muscles and groups of muscles throughout the kinetic chain.

Depending on how the body is constructed (everybody is different) and how it is habitually used determines the complex interactions and compensations within the kinetic chain; and because most people are designed similarly and participate in general activities, there is a list of common tendencies for certain muscles. See Box 1-2 and Fig. 1-3.

These classifications can be combined to form one set of guidelines to be used for evaluating the muscular system.

As seen in Box 1-2 and Fig. 1-3, muscles can be classified by dysfunction (hypo-hyperactive) and function (stabilizer/mobilizer). While each is related to the other, stabilizers are usually hypoactive, and mobilizers are usually hyperactive.

These classifications are, of course, guidelines and not finite rules. Certain muscles, such as the Q.L. and oblique abdominals can act as two different groups (global stabilizer and mobilizer) depending on the situation and fibers used.

Based on this and other evidence that shows how different muscles respond to various stresses, Exercise Progression uses a systematic approach to improving the function and interaction of the muscular system by activating each muscle type in order from deepest to most superficial, or from most stabilizing to most mobilizing. See Chapter 14 for details on progressions.

Stabilizers

A. Local
B. Global

Local Stabilizers

These are mostly deep, small, medially located, segmental, and slower acting endurance muscles that function best in weightbearing postures to maintain joint stability (multifidus, transverse abdominis, interspinales, etc.).[138]

When deloading occurs (decreased weightbearing and sensory input regarding gravity; i.e., sitting, lying, swimming, etc.), the local and global stabilizers tend to atrophy and lose function while the mobilizers hypertrophy. This also leads to less sensory input and, therefore, decreased proprioceptive ability.[138] This may take a lifetime to build up, but its immediate influence is evident once someone tries to perform a balancing exercise after prolonged sitting or lying.

Weakness in these muscles facilitates the over-utilization of the mobilizers and therefore instability. This is a common root of kinetic chain dysfunction due to the common tendencies of society; i.e., sitting, lying, and focusing on physical appearance (arms, chest, back, legs, and other mobilizers).

It is important to notice that the stabilizers and mobilizers tend to respond to pain and dysfunction in opposite manners.

The corrective actions for weak local muscles are to start at ground zero by isolating them and learning to activate them slowly and statically in a variety of positions. This is best done in the absence of other complex exercises; otherwise the hyperactive mobilizers will take over and inhibit the local muscles.

Eventually these isolated actions will be integrated into more functional motions, as in Stage II of Exercise Progression, global stabilization.

Global Stabilizers

The global muscles are similar to the local muscles but differ by being more superficial, larger, and involved with stabilizing *areas* of the body rather than individual segments. They have the same characteristics as the local muscles but utilize more integrated corrective actions, such as weightbearing while utilizing the local muscles to achieve proper joint alignment and stability throughout more functional movements.

Mobilizers

The mobilizers are constantly overactive and trying to manage the duties of the smaller and underutilized muscles, which is a problem because they are not equipped to do so. Their main functions are to create gross movements and co-activate against heavy and unexpected loads in order to enhance stability. Mobilizers are fast-acting muscles that tend to dominate quick, gross, and open chain movements unless trained otherwise.

Corrective actions for these muscles are the initial training of the stabilizers in a closed-chain environment so that gross movements can be performed on a stable body. Then the integration of mobilizers can begin by utilizing faster and larger movements (open and closed chain) while maintaining proper alignment.

Although many of the muscles have not been clinically tested for their weightbearing or non-weightbearing capabilities, these classifications of muscles are helpful for keeping the big picture in mind and knowing where adhesions and trigger points are likely residing, as well as which muscles need to be strengthened and stretched, and how to do so.

It is essential, however, to figure out why these dysfunctions are happening; otherwise results will be short lived.

CNS Control of Lumbopelvic Stability

The central nervous system (CNS) has a tremendous variety of afferent sensory input to interpret in order to maintain stability and efficient movement throughout the body in relation to various situations, as well as numerous pre-programmed muscular interactions at its disposal developed for certain predictable occasions.

The neurological loops involved with motor control of trunk stability will be discussed and generalized here, while their complex neural interactions within the CNS left out of the discussion. There are three main loops that the CNS uses to control motor function throughout the trunk muscles:

1. Feedforward control
2. Feedback control
3. Postural control

Feedforward Control

Feedforward neurological loops are activated in order to stabilize the lumbopelvic area *prior* to *predictable* imposed demands on the trunk.[138] In these situations the CNS predicts the forces that are about to affect the body and dispatches a coordinated neuromuscular plan of attack to neutralize these external stresses. This plan is based on past experiences similar to or equal to the present situation and will stabilize the body appropriately in normal subjects.[138,179,180]

These "planned attacks" utilize different muscles and come in waves of activation, each within milliseconds of one another, and have a unique functional goal.

According to Richardson, et al.,[138] there is a hierarchy of spinal control:

1) Intervertebral translation and rotation
2) Spinal posture and orientation
3) Body control in relation to the environment

Supporting this hierarchy are the following findings and ideas regarding the presence of an inner muscular unit within the lumbopelvic stabilizing system that activates together in unique ways, prior to and during predictable imposed demands.

• The diaphragm[181] and transverse abdominis (T.A.) had tonic or relatively constant activation throughout repetitive arm movement, while the erector spinae had intermittent activation.[172,182]

• The T.A. and diaphragm activate prior to movement as a spinal stability mechanism.[178]

• Intra-abdominal pressure (IAP) and T.A. and diaphragm activity increase in proportion to the velocity, and therefore force, of the reactive moment during repetitive arm movement.[172]

• T.A. activation levels are linked to the intensity of control needed to stabilize the spine.[138]

• When electrically stimulated, the diaphragm can 1) generate a minor extensor moment,[188] 2) increase spinal stiffness against posteroanterior forces, especially at the higher lumbar levels[189,190], (due to the direct attachment of the diaphragm to the upper lumbar vertebrae).

• Although it is difficult to assess, it is plausible that the pelvic floor muscles have a similar effect on spinal stability as the diaphragm.[138]
The T.A. and pelvic floor muscles were the main muscles activated while forming a neutral spine position.[183]

• The T.A. and pelvic floor muscles are often activated as a team.[138]

• The diaphragm and pelvic floor muscles' main role in spinal stability is to create IAP in coordination with the T.A. and restrict movement of the abdominal contents so that the lumbar dorsal fascia (LDF) can be properly tensed.[138, 172,178,181,186]

• Tonic activity of the pelvic floor muscles has been documented during repetitive arm movements.[184]

• The T.A. and multifidus activate independent of the direction of the reactive forces placed on the spine[150,151], as opposed to the direction specific activation of the mobilizing muscles.[150,152,153] This suggests that the T.A. and multifidus are part of the inner unit and feedforward neuromuscular system used to counteract intervertebral instability due to non-direction-specific forces.[138]

• Deep multifidus activity is tonic during repetitive arm movement and in upright postures.[151]

• Multifidus has tonic activity during walking.[187]

• The internal oblique abdominals were activated prior to the deltoid during arm abduction and extension.[176]

It is evident that, during predictable movements, the CNS utilizes an initial activation of an inner unit or local stabilizers to stabilize intervertebral movement, followed by more global stabilizers to control spinal posture and orientation, and finally, or sometimes simultaneously, by mobilizers to prepare the body for predictable situations. See pg. 15 for details on individual muscles of the inner unit.

These naturally coordinated waves of activation are a main goal of Exercise Progression and are best established by 1) eliminating major imbalances and pain, 2) beginning with simple activation exercises and incorporating them into daily functioning, 3) progressing to more complex and faster actions.

Feedback Control

Feedback loops are much simpler than the feedforward loops and rarely, if ever, reach the brain. They consist mostly of simple reflexes, such as the stretch reflex, and are activated in response to unpredictable movements that force the CNS to take action quickly, usually resulting in muscular coordination that involves all influential muscles activating at the same time, deep and superficial.[138]

This type of reaction to the environment can only be trained for once proper feedforward loops have been established; then utilizing increased velocity and unstable surfaces is an appropriate way to train the body for slips, falls, etc.

Postural Control

Postural or tonic control is based on both feedback and feedforward control mechanisms and is in charge of 1) antigravity tonic/postural system, 2) stabilization before movement.[138]

The antigravity system regulates the tone and stiffness of specific postural muscles in order to stabilize the joints, while the "stabilization before movement" system is the same as the feedforward control system mentioned above.

Muscle stiffness controls the forces surrounding joints and prepares/stabilizes them for upcoming stress, even before stretch reflexes.[192] Similarly, trunk stability may be linked to the stiffness of the spinal muscles.[138]

All the complexities of the CNS are not yet understood, such as how, when, and if the different control systems work simultaneously, but the possibility cannot be ignored.[138]

Functional Classifications of Muscles (Fig. 1-3)

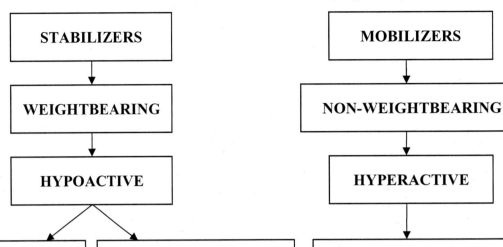

STABILIZERS	**MOBILIZERS**
↓	↓
WEIGHTBEARING	**NON-WEIGHTBEARING**
↓	↓
HYPOACTIVE	**HYPERACTIVE**

LOCAL

- Deep 1-joint muscles
- Maintain segmental stability in all ROM's, especially in neutral
- Activate prior to main action for stabilizing effect
- Control, not produce, ROM
- Endurance/static role
- Activate independent of direction of movement
- High threshold of stimulus
- Continuous activation throughout movement
- Low and slow contraction force
- Local muscles are: deep lumbar multifidus, transverse abdominis, intervertebral muscles,etc.

GLOBAL

- More superficial 1-joint muscles
- Maintain stability and control ROM, especially during deceleration (eccentrically) and rotation
- Lack segmental spine attachments
- Endurance/static muscles
- High threshold of stimulus
- Non-continuous activation throughout movement
- Activation is direction dependent
- Medium contraction force and velocity
- Global stabilizers are: oblique abdominals, gluteus medius, spinalis, etc.

MOBILIZERS

- Most superficial and lateral muscles w/multiple joints
- Long muscles w/multiple functions
- Produce movement, especially accelerating flexion or extension
- Low threshold of stimulus
- Fast, strong, and gross movements, usually concentric
- Non-continuous activation throughout movement
- Activation is direction dependent
- Co-activate for intense or sudden movements
- Mobilizers are: erector spinae, piriformis, etc.

CORRECTIVE ACTIONS

- Compression/weight-bearing Closed-chain exercises
- Local activation techniques 1) lying 2) sitting 3) standing
- Utilize isometric and slow contractions in neutral
- No spinal movement
- Stage 1 exercises

CORRECTIVE ACTIONS

- Compression/weight-bearing Closed-chain exercises
- Integrate local and global stabilizers, progress to rotation
- Utilize isometric and eccentric contractions w/slow to medium velocity
- Increase sensory input
- Stage II exercises

CORRECTIVE ACTIONS

- Both weight and non-weightbearing exercises
- Open and closed chain
- More rapid and ballistic movements
- Decrease sensory input
- Stages III-V exercises

Proper Muscle Activation Patterns (PMAP)

PMAP is similar to, if not the same as, *force couple relationships* and is founded on the principal listed in Box 1-3.

PMAP is only possible if the CNS is properly utilizing all three types of motor control systems (feedback, feedforward, and postural) for lumbopelvic stability.

Box 1-3

> Just about every planned movement should *begin* with a *natural* tensing of the CORE, followed by global stabilization; both in proportion to the forces needed to stabilize the spine and occurring prior to the movement.

Appropriate activation patterns for feedforward control rely on correct postural control of stiffness, while appropriate activation patterns for feedback control rely on precise control of the feedforward system.

In other words, proper movement patterns are based on ideal posture, and efficient reflex arcs are based on ideal posture and normal movement patterns.

According to many studies, the T.A. activates prior to the muscle responsible for the main movement (arm or hip flexion, etc.) and continuously throughout the movement in normal subjects[173-178], while activation of the T.A. is delayed in those with low back pain.[176,177,178]

The pelvic floor[184] and diaphragm also activate prior to and continuously throughout movement.[138,172,178, 181,182,183] This is evidence of the ideal neuromuscular *feedforward* system mentioned by Richardson, et al.,[138] that allows the CNS to control lumbopelvic stability in advance of imposed *predictable forces* with a preprogrammed set of muscular contractions and interactions, which follow the guideline of: the more velocity or stability required, the sooner and greater the abdominal mechanism will activate.[150,172]

Properly activating the inner unit prior to movement or an imposed demand places the body in its strongest and most efficient position, thereby promoting optimum functioning throughout the rest of the kinetic chain.

See pg. 80 for details on abdominal wall activation patterns in spinal stabilization.

Strength starts from within (the center) and then moves outward following the nerve impulses towards their targeted action.

It is noticeable when someone "flows" properly; they have a smooth and natural rhythm. For example, many great athletes have that natural flow.

Even something as simple as lifting a bag of groceries should follow a pattern; the lumbo-pelvic stabilizers, legs, chest, shoulder, and upper arm should activate in that order before the forearm lifts the weight.

If the groceries are lifted before the stabilizing muscles activate, the body will buckle at its weakest links instead of dispersing the tension throughout the "team."

Normal firing sequences (PMAP) for most movements against resistance should be:

1. *Natural* tensing of the abdomen (inner unit - local stabilization)
2. Stabilizers of proximal joints and legs (gross stabilization)
3. The agonist of the movement (outer unit - mobilization)
4. The synergists and stabilizers of the agonist will vary with their timing depending on the direction, speed, and resistance of the movement.

Injuries and pain are known to cause altered patterns of movement due to muscle compensations; this is one reason that *low back pain is one of the greatest predictors of future low back pain.*

Another source of altered recruitment patterns is faulty static or dynamic posture, which creates the same problems as pain, such as: altered joint mechanics, reciprocal inhibition and facilitation, synergistic dominance, and arthrokinetic inhibition throughout the affected areas. These are corrected through the five steps mentioned below.

PMAP is fundamental to obtaining maximum efficiency during simple and complex movements and can be achieved by:

1. Releasing any trigger points, manipulating joints, and releasing tension and pain in the affected and influential areas.
2. Learning to properly activate the abdominal wall and multifidus.
3. Correcting posture by balancing muscle tension around the joints and throughout the fascia network in order to eliminate any neuromuscular dysfunctions.
4. Starting with simple and isolated exercises geared towards stabilization and balance.
5. Progress to complex movements that coordinate the neuromuscular system to efficiently function in all three planes using all three types of contractions (concentric, eccentric, and isometric) along with acceleration and deceleration of movement.

If PMAP is learned, it will reduce future damage to the body and spine, thereby decreasing the intensity and frequency of future problems.

Keys for PMAP training are:

- Know which muscles are involved with the action and where they lie in the body.
- Know what order they should fire in and the appropriate level or intensity of contraction for each.
- Visualize these patterns (where and when they activate) during PMAP training.
- The practitioner can pat the person's stomach while they are exercising to confirm and reinforce the stiffness.

➢ See the muscle testing section in Ch. 12 for assessing important PMAP.

The CORE

The CORE has been defined as many different things in the past, and here's yet another description as defined by this author. *The CORE is three groups of muscles that function together to stabilize and mobilize the lumbar spine and trunk about the pelvis.* It follows the principles mentioned above relating to the three waves of activation and three types of motor control systems.

See fig. 1-4 for more on the CORE.

Figure 1-4 is merely a schematic to help visualize the CORE and how it functions. It is by no means a complete picture. There is much to learn about the CNS and its complexities regarding control of posture and the variety of interactions with the environment.

Classification of Muscle Dysfunction

Classifications of the causes of dysfunction or "non-serious pain syndromes" are described in more detail in Chapters 2 and 12 and will only be briefly mentioned here.

In order to significantly affect a dysfunction, its source must be found and corrected. Three main sources are:

1. Kinetic Chain
2. Physiological
3. Psychological

This is similar to the model used by Chaitow and DeLaney[4,11] to describe the negative influences on a patient's health, which they classify as biomechanical, biochemical, and psychosocial.

Only the physical component (kinetic chain) will be dealt with in this manual, although some notice is given for the other two throughout the text.

A similar way to look at physical symptoms is by integrating all aspects of life, as in the following formula.

$$M + E + S = P$$

M = Mental E = Emotional S = Spiritual P = Physical

This equation shows that our physical self is a manifestation of our inner workings. In other words, "the roots feed the fruits" or "the invisible effects the visible." If one component on the left side of this equation is struggling, then the physical body will manifest symptoms corresponding to that precise struggle.

It is important to know when a non-physical component is affecting the physical body so that the appropriate referral can be made and time is not wasted on inappropriate or even harmful physical strategies.

Health vs. Fitness

The following definitions are as described by the Merriam-Webster's Collegiate Dictionary:[76]

- Health - "the condition of being sound in body, mind, and spirit; *esp* : freedom from physical disease or pain"

- Fit - "sound physically and mentally: Healthy"

- Fitness - "the quality or state of being fit" and "the capacity of an organism to survive and transmit its genotype to reproductive offspring as compared to competing organisms"

It is easy to see why fitness becomes associated with health but oftentimes does not truly promote it.

The above definition of "fit" leaves out the spiritual dimension but is still considered "healthy," while the fitness definitions are based on the degree in which one is fit and competing with others.

These definitions, which are probably the most accepted in society, show that health is three dimensional but fitness is only two dimensional, and if someone has a high level of fitness, then they must be fit and, therefore, healthy.

This type of fitness health is driven by the mind, and without getting too philosophical, is lacking a spiritual component that keeps the body in line with true health as opposed to fitness health.

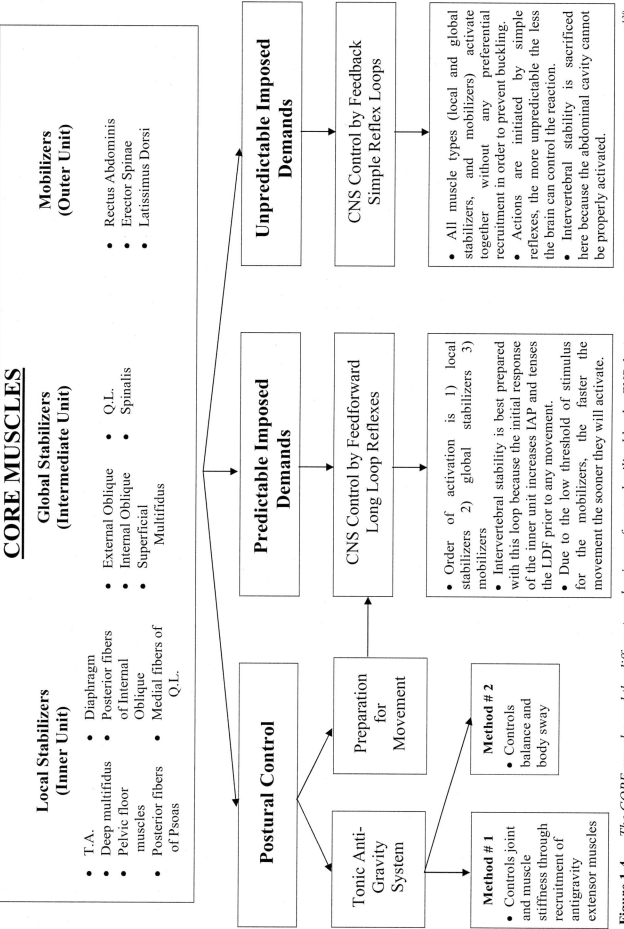

Figure 1-4 - *The CORE muscles and the different mechanisms of control utilized by the CNS during various situations, modified from Richardson et all[138] and Massion.[193]*

The main difference is not spiritual awareness, which is a bonus, but rather enjoying the pursuit of health instead of pursuing results from fitness.

It is rare to find someone who works out the appropriate amount for their body. Most often people exercise too much or not enough, usually out of ignorance or simply ignoring the body's needs; i.e., exercising for the wrong reasons or not exercising due to low health priorities.

Ignorance can be helped through education about the relationship and benefits of health and fitness, but ignoring is a much more complex issue that will not be addressed here, although education can influence a change in motivation.

It is a goal of this manual to encourage health instead of fitness training whenever possible, but it is also this manual's goal to teach athletes and those who are physically active to find a balance between extreme training and health training, and therefore both types (fitness and health) of programs will be described along with ideas about how to alternate between the two.

Health is always in flux and thus requires constant adjustments through nutrition, movement, intensity, and thought process.

There is a point where the amount of exercise or activity is detrimental to health. See graph below.

Health vs. Fitness

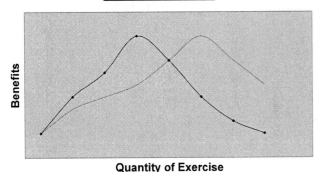

Graph notes:

1. Optimum health requires less exercise than optimum fitness.
2. Too much exercise can be just as detrimental as little or no exercise.

Exercise Goals

- **Health** - To stress the body in a way that encourages *all* of its systems to function most efficiently.

- **Fitness** - To stress the body in a way that achieves specific external results (aesthetics, speed, strength, endurance, etc.).

These two goals can have very different impacts on the body, but ideally they complement one another.

When exercising for health, there is no such thing as a bad workout unless an injury or overtraining results. Understanding this perspective makes it easier to avoid the disappointment of failing to achieve or overexertion to gain specific results (weight, time, repetitions, etc.).

When exercising for fitness, the body's internal functions are often sacrificed to reach external goals. Exercising at too high of intensity and or for too long a time can drain the entire body of its vitality, which can be replenished if treated appropriately, but will eventually have long-term negative effects on overall health if this type of training is habitual.

Unfortunately, those who train at this level either do it on a consistent basis, which doesn't allow enough time for revitalization and speeds up wear and tear, or do it infrequently, which often results in injuries.

These people can look healthy on the outside, but to an experienced observer, their body's systems are noticeably inefficient.

A few things are needed if health is a goal.

1. Patience
2. Knowledge of appropriate exertion levels (mostly intuitive)
3. Understanding that health relies on fitness more than fitness relies on health.
4. Realizing that *health is a state of being* and *fitness is being in a physical state.*

In order to obtain health, the ego must be left out of goal making. The ego wants to protect and maintain the self-image it has created throughout a lifetime.

Examples of some ego images and goals are:

- Looking good (compared to others, of course)
- Being good at something (compared to others, of course)
- Achieving a physical goal, even at the expense of health.

These goals are accepted and encouraged by most of society because of one main idea: succeeding or wining for whatever it takes.

This may be necessary to seriously compete in athletics or extreme activities, but it must be realized that these two examples do not promote health and should not be participated in unless the relationship between health and fitness is understood and accepted.

A wise person will have the ability to achieve both health and fitness goals at the same time. Some example goals for health are:

- Lower resting heart rate, blood pressure, body fat (if obese), and have more daily energy.
- Train for an event, i.e., marathon, race, sport, etc, to the best of my capabilities while listening to my body for signs of overtraining and not be disappointed if I can't compete, because the goal was to train to the best of my capabilities, not achieve results.

With all of this being said, it is possible to be *relatively* healthy if extreme training, like most athletes, is properly utilized.

The point to be made here is that extreme training is not necessary to become healthy, and it is associated with less than optimal health.

The choice is simple; live for the mind (external results), or live for the body (internal results).

Pain and Exercise

In general, if someone has pain or an injury, it is recommended to get their doctor's clearance and advice for exercise before starting an exercise program.

Pain will cause faulty patterns of movement and muscle recruitment in the surrounding areas and eventually create dysfunction throughout the body. Therefore, *people with pain should avoid complex movements or intense exercise because they lack the coordination to properly stabilize the body.*

Even if the body can normally perform a difficult exercise with ease, that exercise is potentially dangerous once the body is in pain. This is very difficult for the mind to accept if health is not the main goal of exercising.

Sometimes during the post-rehabilitation phase of an injury, or even throughout a lifetime, slight pain will be inevitable with or without exercise. Then the goal is as much functional exercise as tolerable so the body can better handle daily (housework) and not so daily (skiing) activities.

The following guidelines were established by the American Academy of Health, Fitness and Rehab Professionals (AAHFRP)[5] and are useful for determining who should and shouldn't workout with pain.

On a scale of 1-10, if pain is:
- 1-3   Exercise may be tolerable
- 4-5   Activity should be modified
- 6-10   Stop activity

Stress can be physical or mental, and the more the body is "stressed" with exercise (in a productive manner), the more prepared it will be to combat the stresses of everyday life, including mental and emotional stress.

Improving Injuries

There are a number of ways to improve during a post-rehabilitation exercise program. One is by coincidence, which happens from doing exercises and activities that don't irritate or directly affect the injury and, therefore, let the body heal by using its own internal resources.

Another way is from utilizing exercises that correct or positively influence the injured structure and its surroundings, not necessarily by focusing on the injured area. This way can also speed up recovery time compared to "coincidence" as well as correct the imbalances that cause re-injury.

Improvement should be based on pain levels and daily functioning more than how much or how many times a weight can be lifted.

If gym strength increases but ease of daily living doesn't, different exercises are needed. Determining who should be challenged with exercises and who should go easier is an important factor and delicate balance.

The feeling of accomplishment rather than being overwhelmed with exercise can be the deciding factor in improvement, mentally and physically.

Exercise naturally causes some discomfort and irritation. If the tissues being exercised are already irritated, then a lot of discomfort will obviously follow. If this response can be minimized to 2-3 days while functional ability is maintained, then the workout was a success.

Obviously, individual tolerance levels must be kept in mind, but sometimes, with some education and encouragement, healthy tolerance levels can be increased.

Progressing

The progression variables described in Chapter 14 are in such an order and magnitude that they promote optimum growth. Progressing through the stages too quickly or in an altered order can lead to underutilization of the neuromuscular system, injury, improper recruitment patterns, decreased potential for strength and power, and even more undesirable results.

It should be up to a professional to decide which parts need to be focused on and which can be ignored or worked less.

Re-evaluations and progress reports should be done every four weeks.

Amount of Exercise

Main Factors affecting the Amount of Exercise:

- Age
- Health/Fitness level
- Available time to exercise
- Stage of recovery from injury
- Type of injury
- History of exercise
- Goal

The exercise routines in this manual give the maximum amount of exercise desirable for most individuals. Some people will have conditions that limit their amount of exercise to well below what's given in routines.

Only experience and good judgment can determine the proper amount and type of exercise a person should have, especially those with injuries.

A protocol can hurt as many people as it helps, so the exercises in the routines are more of a guideline than set of rules, and utilizing quick thinking is essential in therapy and gym settings.

The guidelines below (Boxes 1-4 and 1-5) are for determining what exercise level someone is currently at and how much exercise is recommended for that individual. Exceptions are common.

Don't let the high number of times per week in Box 1-5 for each component seem overwhelming, because many of the corrective exercises are simple and take only a few minutes each day.

In general, strength training only needs to be done a maximum of three times a week, but with the addition of crucial corrective exercises, which should be performed by most people throughout the week no matter what level they are at, the number of times per week increases to five or even seven for some of the important exercises.

Health changes cyclically and randomly, as do the body's requirements for exercise, exercise intensity, and nutrition, so breaks from certain activities and routines should be taken accordingly.

This should be taken into account when the ego will not allow a lighter weight to be lifted on days when the body seems weak, or taking a day off when energy is depleted.

Box 1-4   Determining Fitness Levels

Beginner	Intermediate	Advanced
1. No regular strength exercises in the past six months 2. Sedentary lifestyle for the past six months	1. Strength and cardio exercises 1-2x per week for the past six months **or** 2. Semi-active lifestyle • Manual labor job • Participates in a sport, aerobics, yoga, etc.	1. Strength exercises at least 2x week 2. Cardio at least 3x week 3. Overall intensity at least 75%, 2-3x per week 4. At least 6 months at this level

Box 1-5   Recommended Amount of Exercise

	Beginner (Initial Stage)	Intermediate (Improvement Stage)	Advanced (Elite Stage)
Cardio	3-4x wk/15-30 min*	3-5x wk/25-40 min*	3-7x wk/30-90 min
Stretching	5-7x wk*	5-7x wk*	5-7x wk*
Proprioception	0**-5x wk	3-5x wk	2-3x wk
Strengthening	3-5x wk***	3-5x wk	2-5x wk
D.A.M.'s	As needed	As needed	As needed
Exercises per Body Part[****]	1-2	2-3	2-6
Sets per Exercise[****]	2-3	3-4	6-12
Total sets per Body Part[****]	3-4	3-5	9-20

*   As recommended by the American Academy of Sports Medicine for sedentary low risk persons.[33]

**   0 times per week are for those in Stage I who need to focus on isolated, not integrated contractions.

*** Strengthening exercises are very simple and focus on isolated contractions and PMAP.

**** As recommended by the National Academy of Sports Medicine (NASM).[13]

Chapter 2   Assessment Guidelines

Assessments vary as much as the professionals who use them. The more assessments that are utilized the greater chance there is for successfully categorizing someone and progressing them towards health. *A good assessment utilizes a person's history to choose the appropriate tests and then looks at the relationship between all failed tests and their possible causes. A progressive program is then created to meet the needs of the individual, which ideally incorporates the entire body and roots of any dysfunctions.*

One failed test does not create a program, it only points to an isolated dysfunction and requires direction from other tests to establish the whole picture of interrelated dysfunctions. For instance, a failed muscle test could be caused by weak and imbalanced muscles or from a nerve root problem, and thus both areas should be assessed. Sometimes the assessments can take longer than the manual therapy or exercise session, but a shorter and more precise treatment has more benefits than a longer and more non-specific treatment. For this reason, Exercise Progression places people into four different assessment categories and uses nine different assessment skills that in the author's experience will find the cause of most aches, pains, and dysfunctions, as well as build the foundation for a corrective exercise and manual therapy program.

There are a few different types of people that are important to differentiate in order to efficiently assess their condition and needs; mainly asymptomatic and symptomatic. Each of these individuals requires unique assessments of their abilities and conditions. It is the responsibility of a doctor or specialist to diagnose those with disease, pain, or injuries, but, unfortunately it is not easy to find someone who can diagnose the condition of the muscles or what is causing pain.

The reason that there are not separate assessments for more advanced individuals and athletes, is that all compensations made during a dynamic or sport specific evaluation are due to simple, isolated, and local dysfunction. Therefore, finding faults in complex movements and then trying to correct them by perfecting that movement or incorporating other complex tasks, will be just as effective as building a nice strong house on top of a weak and crooked foundation. Isolation, and then integration, is the goal; otherwise the body will always be limited by the CNS inability to control segmental stabilization.

The following assessment protocols have been developed to use as a tool for *learning, not diagnosing*, the condition of a person in as many aspects (soft tissue, structure, and function) as are relevant to building an exercise or manual therapy program. The professional should understand and practice within their ability and use the results of the assessments as guidelines for creating an exercise program, not for diagnosing someone with pain or injuries.

The assessments are important for showing a person where they are deficient in ROM, posture, and function, but not the condition of their underlying injury, unless the professional is properly qualified. These assessments are essential for fitness professionals because people often come into a gym setting with aches and pains that have already been treated by a specialist to no avail, and they will do anything to improve their condition. This is a precarious situation since the person often has a vague diagnosis, or has even been told that nothing is wrong and if the pain doesn't go away in a couple of weeks to come back to the doctor for a shot or some medication.

Advice like this and lack of diagnosis is creating a population that is basically treating themselves with whatever they feel or hear is best, which commonly comes from friends or anyone else that has had a similar experience. These populations will then most likely resort to the next level of help, such as massage therapists, personal trainers, etc. This next level of professionals must adapt to the population that is being created by the lack of functional and muscular diagnosis derived from the general health practitioner if they are willing to work with these populations. The adaptation should be learning to recognize the dysfunctional patterns that are detrimental to exercise and daily living, while at the same time adhering to their professional responsibilities of working *with* the doctor on a referral basis for special needs people and not diagnosing or creating treatment plans for special cases without the proper licensing or guidance.

Guidelines for Assessing Asymptomatic and Symptomatic Populations

In order to learn the needs and health of a person in the most time efficient manner, the assessment must be tailored to the quality of each individual's condition.

First, it must be noted whether the person is asymptomatic or symptomatic. Second, if they are symptomatic, what stage of healing are they presently in; acute, subacute, or chronic? Then, use the variety of assessments to discover which tissues and dysfunctions are involved so that a general classification can be given to describe the condition and needs of the individual. Note that the classifications of acute, subacute, and chronic here are different than the stages of soft tissue healing (see pg. 76), which deal with recovery from traumatic injuries; the stages that follow refer to pain caused by repetitive strain (cumulative micro traumas), not traumatic injury, and respond well to corrective exercise, which is the focus of Exercise Progression. As Craig Liebenson[41] states; *"exercise and active care are crucial to the management of subacute, recurrent, and chronic conditions"*.

Asymptomatic, subacute repetitive strain, and chronic pain individuals are the target population for Exercise Progression. Acute and subacute injury traumas are best suited for a licensed practitioner until Stage II of healing has finished, then with guidance from the doctor Exercise Progression can complete the recovery.

Exercise Progression places people into three different groups in order to facilitate the assessment; 1. Asymptomatic 2. Symptomatic, repetitive strain 3. Symptomatic, traumatic injury. The symptomatic population can then be further categorized by which stage of healing they are in. The following descriptions give do's and don'ts and helpful hints for asymptomatic and symptomatic assessments. See fig. 2.1 for a flow chart on assessment progression.

Asymptomatic Assessment

This population can be classified as pain free or having minor aches and pains, i.e. an occasional sore neck or back, caused by the repetitive stresses of daily living. Assessing the needs of this individual will utilize six of the nine categories (see pg.'s 25-29 for detailed descriptions of each category), with the *exclusions being the neurological, structural, and palpation assessments*. These last three tests are optional and often unnecessary for an asymptomatic person, although instances occur where they are helpful.

The objective here is to uncover any major imbalances that will interfere with exercise and to create a program that meets the goals of the individual and yet restores function in the kinetic chain. This can take a lot of educating and insisting to get someone without symptoms to believe that a corrective exercise regimen is the most efficient way to lose weight,

improve strength and stamina, etc.

Symptomatic Assessment

Pain creates altered movement patterns and inhibitions that are not always present in the person when they are pain free, for this reason it is difficult to truly assess the function of an acute or painful dysfunction if an active test causes pain. The clinical wisdom of Vladimir Janda[43] teaches us that; *"A precise evaluation of tight muscles and movement patterns can be performed only if the patient is or is almost painfree"*. Of course, the tests will show the current capabilities of the person, but not their condition before the injury, which if it is a new injury or pain, is very relevant for exercise programming.

In chronic situations, active tests produce reasonably accurate results because the body has "become" the compensations, but acute conditions can cause false-positive tests because they often hide the body's true ability. For instance, an athlete with low back pain from a recent injury can fail a functional test due to pain, trigger points or ischemic conditions, but before the injury they could have easily passed the test. They obviously don't require special training to improve the failed test, instead they need treatment to improve the injury. *Thus, for acute or painful situations, active or functional tests should not be performed unless the results are used as guidelines for improvement, not for program planning.*

Acute Assessment

The acute stage for repetitive strain syndromes will last about 2-3 days[41] and should be rested appropriately until the symptoms reduce greatly. If the symptoms do not reduce greatly then referral to a specialist is indicated. Once the swelling and inflammation subside it can be considered subacute and an assessment is then appropriate once the doctor approves exercise. An acute injury should not be assessed unless the professional is properly licensed. Acute assessments will not be described in this manual because exercise is contraindicated.

Subacute Assessment

The subacute stage for repetitive strain syndromes and moderate injuries lasts 6-8 weeks and up to 16 weeks for severe injuries[41]. Once a doctor has cleared the individual for exercise, repetitive strain injuries in this stage can be assessed by *using the nine categories* described below, although the functional assessment will not occur until Stage I is completed and pain has improved.

Traumatic injuries in this stage should be assessed by a licensed practitioner who then prescribes the appropriate corrective strategies, which is usually physical therapy.

Chronic Assessment

Symptoms lasting past 16 weeks are usually considered chronic[41]. This stage is the most complex of all because psychological stress often plays as big a role as physical stress in the manifestation of symptoms. Never the less, all causes must be taken into account and assessed for relevance and priority involvement. While it is commonly believed that mild soft tissue injuries should be healed by 16 weeks and considered chronic if otherwise, many situations are such that the entire 16 weeks of "healing" are spent repetitively straining the tissues due to a job or other daily activity obligation. In these cases it seems more beneficial to classify the injury as subacute, even though it might be 12 months since the original onset of symptoms.

If after 16 weeks inflammation or swelling is considered chronic, then the condition of the tissues will not be taken into account with the typical chronic protocol, which focuses on functional restoration. This leads to overtraining that could be avoided if a subacute corrective exercise strategy is employed. The above situation is obvious when a relatively minor injury has symptoms that worsen or don't improve over a long period of time. If either inflammation or swelling is present after 16 weeks and repetitive aggravation is suspect, then it is fair to assume that a change in routine is necessary for proper healing to take place and that corrective exercise is a priority over functional restoration.

Always refer to a specialist if the source of pain is unknown, there is a chance that an underlying disease could be the cause of chronic pain.

The chronic assessment involves the same format as the subacute repetitive strain assessment, which is *utilization of all nine categories.*

Classifying Assessment Findings

Once a complete assessment has been performed, it should be clear which areas need to be worked on and what classification(s) fits best. When combining the sub-classifications, *always begin naming with the most influential problem.* For instance, if a lax ligament is causing structural hypermobility, a lack of functional stability, and it was a sub-acute repetitive trauma, it

would be classified as; Repetitive trauma/sub-acute: soft tissue (ligament), structural (hypermobilty), and functional (instability).

The following classifications help to concisely summarize the condition and needs of the individual and are to be used as an aid to exercise programming and informing a person about their functional deficiencies, not diagnosing their problems.

Asymptomatic Classifications

Box 2-1

Soft tissue	Structural	Neuromuscular

Box 2-1 is all part of the kinetic chain classification used below in Box 2-2.

Classifications of Non-Serious Pain Syndromes
Box 2-2

Kinetic Chain	Physiological	Psychological
Soft tissue* Structure* Neuromuscular	Nutrition Cardiovascular system Internal systems etc.	Somatization Depression Fear/Anxiety Inability to cope etc.

* These are further classified by cause (repetitive strain or traumatic injury) and phase (acute, subacute, or chronic).

The following are descriptions of each classification and its sub-classifications. Note that the causes and phases for soft tissue and structural classifications are already described in the symptomatic and asymptomatic assessment descriptions, pg. 21.

The Kinetic Chain

Soft Tissue

These tissues are tested throughout most of the assessment and are commonly involved with structural and functional dysfunctions. See the individual assessment categories to learn how to assess them.

o   Muscle (strain, adhesions, shortness, elongated, trigger points, etc.)
o   Nerve (peripheral entrapment/sciatica)
o   Ligament (sprain or laxity)
o   Tendon (strain, tendonitis, or trigger points)
o   Bursae (bursitis)
o   Fascia (strain, restricted, or adhesions)

Structure

These three sub-categories are general structural abnormalities that will be added to in the low back assessment in chapter 12.

o Joint degeneration
o Hypermobility
o Hypomobility

Neuromuscular Function

o Biomechanics/ PMAP dysfunctions
o Muscular endurance (not cardiovascular)
o Strength
o Proprioception

Physiological

Physiological refers to the organs, blood, lymph, energy, cardiovascular system, nutrition, and inner systems of the body and how they are functioning, i.e. swelling, inflammation, stagnant, high blood pressure, etc. It is out of the scope of this text to discuss physiological influences other than the cardiovascular system's endurance and certain nutrition facts, but it is useful to mention that in Eastern medicine the different systems can be related to different emotions, attitudes, and attributes that can in turn influence the function of the corresponding system and any related body parts. In the case of emotions affecting an inner system, the problem could be considered psychosomatic, as opposed to a physical abnormality in an organ, such as gallstones.

It is also useful to note that certain practices, such as Yoga and Qi gong, utilize different movements with a specific mental focus in order to improve the energy of specific internal organs and systems.

Psychological

Assessing for psychological involvement is best suited for a specialist, but there are certain things to look for that can indicate a need for referral, such as maladaptive tendencies (overreactions, negativity, low self esteem, etc.). These types of behaviors can contribute to or cause non-serious pain syndromes and also negatively influence an exercise or manual therapy program.

Unless it is obvious that psychological involvement is the main cause of pain or dysfunction, a corrective exercise program can often improve the overall function of the body as well as any minor psychological distress regarding the issue being corrected.

How and What to Assess

Deciding on how involved an assessment should be is a matter of personal preference and varies greatly depending on the specialty of the evaluator and goals of the individual. There are two main types of assessments used in Exercise Progression.

1. The total assessment
2. The concise (lazy) assessment

Total Assessment

This type involves assessing as many variables as the professional is capable of and will take a total body approach for the assessment and corrective actions program. It will include nutrition, attitude, and analyzing all of the possible influencing factors mentioned in this text, even if they don't seem relevant at the time. The 'total' approach is best used on those with chronic problems, those who haven't improved with conventional care, or those who seek a complete recovery or program.

Concise Assessment

The term 'lazy' does not indicate that this is a bad approach, but it does imply that it can be used inappropriately. A concise assessment is one that evaluates the most influential factors which can also be promptly dealt with and improve symptoms or dysfunctions quickly, i.e., a quick fix. Deciding on which factors are the most influential is of course up to the clinical wisdom of the evaluator.

This type of assessment is ideal for someone who lacks the proper time or money needed for a complete exercise or manual therapy program, such as someone in town for only a few days visiting, or for those who are not willing to put in the time and effort that is required to improve their situation, i.e. wanting only a quick fix. Ample time must go into educating the latter population about the negative aspects of a quick fix, but in the end, the individual should get what they want and are paying for, which is often relief from symptoms.

This may go against many professional's ideals or style, but it is the author's experience that the quick fix population responds well to having their needs met and respected and has a better chance of slowly converting to a 'total' approach by being educated and having their recurrent problems repeatedly treated successfully, albeit by quick fixes.

The concise assessment and quick fix corrective actions are great tools to help specific populations, but it is wrong to think that this approach is for everyone. Be careful of falling into the trap of giving people what

Assessment Progression (Fig 2-1)

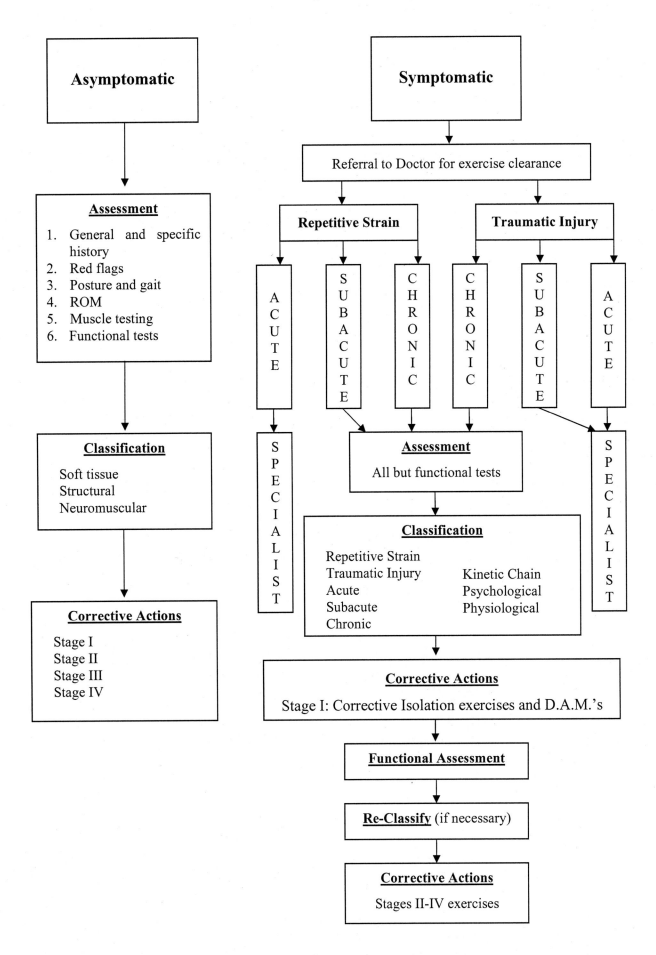

they want without educating them about what is best for their body in the long run.

Assessment Flow

Each category (ROM, posture, etc.) of assessments should be tested for all of the muscles and areas one at a time, rather than assessing one area or muscle at a time with each category and then moving on to the next muscle or area. The latter strategy can cause false negative or positive tests, for instance, if the hip flexors are palpated, stretched, and tested for strength all in the same minute, it can over stimulate the muscle and make it react poorly to the final tests. The approach employed here allows the muscle or area to recuperate after each assessment while the other areas are being assessed, this will lead to more accurate test results. As seen in the flow chart, the functional assessment for a symptomatic population comes after Stage I has been completed.

Finding Key Links

Finding key links is always a priority of assessing and is essential to long term results. Once a dysfunction has been found, its cause must also be found; otherwise certain corrective actions might resemble plugging one's ears when the music is too loud instead of turning down the music, i.e. focusing on the symptom. Often times correcting a key link will correct or improve many or all of the related dysfunctions. Key links are similar to the key trigger points mentioned by Travell and Simon's[7] but also include influential habits and dysfunctions. If these links are not identified and improved, then progress will be slow, if at all for pain improvement. The key links for the low back are described on pg. 148.

The following are general descriptions of each assessment category. The individual low back assessments are located in chapter 12.

Assessment Categories

1. General and specific history
2. Red flags
3. Neurological tests
4. Structural tests
5. Posture and gait
6. ROM
7. Palpation
8. Muscle testing
9. Functional strength tests

➤ This is the order that they should be tested in.

Fig. 2-2 Another way to look at it;

Static Function	Non-Dynamic Function	Dynamic Function
• Posture • Palpation	• ROM • Structural • Muscle tests • Neurological	• Functional strength tests

Main Goals of the assessments:

1. Discover any red flags that contraindicate exercise or require referral to a specialist.
2. Find the *key link* causes of repetitive strain or pain, i.e. structural, soft tissue, neuromuscular, nutritional, emotional, etc.
3. Create a picture of the kinetic chain in terms of weakness, tightness, and dysfunction.

History

A general history is an overview of all injuries, surgeries, medications, diseases, goals of treatment, and current and past lifestyle. A specific history is about the problem in question and can vary for each body part. The history can give an idea of the condition of the tissues and structures if an understanding of biomechanics and injury mechanisms is had by the evaluator. *History is the single most important assessment tool.* The history should be taken in a manner that promotes an easy conversation to get to know the person. Questions that lead a person into answers, judgments, and inappropriate questions can hinder the assessment taking and therefore the entire program. The following are general questions that get to the point and reveal a detailed picture of the person.

General Questions

- Age
- History of jobs and activity level
- History of traumatic events
- All major injuries (past or present)
- Any diagnosis of disease or dysfunction?
- Symptoms (in order of importance)
- Any conditions or medications that limit exercise?
- What are your goals in regards to your condition?
- Nutritional intake form
- Sleep quality

General Questions about Pain

- Did one incident start the pain?

- If so, what?
- How long have you had the pain?
- Have you ever had the pain before?
- When and where is the pain worst?
- Is the pain constant?
- Does it radiate?
- Describe the pain.
- On a scale of 1-10, where is the pain?
- Does it affect daily routine?
- Does activity help?
- What helps the pain?
- What makes it worse?

Red Flags

These are mostly signs that serve to alert the professional of any problems that are serious and might require a referral to a specialist. A red flag contraindicates exercise but can often benefit from the appropriate manual therapy. *Red flags should be assessed first, following the history*, and referred to a specialist whenever appropriate.

Neurological and Structural Tests

These are very useful to be aware of even if the professional is not a doctor or able to diagnose because they can detect very specific and serious dysfunctions that will drastically alter the course of the program if they are not taken into account and referred to a specialist. The main goal here is to find any red flags, such as nerve root involvement or peripheral entrapment. Joint and muscular dysfunction or injury can also be narrowed down on these tests.

Posture and Gait

Posture is viewed at the beginning of the hands-on assessment because it gives a picture of the entire body and its musculoskeletal interactions all at once. There are specific postural faults that point to probable muscle imbalances which can lead the evaluator to focus on important areas. A good postural assessment is essential to finding *key links* of dysfunction and not over focusing on a problematic area. As Karel Lewit[42] reminds us; "he who applies treatment to the site of pain is usually lost".

Ideal posture and alignment allows for ideal structural and functional efficiency in the body and is essential to good health[14,41,101.] Posture requires the combination of muscles, fascia, bones, joints, and the neurological system to keep the body moving and standing properly. There are two types of posture:

Static Posture

Sitting or standing (not moving): Static posture is a foundation for functional posture and should be improved before focusing on dynamic positions. The static posture findings do not give the reasons for any imbalances or show how the person has functionally adjusted to them; these are best investigated through the other assessment tests. In other words, muscle testing, ROM tests, and functional tests are needed to confirm the observations of static posture, just as static posture observations are needed to narrow down which other tests should be performed in order to efficiently find key links and dysfunctions.

Dynamic Posture

Walking, bending, exercising (moving): Dynamic, or functional posture operates on the limits of static posture. *While coordination and neuromuscular efficiency are essential to function, good static posture is essential to neuromuscular efficiency.*

These two postures (dynamic and static) are evaluated while standing, walking, and performing various movements that are mentioned throughout the assessments.

Gait analysis can be broken down into intricate phases, each with many interactions to be observed. For a detailed description of gait analysis, refer to Chaitow and DeLany[4.] Otherwise, practice by observing the body as a whole during walking, from the back, front, and side, and noticing where movement seems inefficient and varies from right to left. There should be a natural rhythm to walking, but tightness, fatigue, pain, weakness, habitual carrying of objects and joint abnormalities can create observable patterns of dysfunction which can be traced back to a single fault.

A keen eye will find where the compensations take place and therefore where to focus the rest of the hands on assessment. It is often a good idea to observe the gait cycle with and without shoes, especially if the person frequently walks around barefoot.

Hyperlordosis and insufficient hip extension or toe off movements are common dysfunctions during the gait cycle. Many gait and posture dysfunctions stem from repetitive uneven carrying of objects, i.e. heavy bags or children, and thus bad habits should be improved before focusing on gait corrections.

There is also an emotional posture. Posture has even been defined as "the attitude of the body"[103.] This type of influence will not be described in detail here because it is a whole other topic. But it is useful to mention that if exercises don't seem to improve a posture or psychological issues seem to be limiting improvement, then education about the importance of a positive attitude in relation to good posture can be a determining factor in improvement. It is not unusual for someone to go through professional counseling and have their posture improve as a byproduct of the therapy. The lesson to be learned from this is don't beat your head against a wall trying to correct an individual's posture with exercises if what is needed is an attitude adjustment.

ROM

ROM tests show the ability of the body in regards to flexibility and quality of movement potential. If the person being evaluated is known to use specific movements on a routine basis, but cannot pass the related ROM tests, then it can be assumed that compensations take place in order to perform the movements. These compensations can be figured out by learning which agonists, synergists, and antagonists are most likely to work harder to make up for the decreased movement. Therefore, it is important to know what type of flexibility the person requires in order to get an idea of the compensations that relate to certain failed ROM tests.

For example, a baseball pitcher can have low back tightness that is caused by decreased external rotation of the pitching arm because the torso and hips will compensate by over rotating. In this case focusing on increasing external rotation in the shoulder will benefit the low back.

The compensations found in the ROM assessment should add to and reinforce the postural findings and can be furthered defined with muscle testing.

Palpation

Descriptions and pictures of palpation methods will be mentioned in chapters 12 and 13. Palpation methods are best suited for those who utilize manual therapy in their practice and feel comfortable with touching strangers. It is essential to feel comfortable with palpation; otherwise the client will feel uncomfortable and tense up.
There are three general rules to palpation;

1. Short fingernails
2. Knowledge of anatomy and landmarks
3. Permission to palpate

When palpating trigger points (TP'S); only palpate ones that can be treated during the same visit, otherwise severe exacerbation of the person's referred pain can

result for up to two days[8]. To locate a TP, palpate for *a nodule within a taut band that elicits extreme tenderness* and often times a characteristic referred pain pattern[8]. Palpation can also be used to find swelling, inflammation, heat, tension, trauma, hypersensitivity, pain, taut bands, restricted fascia, and dehydration.

These symptoms should be assessed for in the problematic areas, as well as in the muscles that refer pain to the symptomatic area. Knowledge of the hierarchy of TP chains (a TP in one muscle can cause TP's in another) can lead to the discovery of the key link, which will improve or even correct the related dysfunctions.

It is important to note any related TP's, restrictions, hypersensitivity, inflammation, or referred pain that come up in the palpation, even if it was released in the process. This will ensure keeping an integrated picture in mind and utilization of the kinetic chain for corrective actions.

Muscle Testing

Manual muscle testing is essential for learning the capabilities of an isolated muscle as well as certain activation patterns, such as hip extension and abduction, trunk flexion, and scapula rhythm. Specific tests are described in the low back assessment section.

Muscle testing is used here to solidify results from the ROM and posture exams, as well as learn if there are any other causes of weakness in the area. In some cases of weakness, the muscle test does not exhibit true function of the muscle, such as when a seemingly normal muscle tests weak. Instead, it can show that an influential factor or factors is disrupting the motor patterns of the tested muscle and probably other muscles nearby. Poor posture is a common cause of motor disruption.

Muscle Grading

0   No ROM or contraction felt in the muscle
1   No ROM, yet a slight contraction can be felt
2   ROM present in non-gravity position (Poor)
3   ROM and ability to hold against gravity only (Fair)
4   Ability to hold against slight resistance (Good)
5   Ability to hold against max* resistance (Normal)

* Max resistance varies depending on the size and location of the msuscle.

Interpreting manual muscle testing results

If a muscle tests weak, then the source of weakness can be narrowed down with the following observations.

- If the weakness is gradual, then the muscle is most likely weak.
- If the weakness is extreme or pressure cannot be resisted at all, then other actors are usually involved, i.e. inhibition, associated joint dysfunctions (arthrogenic weakness), nerve involvement, improper muscle activation patterns, etc.
- If a muscle tests short and weak, then the cause of weakness must be determined to see if stretching is indicated. Causes of weakness could be associated TP's or joint dysfunctions, pain, nerve involvement, etc.
- If any pain is present the test is no good for assessing strength.
- *If a muscle initially tests strong but is suspected to be dysfunctional and elongated, then an endurance test is needed to find the weakness.
- If a muscle fails the endurance test but passes the original strength test, then it is not so much inhibited as it is in a state of decreased functioning due to its overloaded posture.
- If a muscle tests short and strong, then stretching it is usually indicated.

When manual muscle testing, the pressure can be applied in a manner that tests the individual for a specific outcome, such as *endurance, strength, or power*. Muscle testing can be misleading if the wrong function is tested for. For example, an athlete with LBP who utilizes explosive forces can often pass an endurance or strength test but fail a quicker and more intense test because their body doesn't become overloaded until explosive strength (power) is activated. This kind of power testing should not be done for all muscles, those in pain or with major imbalances, or those who are obviously not athletes or well conditioned.

- To test for endurance, (1) apply a moderate amount of pressure for up to ten seconds, (2) apply 1-2 seconds of pressure and repeat for ten repetitions, or (3) have the person isometrically hold the muscle in its shortened position for up to 30 seconds.
- To test for strength, apply a stronger force (the muscle being tested will determine the force necessary) for only a few seconds.
- To test for power, apply a gradually increasing pressure until a strong amount is exerted (isometrically) and then ask the person to quickly contract through the resistance barrier given by the practitioner without exceeding the controllable range of the muscles. The most important factor in explosive testing is not how the one muscle performs, but how the core and other stabilizers are activated before the power is utilized.

This means that detailed observation is necessary while feeling for function.

Ideal tests for power assessment are the sit-up, psoas, back extensors, gluteus maximus, and gluteus medius abduction muscle tests. Experience in muscle testing is a must before attempting power assessments.

Isolated muscle testing takes years of practice and study to obtain accurate results of strength, weakness, and dysfunction. Kendall and McCreary[49] and Hislop and Montgomery[53] give detailed descriptions and examples of the trials and tribulations of muscle testing and are recommended readings prior to any practicing of muscle testing.

The muscles tested should coincide with the muscles that were most often indicated in the assessments leading up to this point of the assessment. Results from the testing should be weighed with all other findings from the previous assessments in order to determine the true cause of a weakness or dysfunction. Muscle testing is also useful after a session of manual therapy to show improvement or lack there of. It is a great tool to physically demonstrate that the work being done is helping.

Functional Strength Testing

Functional testing shows an individual's basic functional capacity as well as identifies areas in need of restoration. Re-evaluation of these tests along with the ROM, posture, proprioception, and cardio tests every four weeks gives the ultimate progress report and is ideal for work hardening programs because some of the results are quantifiable, such as repetitive squatting while picking up a weight. Many of the functional tests can also be used as an exercise to improve that specific task.

Analyzing results from functional tests should take into account the physical demands that the person goes through on a daily or frequent basis. For instance, a construction worker or athlete should meet higher standards on many of the tests than a computer analyst. Individual variations are noted for the appropriate tests in the low back functional assessment section.

Functional tests are great for showing how isolated imbalances work together to create widespread compensations. It is important to note when people have static posture or ROM imbalances but can perform dynamic actions with good form. These individuals are usually well trained and have overcome their imbalances with superior strength and control, but further testing will often find that endurance of dynamic stability is lacking due to the static imbalances. For this reason the functional tests here do not involve evaluating advanced or complex movements. In other words, *even if there is dynamic dysfunction, it is the isolated or static imbalances that need to be corrected first in order to establish a foundation for all movement.* This is also why the functional assessment should not be performed by symptomatic populations until Stage I is completed, (see flow chart), by then some of the functional deficiencies may have improved in response to the corrective activation exercises.

Chapter 3   Cardio

The cardiovascular system is the engine that runs the body. The more efficiently it works, the more efficiently the entire body functions. If it is trained appropriately, the heart (at rest) will pump more blood with each beat, while utilizing fewer beats per minute.[33,34] This decreases the demands on the heart at rest and during exercise.[33,34] But if it is over, or under trained, the heart can also limit or decrease health throughout the body.

There are many different ways to assess cardiovascular fitness, and most involve special equipment, equations, and tables to calculate VO2 max. Exercise Progression will use a simple and effective method to assess cardiovascular training, but an experienced practitioner is vital to assessing the individual's effort and pushing them within their health limits.

Some people will not be comfortable exercising at 60% of their heart rate reserve (HRR), but with some education and encouragement they can achieve increased confidence, fitness, and health.

In order to assess a person's effort and reaction to exercise, their heart rate needs to be taken. The feedback will be from conversation and a heart rate monitor. The *key factor determining maximum effort is whether the person can hold a conversation without struggling for breath.* But, both a heart rate monitor and conversation are needed because some people are:

• So deconditioned that their target heart rate (THR) is much too difficult to reach or maintain, and therefore a strenuous conversation is a better sign of excess effort.
• Highly trained and can converse easily at higher heart rates, and thus need the conversation limit.
• Accustomed to overexertion and can sustain injuriously high heart rates for a prolonged time, these individuals need a heart rate monitor and THR to avoid deterioration and achieve health.

The formula used here to obtain a target heart rate range for a low risk male or female will be the HRR, or Karvonen Method, as used by the Amereican Academy of Sports Medicine (ACSM).[33] This method consists of subtracting the resting heart rate (RHR) from the maximum heart rate (MHR = 220- age), and then multiplying that number by a percentage (usually 60-80%), and finally adding the RHR back to the number to obtain a healthy range. For example, an average thirty year old with a resting heart rate of 50 beats/min would use the following formulas;

Target Heart Rate range = [(MHR-RHR) x percent intensity] + RHR

THR range (60% intensity) = [(190-50) x 0.60] + 50 = 134 beats/min

THR range (80% intensity) = [(190-50) x 0.80] + 50 = 162 beats/min

THR range (60-80%) = 134-162 beats per minute

The MHR (220-age) is only an approximation and has a variance of plus or minus 10-12 beats per minute.[33] The HRR formula is more accurate than simply taking a percentage of the MHR, especially when dealing with beginners and those training in lower heart rate zones; it is also more closely linked to the %VO2max and %VO2R than the other formula.[33]

If there are any medical conditions that limit exercise, always check with the doctor for a proper THR.

In order to increase cardiovascular fitness for low risk individuals, it is recommended[33] that one must:

1. Exercise 3-5 days per week
2. Exercise for 25-40 min per session
3. Sustain 60-85% HRR
4. Do aerobic exercises (walk, jog, swim, dance, etc.)
5. Engage in enjoyable aerobic activity

Choosing an appropriate cardio exercise can be a difficult task with such a variety of options to choose from. As far as the cardiovascular system is concerned, as long as the heart rate is where it's supposed to be, it will get the appropriate benefits. But for the muscles and bones, each machine is very different.

Walking, jogging, or running, are the *best over all exercises*, injuries permitting, for the entire body. They create an impact force on the feet that strengthens the bones throughout the body, unlike swimming, biking, stair steppers, rowing, or elliptical machines that do not stress the bones enough. A mixture of non-impact and impact aerobic activity can be done for a variety of purposes, but impact is essential for bone density, especially for females.

The treadmill is one machine that this author does not recommend for daily use unless it is the only option for walking or jogging. Two reasons being are;

1. The movement of the belt swings the leg into extension, therefore removing that responsibility from the leg extensor muscles, which are very important for posture and low back functioning.

2. It forces the hip flexors to alternate between decelerating leg extension and flexing the hip. Meanwhile the hip extensors are not getting the workout they should, if at all, which leads to the already too common faulty posture of an anterior tilted pelvis and dominant hip flexors.

Walking, jogging, or running on the ground is ideal because it forces the leg extensors to work and promotes a more natural pattern of movement. Most other cardio machines are relatively effective, but sitting on a bike to exercise makes little sense if the rest of the day also involves a lot of sitting.

While the whole body benefits from cardiovascular training, there are specific adaptations (increased VO2 max or decreased submaximal exercise heart rate) that occur more profoundly in the areas being used, for instance, upper or lower extremities.[33] This is important if someone wants to have endurance capabilities in their arms. This person should work the arms as well as the legs during cardio training.[33] Rowing, cross-country skiing, swimming, and arm ergometers are all suitable for upper extremity endurance training.

The amount of recommended exercise is constantly changing and creating confusion about how much exercise is healthy. While engaging in aerobic exercise more than five times per week is not associated with improved cardiovascular fitness, common sense reveals that movement is life, and *moderate activity* of at least a half hour on a *daily* basis is essential for a healthy body, especially if the majority of the day is spent sitting.

❖ Intense aerobic activity should not be done during the same workout as intense weight lifting, due to the high demands it places on the heart. The heart is a muscle and needs proper rest.

Exercise should be stopped immediately along with a referral to a medical professional if the person develops any of the following red flag symptoms.

Chest pain
Dizziness
Numbness and tingling
Radiating pain
Shortness of breath

Stages of Cardio Training

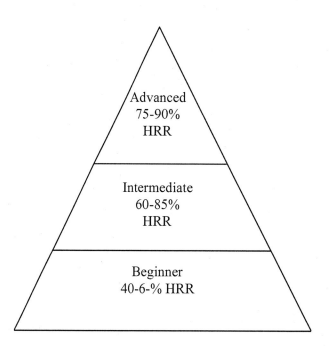

Stage I   **Beginner** (Unfit)
Stage II   **Intermediate** (General Health)
Stage III   **Advanced** (Athlete/Extremist)

Cardio Progression Stages I-III
Beginner to Advanced Exercises

Description

The cardio progressions are the simplest stages to follow in Exercise Progression. All that is needed is a THR range, heart rate monitor, mode of exercise, and a goal time of duration. This simple format even works for athletes and advanced persons. In general, when training for a specific result, the more the training resembles the goal performance, the better the results will be. For serious competitors, a special coach or training regimen should replace the cardio progression stages in this book.

Guidelines

- If health is the goal, find a comfortable intensity that is within the accepted scale and stick with it. There is no need to push past the comfort zone if that zone already promotes health. Focusing on numbers can lead the body down the wrong path.
- If losing weight is a goal, then intense cardio is not recommended. Although it may be counter-intuitive, if the body is working very hard it will not burn as much fat as it would if it was exercising at a steady rate, usually around 60-80% HRR. For fat loss goals it is best to stick with less intensity and a longer duration.
- Proper hydration and nutrition are essential before and after exercise to avoid sudden fatigue or dizziness.

Priorities

- Utilize impact training (walking, jogging, or running) to strengthen the bones and stabilizing muscles.
- Pay attention to the heart, don't overdo it.
- Whenever possible, train outdoors in the fresh air.
- Stretch after cardio sessions.

Variables

- Duration   Each stage is completed when the following can be done comfortably.
- Frequency   3-5x week
- Intensity   Stage I (40-60% HRR) Stage II (60-85% HRR) Stage III (75-90% HRR)
- Time Stage I (15-30 min)   Stage II (25-40 min)   Stage III (20-60 min)

Choosing Exercises

- Choose from upper extremity machines, lower extremity machines, a combination of both, or any enjoyable activity that increases the demand on the heart in an appropriate manner.
- Seven times a week is not too much if it is simply brisk walking, although occasional days off should be taken.

Chapter 4   Stretching

Before we talk about stretching, the reader should know that this chapter is about stretching as its own component. It is possible however to never really set time aside to "stretch" and still stay flexible and balanced. This is done by incorporating dynamic movements with stretch-like exercises throughout the workout.

For example; lunges stretch the hip flexors, front kicks stretch the hamstrings, cable presses with full ROM stretch the chest, rotating one-arm rows help mobilize the thoracic spine, etc. But because this is a low back disorder manual, we will talk about how to take time out and stretch to relax the body, increase body awareness, and ease tension.

With that being said, stretching is unlike strengthening because it requires precise techniques in order to reap the benefits. Muscles will grow stronger if enough weight is lifted, regardless of technique, of course proper techniques and progression will yield better results. But if stretching is done incorrectly, more often than not that time was wasted and there will be little to no change produced in the length of the tissues. This is one reason why people give up on stretching; it's difficult to produce results! There needs to be a total body stretching and strengthening *strategy* in order to create the appropriate changes, otherwise problem areas will cause related muscles to tighten or compensate. There are many sections throughout this manual that deal with these strategies.

In Exercise Progression stretching is similar to strengthening in that it begins with simple posture correcting stretches, and then progresses to complex dynamic actions. Advanced stretching requires more than just flexibility; it requires strength, stability, coordination, and balance to place the body into the positions necessary for dynamic flexibility. For this reason, a systematic progression is needed to avoid injury.

Connective and contractile tissue both progressively shorten if they are not stretched regularly.[10] Therefore, stretching must be frequent in order for the body to avoid tightening up into a constricted mass of rigidity. But before stretching, it's necessary to know *what, when, why, and how* to stretch. There are many different techniques of stretching, but none are very effective unless:

- Enough *time* is spent stretching
- Proper *breathing* is used
- The muscles are *warm*
- The stomach is not full
- It is known how much or how little movement is needed for a *safe stretch*
- It is known *what* is being stretching
- The movements are smooth, *no bouncing*
- The *mind is focused* on stretching
- The resistance barrier of the tissues is respected so that the stretch reflex is not a limiting factor.

Benefits of stretching

- Correcting muscle and posture imbalances that can lead to many problems
- Enhanced physical fitness
- Facilitated daily movements
- Improved mental and physical relaxation
- Decreased risk of injury
- Decreased muscular soreness and tension, especially post-exercise soreness
- Helps body's systems function smoothly by increasing blood flow and nutrients, and decreasing tension.

Types of Flexibility

Non-dynamic

Passive, self-myofascial release, active, isometric, and active assisted stretching techniques are all non-dynamic. This type of flexibility is less complex and usually achieved in one plane, sometimes two, and is best used to correct posture imbalances and elongate muscles because of its relatively simple methods. It does not transfer very well into dynamic or multi-planar flexibility because it lacks the neuromuscular coordination. Non-dynamic flexibility is the foundation of stretching and should be the first goal of any novice or injured person.

Dynamic

Dynamic techniques, like Yoga movements, are the only way to achieve dynamic flexibility. This type of flexibility is controlled by the neuromuscular system and allows the muscles to elongate while controlling the body's speed, direction, balance, and coordination. Therefore, neuromuscular and postural efficiency are required to avoid injury. All three planes of movement should be challenged in a way that prepares the body for real life situations, such as reaching behind the washing machine to pick up fallen clothing. Dynamic flexibility cannot be totally converted into non-dynamic flexibility because the maximum length allowed by the muscle is rarely reached in a dynamic stretch.

➤ Both types are needed for overall flexibility.

Example: An athlete has a daily routine of non-dynamic stretching for the entire body and can pass every basic ROM test there is, but he/she does not do any dynamic stretching. If they are blessed with great coordination and flexibility it is possible to escape wear and tear or clumsy injuries. But, if they are like most people, they will need to practice dynamic flexibility, otherwise a situation will eventually occur that puts the body into a position it has neither the strength, flexibility, or coordination to control, all of which could have been trained through dynamic stretching.

Mental

A flexible mind is an open mind which transmits its energy into the tissues, leaving them supple and adaptable to change. A closed mind equals a rigid attitude which can lead to a rigid spine and body that is not flexible to change. Often times changing an attitude will soften tissues and leave them more pliable and healthy, as well as improve many systems and their functions in the body. Mental exercises are out of the scope of this text, but in general if one can be aware of their attitude then one can practice to be more flexible and open to ideas and situations, most importantly the ones that we disagree with or hide from. A key to success of course is the desire for improved health.

Important Reflexes

Stretch Reflex (muscle spindles)

Sudden or excessive stretching of a muscle causes that muscle to contract and resist the stretch.[18,19,27] This is the main reflex involved in stretching.

Reciprocal Inhibition

As a muscle contracts it forces its antagonist to relax.[19] And, a tight muscle creates decreased neural drive to its antagonist.[27,41,101,102]

Autogenic Inhibition (golgi tendons)

If the neural impulses that sense tension are greater than those causing the muscle contraction, then the contraction will be inhibited (the contracting muscle is inhibited by its own receptors).[27] Sustained golgi tendon stimulation will also cause inhibition (autogenic) of the muscle spindles in the agonist.[27] This is the reason that a stretch should be held for at least 20 seconds. For example, once the resistance barrier is reached for a stretch the muscle spindles in the stretched muscle will initiate the reflex to contract and shorten that muscle to protect it, but if the stretch is held at this barrier for a certain time (about 20 seconds) the golgi tendon reflex will inhibit the muscle spindles and allow the stretch to progress into new lengths that can become easier to maintain because the muscle spindles adapt by becoming desensitized and requiring a greater length/stretch to activate their reflex.

➤ See pg. 46 for descriptions of golgi tendons and muscle spindles

Stretching Techniques

Most stretching techniques are ineffective unless the resistance barrier and reflexes of the tissues are respected. The *barrier* refers to the first point of sensed or palpated resistance to movement and always comes well before the limits of the tissue. This barrier must be perceived and utilized in order to work with and not against the reflex systems. The main error in stretching comes from treating a muscle like it is a physical object that needs to be lengthened. In reality it is a physical object that is controlled, and therefore lengthened, by a higher system, i.e. the neurological system and its reflexes.

The following techniques are starting from the easiest (Passive) and progressing to the most difficult (Dynamic). See Exercise Progression Vol. II for pictures and descriptions of the stretches.

- *Passive*
- *Self-Myofascial Release*
- *Active*
- *Isometric*
- *Ballistic*
- *Active Assisted*
- *Dynamic*

Passive (static)

A part of the body (usually the hands and arms), a partner, or an object is used to hold the muscle in a stretched position at the first barrier for 20-30 seconds. An example is lying on your back with the feet up on a wall. This type of stretching is used for *cooling down* after activity. It is also ideal *for beginners* and isolating muscles to *correct imbalances.* This is the easiest and safest type of stretching.

- Hold for 20-30 seconds each, repeat 2-3 times, up to 4 times per day

Self Myofascial Release

This technique uses small balls, foam rolls, or massage devices to put direct pressure on the muscles and fascia, moving from one spot to the next. The rolling techniques (volume II) are used to find tender points on the muscle. It affects muscle length indirectly by rubbing out the trigger points and adhesions in the muscle that stretching sometimes misses.

Experience is needed in order to properly release the tension spots, otherwise it is possible to "wake up" and aggravate painful areas that weren't noticeable before the treatment. This type of stretching is ideal for those who have to limit their range of motion or who have soft tissue adhesions, and can be used in conjunction with other stretching types. It can be done *before and or after activity*, depending on the severity of the adhesions.

- Hold each point for 20-30 seconds, 1-2 time per day, up to 4 times per week per body part

Active

This technique contracts the muscle opposite of the stretch, thereby utilizing reciprocal inhibition to relax the muscle. It works by contracting a muscle to put its antagonist into a lengthened position, i.e. the quadriceps contracting and pulling the hamstrings into a stretch.

Active stretching is great for correcting posture because it can work on strengthening a weak muscle (rhomboids) while simultaneously stretching a tight muscle (pectoralis major). This brings balance and stability to the surrounding joints and area. Active stretching is also great because it keeps the joint(s) and tissues being stretched in a position of relative safety due to the fact that the areas being stretched will only go as far as the contracting muscles can take them, and any sort of pain or dysfunction will result in a stretch reflex that causes the muscle being stretched to contract, therefore stopping the stretch. As long as the muscles are warm and stretched slowly, no injuries should occur. Care should be taken with stretches that use body weight to influence muscle length because the weight can be too much for the stretch reflexes to overcome. The active stretching technique is best used as a *posture correcting exercise, muscle activation*

exercise (reversing reciprocal inhibition), or a *warm-up*, rather than as a warm-down.

If the contraction is held for too long it can cause muscle fatigue and decreased oxygen in the contracting muscle, therefore contractions should be limited to 10 seconds.

- Contract for 6-10 seconds each, repeat 5-10 times, 1-3 times per day (moderate contraction)

Isometric

This technique contracts and stretches the same muscle. Passively stretch the muscle to the first resistance barrier, then use the arms or an object to resist a moderate contraction of the muscle being stretched, contract for 6-8 seconds without movement (isometric). Finally, relax the muscle at least 20-30 seconds in the stretched position and repeat until no further progress is made. An example is the supine hamstring stretch against the wall. This type of stretching has a greater risk of injury than a passive stretch and should be done *at most every other day* because of the demand it puts on the muscle

- Contract for 6-8 seconds, relax it in the stretched position for 20-30 seconds, repeat 1-5 times, 1 time every other day

Ballistic (bouncing)

This is considered *more dangerous than useful*. It can actually cause the muscle to tighten up from repeatedly activating the stretch reflex. The more sudden the change in muscle length the stronger the reflex is. Although ballistic is a type of stretching it is ***not recommended***.

Active Assisted (neuromuscular stretching)

Over the years there have been many contributors to the improvement of neuromuscular stretching and techniques. This book describes what has worked for the author, which is a mixture of muscle energy techniques (MET) and proprioceptive neuromuscular facilitation (PNF). Therefore, the following techniques are modifications of both, with brief descriptions of their applications and techniques. A detailed description of neuromuscular stretching requires a book all in itself, so further reading is recommended on the subject to fully comprehend the mechanisms and applications of the techniques. Active assisted stretching is the ultimate way to stretch because it utilizes the reflex mechanisms of the body and the experience of a good practitioner to safely and effectively stretch, strengthen, or re-educate muscles. A partner allows for a varied resistance against isotonic and isometric contractions in specific directions.

Isometric contraction – a muscle, or group of muscles, contracts against an equal force which allows no movement to take place.

Isotonic contraction – a contraction that produces movement. There are two types of isotonic contractions, concentric and eccentric.

Concentric - the force of the contraction is more than that of the resistance, creating a shortening of the muscle fibers which is good for toning weak muscles.

Eccentric – the force of the contraction is less than that of the resistance, so the muscle is overpowered which lengthens the muscle fibers. This type of stretch is beneficial for altering soft tissue adhesions[4,11,12] but is detrimental to injured tissues because it causes microtraumas.

Active stretching techniques are successful because of two neurological reactions.

1. *Postisometric relaxation* (PIR)
The tissues involved with the isometric contraction are more easily stretched during the 15 seconds that follow the contraction due to Golgi tendon reflexes.[4,11,15]

2. *Reciprocal Inhibition*
An isometric contraction of a muscle results in the relaxation of its antagonist which allows it to be stretched with less resistance.[4,11,12]

Guidelines

• Active assisted stretching is for advanced and experienced persons only and should be done *at most every other day* on a given muscle because of the high demands it puts on the tissues. It should be done very carefully on kids, those who are pain sensitive or osteoporotic, the cervical region, and the elderly.

• The person should be relaxed with the body well supported.

• Slight discomfort is acceptable, pain is not.

• If the person is able, without pain or excessive effort, gentle active assistance to and through the barrier is beneficial because it creates reciprocal inhibition in the stretched muscle.

• Light to moderate contractions are used, 20-50%. Always start with a light contraction and progress only if needed.

• All contractions are built slowly and smoothly and held for 6-8 seconds, with a 10 second maximum in

order to keep a sufficient supply of oxygen in the muscle.

• The initial contraction should be made at or just before the barrier.

• The muscle is stretched gently past the barrier after a contraction and then held for at least 20 seconds, it should be eased back slightly before the next contraction is made. This is to protect the muscle from contracting in a vulnerable position.

• A resting period of 2-5 seconds along with a slight let up of the stretch is beneficial following the contraction to ensure complete relaxation of the muscle before moving it past the barrier and into a stretch.

• One cycle of a stretch (contract, relax, and stretch) is repeated 3-5 times or until no further length is gained in the muscle.

• Each stretch is held for at least 20 seconds.

• When *pain or injury* is present in a muscle, the barrier is the farthest that the muscle should be pushed. Then 3-5 isometric contractions can be used along with a progression to a new barrier (without a stretch past it) made after each contraction. Each barrier should be held for 10-20 seconds.

• Breathing is essential to muscle lengthening and is best if done as follows.[9]

1. Inhale as the isometric contraction begins.
2. Hold breath for the 6-8 second contraction.
3. Release the breath and contraction slowly.
4. Inhale and exhale slowly once more.
5. This last exhalation should coincide with a stretching of the muscle to or past a new barrier.

• Eye movements are also useful in facilitating a stretch. Karil Lewit MD[14,15] found a relationship between eye movements and isometric stretching exercises that is as follows. During the contraction phase, one should look in a direction that is away or opposite of the direction of the stretch, and during the relaxation or stretch phase the eyes should look towards the direction of the stretch.

Active Assisted Techniques

Isometric Contract and Relax

A partner passively stretches a muscle until the barrier is reached, then that muscle or its antagonist is isometrically contracted against resistance for 6-8 seconds while holding the breath and coordinating the eyes' movements. This is followed by 2-5 seconds of relaxation, and then the partner passively stretches it to the next resistance barrier and a little beyond, in unison with the exhalation and eye movements. If possible, the person should assist with the movement into the stretch. This stretch is held at least 20 seconds and then repeated until no further progress is made.

Isometric contract and relax technique is very effective for most stretching situations.

Contract-Relax-Antagonist-Contract (CRAC)

A partner passively stretches a muscle until the barrier is reached, then that muscle is isometrically contracted against resistance for 6-8 seconds (just like the previous method). Next, that muscle is relaxed and its antagonist is immediately contracted isometrically for 6-8 seconds. Finally the muscle is relaxed into (not past) the next barrier for at least 20 seconds, and then repeated if necessary.

The *CRAC* technique is effective but not always applicable because of the shortened positions the antagonist can be put in during a stretch. For example, the hamstrings will commonly cramp if contracted while in the shortened position of a quadriceps stretch. On the other hand, the quadriceps are a perfect example of an antagonist that can be isometrically contracted, such as in a hamstring stretch.

Eccentric Contract and Relax

This method of stretching is used to break down adhesions[4,11,12] in the tissues that build up with age or overuse and can sometimes be uncomfortable, so the person should be told to contract only as hard as they can tolerate. Their contraction is slightly overcome by the practitioner's effort, therefore creating an eccentric or lengthening contraction by the person. The contractions start easy and build up to a maximum pain free effort (provided the practitioner can resist that effort) with each ensuing contraction. The practitioner should stretch (overpower) the muscle only as far as the muscle can maintain a contraction without compensations elsewhere.

A maximum of five contractions should be made, with each contraction lasting at most five seconds. This technique requires at least three days of rest in between sessions on the same area, and is not for the delicate, pain sensitive, or cervical regions of the body. Manual therapy techniques are sometimes useful prior to 'eccentric contract and relax' methods in order to reduce the discomfort of the contractions.

Dynamic (functional)

Dynamic stretching incorporates multiple muscle groups to stabilize, balance, accelerate and decelerate the body through multi-planar movements, and at the same time take the joints through their greatest and safest ROM for that particular position. It's not often in a daily routine or sport that simply one muscle is used, so stretching one at a time should be integrated with stretching many at a time. Dynamic flexibility training should;

1. Sufficiently challenge the neuromuscular system.
2. Involve complex movements and muscles acting as a team.
3. Utilize proper alignment of the joints to obtain a *healthy* ROM.

Dynamic stretching is the best way to stretch in order to prepare the body for working out or other physical activities because it warms the body up (temperature and neuromuscular coordination) and lengthens the muscles without causing the post-stretching weakness and decreased performance that static stretching does. Unfortunately, it is common for people to injure themselves during some of the advanced stretches. Therefore it is important to systematically progress the body's tissues and neuromuscular system in a way that keeps the body in control of its movements. This control is difficult to achieve without first correcting the major imbalances and learning proper muscle activation patterns (PMAP).

Dynamic stretching can be done as a progressive sequence of stretches or on an individual basis. The progressive sequence follows the principals of yoga which challenge the entire body through coordinated patterns of movement starting off easy and ending up more difficult. Throughout the progression the body will use proper breathing to become warmer and warmer, further enhancing the stretching potential of the muscles. Towards the end of the progression is when long-term increases in muscle length are achieved. There are many ways to develop a progressive stretch routine, as is evident by all the different yoga books. The progressive routines in this book have been developed from the author's experience of working with injured and healthy populations as well as his own injuries and sports career. The best way to create a personal program is to try as many routines as possible and then mix and match the movements that help the most and put them in an order that flows from simple to difficult.

Dynamic stretching is advanced and requires strength, balance, coordination, flexibility, and stability; it is not for beginners or people with major imbalances. Following the complete routines described in Exercise Progression is recommended before starting any dynamic stretching.

Dynamic stretching is *great for warm up* if it's limited to a duration that won't cause pre-activity fatigue. It's also great as its own workout when done for longer periods of time. Some benefits of dynamic stretching are *increased strength and overall neuromuscular efficiency.*[20,22,23]

- *Within a progression*: 1 rep, hold for 20-30 seconds*, continue on to a given number of complementary and progressive stretches, repeat this cycle 3-10 times. A progression can have any number of cycles, depending on the goal. 1-7x per week
- *Individual Basis*: 1 set of 5-10 reps, hold for 20-30 seconds each*, 3-5x per week

* Some dynamic stretches use fluid movements and therefore are not held for very long.

Time (frequency and duration)

Stretching will not be very beneficial if seconds being counted are the focus; the focus must be on the tension of the muscle and relaxing it. There is no one time (frequency or duration) that is agreed upon to be the most beneficial for increasing muscle length, this must be attributed to the uniqueness of each person's condition.

Ideally stretching is done at least ten minutes a day with a longer 30-60 minute progression session performed at least once a week. In general, 20-30 seconds is the recommended time to hold a stretch and inhibit the reflexive muscle tightening that a stretch causes. There are no permanent results from stretching, in other words the muscles will shorten if they are not lengthened regularly. Depending on the reason for the tightness it can take seconds, minutes, days, or even weeks of stretching before a muscle relaxes and a new length is established. How often stretching is needed will depend upon each person's daily routine and health. The less movement throughout the day the more need there is to stretch and exercise. Most people need to stretch everyday.

Breathing

If breathing isn't relaxed and synchronized with the stretch, then results will be poor. The exhalation helps relax the muscle and is most beneficial during the elongation phase. While holding a stretch for the appropriate time the inhalation should be similar to the exhalation in force and duration (3-5 seconds in, 3-5 seconds out, with a pause in between). This isn't always possible at the beginning of a difficult stretch, but by the last few seconds a rhythm should be achieved, otherwise the muscles won't completely relax

and *accept* the new length. At first it will seem impossible to relax in some of the new positions, but by focusing on proper breathing it is possible to reach the muscle's greatest stretch potential.

What is being stretched?

Muscles/tendons: See techniques in previous pages.
Nerves: Nerves are already being stretched when muscles are stretched, but to fully stretch them they must be stretched across their entire length, which is from head to toe, pelvis to toe, and from head to finger. Nerves can **easily** be **overstretched** and inflamed if the duration or intensity is too much. They should be stretched gently and slowly in a relaxed manner. *Talk to your doctor before stretching nerves.*

- Hold for 2-3 seconds, repeat 5-6 times, 1-2 times per day

Joints (cartilage, synovial fluid, bursae, etc.): Joints are also already being stretched when muscles are stretched, but sometimes adhesions or scar tissue limit the joint's range of motion and special techniques from a professional are needed to free it up. It is usually obvious when a joint is the limiting factor during a stretch because the range of motion comes to a sudden stop instead of a gradual one. This can be painful or not. Professional help, such as mobilization techniques, is recommended when stretching joints.

Fascia: Stretching fascia is more subtle than stretching muscle because of the superficial and deep layers that intertwine from head to toe (see pg. 130 for a description of fascia); it requires experience and a "feel" for the body's tension. It's less like a muscle stretch and more like an interaction with the body's network of physical strain in a way that unlocks tightness throughout the entire body, not just a small area.

Self-myofascial release can be used in conjunction with the other fascia stretches if necessary. Fascia stretches (not self-myofascial release) should be held 90-120 seconds, just as in the manual therapy techniques for myofascial release, in order to open up hyrdo-attractive channels of flow that alter the extra-cellular matrix from a gel-like substance to a more liquid state, thereby leaving the tissues more resilient.

How far is enough to get a good stretch?

The goal isn't to go as far as one can, rather as far as one should. The end-feel of a stretch is the best guide to how far and even if stretching should be done. If the end-feel is a structural blockage or sharp pain, then stretching can do more harm than good. But if the end-feel is a leathery restriction, like muscle, then stretching should help the limitation.

Stretch the muscle to the barrier (*first point* of moderate tension), hold until the muscle "let's go" or about 20-30 seconds is reached, then, relax it or gently stretch it to the next point of noticeable tension. More is not always better when it comes to twisting, bending, pulling, pushing, and everything else that is possible to do to the body. It can be a fine line between injury and improvement depending on the condition of the surrounding tissues and the stretching techniques used. Stretching to the limit will often create instability in the involved joint(s) due to surpassing the ability of the antagonist to stabilize the joint(s). A great way to prevent overstretching is to stretch slowly and smoothly, get the muscles warm, and *make sure the surrounding muscles (especially the antagonist) can support the joint in that position.*

What muscles should be stretched?

Most often people tend to stretch the areas that feel the tightest, this may help momentarily but that tightness is often coming from other disturbances, such as bad posture. For example, the benefits of neck stretching will last only until the head starts to fall forward again from bad posture, therefore the chest needs to be stretched and the shoulders pulled back in order to keep the neck muscles in a position of ease.

Ideally an experienced professional checks posture, ROM, and other things to find imbalances and creates a plan of what to stretch. Sometimes one muscle must be strengthened for another to fully stretch. Since not everyone is so lucky to have the option of a detailed assessment, a *general* approach can be taken to stretching the muscles that are most commonly tight, see Box 1-2.

When stretching, remember that just because a certain muscle isn't tight today doesn't mean it won't be tight tomorrow or the next day. So "scanning" the whole body on a weekly basis is very valuable and takes less than 10 minutes once familiar with the stretches; use the cool-down stretches that are in the appendix.

What order is best to stretch in?

As long as the muscles are properly stretched, most of the benefits will be had. But to *best* stretch a muscle, other muscles and more importantly *fascia* must

sometimes be stretched first. Because the fascia intertwines throughout the muscles it can limit their stretching ability. The fascia also is not greatly affected by individual muscle stretches, and therefore must first be 'unlocked' by stretches that incorporate the different layers and directions of fascia, then the muscles will have a freer environment to stretch in.

Progressive routines are ideal for this if designed properly. When stretching specific areas of the body it is beneficial to start first with the surrounding fascia (larger areas and more general stretches), and then with the muscles that are tight and have the greatest influence on the surrounding structures, and therefore the surrounding muscles.

When should stretching be done?

Before exercise

Stretching before exercise is tricky and gets mixed results from many studies. It can be ill-advised to change a warm-up routine that has been successful in the past, no matter how unorthodox it seems. When the mind is relaxed, the body is relaxed, so unless the person can be convinced that a new warm-up routine will be better, it is best to stick with what works.

Acute stretching has been shown to *decrease strength and power*[21][22], for at least ten minutes[21] and up to one hour[23] after stretching. Although stretching does seem to decrease injury potential, it may also decrease performance.[20] It seems obvious that one shouldn't try to *simply* lengthen a muscle soon before it needs to shorten and produce great force, even though the lengthening may contribute to some degree of injury protection for the muscle. Goals for warm-up stretching should be;

Goals of Warm-up Stretching

1. Activity specific
2. Utilize active control by the neuromuscular system
3. Correct major imbalances
4. Do not hold stretches for long periods of time (over 5-10 seconds).

These goals will prepare the neuromuscular system for action while preventing injury by lengthening the muscles and improving dysfunctions caused by compensations.

With all that being said, sometimes there are certain muscles that need to be passively or if possible actively stretched and thus weakened before exercise in order to improve major imbalances and reciprocal inhibition. For instance, if the gluteus maximus was going to be strengthened, it could be facilitated by stretching the psoas (if they were tight) before the exercise. Tightness in muscles causes decreased neural drive in their opposing muscles (reciprocal inhibition), and using muscles that have decreased neural drive will lead to less than optimal results. Therefore, people with inhibited muscles should stretch the antagonistic muscles prior to exercise, while people without major imbalances can prepare for exercise with more activity specific movements. A few of the benefits gained by pre-activity stretching of specific muscles involved in major imbalances are:

1. Activating inhibited muscles.
2. Inhibit overactive muscles, making them more like the others.
3. Creating better joint mechanics and thus reducing wear and tear.
4. Improving dynamic strength by increasing muscle recruitment and force couple efficiency.

This type of specific warm-up stretching prepares the body for dynamic movements (sports and exercise) as well as isolated exercises. When stretching before exercise a few options are useful:

• If time permits, total body stretching at least one hour before the activity will lengthen the muscles without causing a decrease in strength by game or workout time. Then, soon before it's time for action, activity specific movements along with dynamic stretching should be used to warm-up the neuromuscular system, along with *active* stretches that improve influential dysfunctions.
• If time doesn't permit, strategic *active* stretching can be done on muscles that cause inhibitions and postural distortions, while the rest of the warm-up is focused on activity specific movements.

When injuries and major imbalances are a concern, it is more important to correct dysfunctions before activity with stretching than have maximum strength in the muscles. For those with major imbalances or injuries, start by getting the muscles warm with 5-10 minutes of cardio, jumping jacks, shooting a basketball, etc., and then prepare the area with the movement stretches (see below). Once the muscles are warm and the structures have been loosened, specific *active* stretches should be used for correcting any major imbalances and reciprocal inhibitions in the muscles targeted for exercise. This will improve function in the area opposite of the stretch (due to the antagonist

contraction), as well as overall posture, therefore allowing a more efficient workout.

Dynamic stretching can also be used before exercise as long as no major imbalances are present and sufficient coordination is possessed. See appendix for dynamic stretching routines.

In conclusion to pre-activity stretching, it seems like general flexibility and neuromuscular coordination are the keys to avoiding injuries. However, this flexibility should come from a regular stretching routine that is performed on its own time, away from serious exercises or activity. Stretching in general will increase flexibility and therefore increase the length a muscle can be stretched before it is injured, but balance and coordination are what keep the body out of these dangerous positions in the first place.

❖ Prolonged or passive stretching should not be done immediately prior to exercise on muscles that are going to be the focus of strengthening or used for stabilization.

After exercise

Use passive or gentle active assisted stretches to reduce post exercise soreness and cramping, this is the muscle's reward for working hard, along with proper nutrition and rest.

By itself

Dynamic stretching can be a total body workout when done in a progressive series that lasts over 15 minutes. In general, stretching can also be used for correcting imbalances and relaxing.

Time of Day

The muscles and joints are most susceptible to injury soon after waking due to the decreased functioning of the neuromuscular system. The spine is especially at risk in the morning because of the increased fluid in the discs after lying down all night.[85] For these reasons, only *gentle* stretching is recommended in the morning. In the author's experience, *advanced* stretching and exercise is best done in the afternoon or early evening, and at the earliest three hours after awakening.

What if there's **not enough time to stretch?**

If time is limited then optimum results will not be achieved and the risk of injury will be greater. But, by learning what areas are tight, time can be saved by only stretching the muscles that are a priority. Also, being very specific with the dynamic warm-up will take time off of the total stretching program. If stretching is always done in this manner then muscle balance will be difficult to obtain.

When time is a factor in each workout, do the minimum amount of stretching required before and after exercise, but then dedicate one entire workout per week to only stretching (and maybe cardio), if done correctly it can be a great workout.

The **Tight Hamstring**

Why are so many people's hamstrings tight and non-responsive to stretching? It is often times because of a misunderstanding of the 'tightness' felt in the hamstrings. Most hamstrings are not short, they are overloaded or strained, which creates a tight feeling, and it is the hip flexors that are tight/short. The hip flexors are the most dominant muscle in the pelvis due to prolonged sitting and the fact that most aerobic exercises emphasize them. This dominance tilts the hips too far forward which shortens the hip flexors and lengthens the overpowered hamstrings and gluteus maximus muscles.

The hamstrings and gluteus maximus contribute to posterior tilting of the pelvis while the hip flexors help tilt the pelvis anteriorly. This constant tug of war is easily won by the hip flexors and eventually weakens (reciprocal inhibition) the gluteus maximus and causes the hamstrings (and lumbar erectors) to strain and tire from synergistic dominance (picking up the slack for the inhibited gluteuls). Even though stretching the hamstrings feels good and takes the edge off the strain, it doesn't help the imbalance at all, it actually promotes it. *The key is stretching the hip flexors and strengthening the gluteus maximus,* among other things that may be noticed from a detailed evaluation. Once a certain balance is achieved, the hamstrings should be less strained and ready for some strengthening exercises.

It is still appropriate to stretch the hamstrings, if it's done gently. Extreme stretching can further strain the muscle, increase anterior tilting of the pelvis, and therefore increase anterior shear forces on the lumbar spine. This tug of war is very similar to that of the neck, where the pectoralis muscles and SCM act like the hip flexors, the rhomboids like the gluteus maximus, and the posterior neck muscles like the hamstrings. Thus, stretching the chest and SCM, strengthening the rhomboids, and eventually strengthening the posterior neck muscles will help many neck problems.

Stretching to Reduce Muscle Tension

One study showed that a four week stretching program increased ROM without changing the stiffness in the muscle.[24] Another study found that a short stretching program resulted in increased ROM but no change in resting muscle tension.[25] These studies provide evidence that increasing ROM should not be the focus of stretching if decreasing muscle tension is a goal. Instead, relieving muscular tension should be done by balancing the tension of influential areas and correcting faulty postures. This will allow the tense muscle(s) to relax in a more natural position. When general stretching fails to reduce tension, breathing exercises and corrective stretching and strengthening may be the missing factors to relieving tension.

ROM and Weakness

Flexibility is often limited by a weakness in the antagonistic muscle(s) at that specific ROM.[127] This weakness cause's instability of the joint in that position which causes a protective reflex (tightness) that keeps the joint out of injurious positions (unless an extreme force is present). Therefore, stretching a muscle past this point without strengthening the weak antagonist will promote instability in the joint at that ROM. For example, if someone has limited shoulder external rotation (due to short internal rotators) along with weak external rotators, then they should strengthen (by using active stretching of the internal rotators) the external rotators of the shoulder in the position of limited ROM. This will create stability in the shoulder and increase ROM safely.

An obvious sign of ROM beyond the muscle's control is the hypermobility seen in gymnasts or other athletes after they have been out of competitive training for a while. Their muscles are not as strong as they used to be but the ligaments are still (and always will be) very loose, this combination creates a lack of stability in certain ROM's, i.e. hips or shoulders dislocating regularly. In this situation the person must learn that they are vulnerable to injury in certain positions and will have to control their ROM within the limits of joint stability. This can be hard for those who habitually stretch and exercise with their old athletic mentality. A new approach of stability first and then controlled ROM needs to be adopted if wear and tear is to be avoided.

To stretch muscles that overlap a hypermobile joint, massage and myofascial release will get the muscles loose without going through the extreme ROM needed to stretch the muscle and subsequently degenerate the joint. Of course some people need extreme stretching to maintain this extra mobility in order to compete in sports, so strengthening the antagonist is imperative, but once they stop competing and health is the new found focus, then the ROM should be limited to prevent any further deterioration in the joint. Stretching is still appropriate, but the goal is not increased ROM, it is increased blood flow, releasing adhesions, dynamic flexibility, and stress relief.

Stretching injured areas*

Injured areas should be stretched in a manner that increases blood flow to promote healing but doesn't overstretch and cause further damage. It can be a little uncomfortable (an injury is already uncomfortable) but should be without sharp pain. Some injuries can momentarily or permanently limit ROM and will be further damaged by trying to stretch it to its normal length. Injury stretching is very subtle with increased blood flow, not length, being the goal, therefore, stretching past the muscle's barrier (first sign of resistance) is not recommended.

By recognizing there's an injury and knowing *what and how* to stretch, often times a myofascial release or massage technique on the surrounding tissues, not directly on the injury, is best to increase blood flow and promote healing and flexibility without adding unneeded stress to the area from too much ROM.

*Make sure you **check with a doctor** to see if it's appropriate to stretch the injury. **Stretching injuries can cause further damage to the tissues**, especially muscle, tendon, and ligament tears.

Movement Stretches

Movement stretches can be used as a warm-up (after a general warm-up) for stretching or mobilizing an area and involve movements rather than holding a stretch; this loosens up specific tissues and structures that are related to the areas about to be stretched. The following movement stretches can be used to warm-up a particular area.

Upper Body

1. Mini horizontal arm circles (30 seconds each direction)
2. Full arm circles (30 seconds each direction)
3. Standing torso rotations (10-20 each direction)

Low Back, Hip Complex, & Lower Body

1. Standing leg swing (15-30 seconds each leg)
2. Supine hip twist (10-20 reps each side)
3. Pelvic tilts (6-10 reps lying, sitting, or standing)

How to stretch

The physical aspect

Thinking about it energetically, the brain sends impulses to the muscle telling it to move, receptors in the muscle are constantly sending impulses back to the brain informing it about the muscle's position, speed of movement, length, and tension.[18,19] Receptors in the muscle also send signals back to the spinal cord that shoot right back to the muscle, totally bypassing the brain, these are reflex arcs, the simplest being the *stretch reflex*.[18,19]

The stretch reflex *increases* tension in the muscle being lengthened, and has a static and dynamic component[16,27] so as long as the muscle is moving it will have some tension in it that interferes with its passive stretch potential. This tension will increase proportionally with the speed of the stretch.[16,27] Therefore, *a slow stretch should be applied to inhibit tension in the muscle* (autogenic inhibition) and facilitate its elongation.[17] Also holding the stretch for at least twenty seconds will stimulate the golgi tendon reflex and inhibit the muscle spindle's stretch reflex, which will create an adaptation in the muscle spindles and allow the muscle to stretch further without initiating the stretch reflex.[27]

These reflexes help the body function on a daily basis (maintaining posture and muscle tone)[18,19] but can limit stretching if they are not understood. If the reflexes are not taken advantage of, then stretching is just like any other movement, it will move the muscle without any affect on its long term length.

Experience leads the author to believe that the reflex arcs are hypersensitive when the mind is busy, therefore allowing a smaller stimulus to activate the reflex and decrease the muscle's stretch potential. In order to best override the stretch reflex the mind must be relaxed. When the mind is focused on body awareness the muscles can relax along with the reflex arcs, allowing for a maximal stretch. Injuries and sharp pains are exceptions, even if they can be tuned out, they shouldn't.

While relaxation is often a goal of stretching, the rest of the body should not be limp during the stretch. For instance, while stretching the low back it is often beneficial to activate the abdominal muscles in order to stabilize the intervertebral segments against excessive motion.

The mental aspect

Stretching is best done with a quiet mind and some knowledge of how the muscles respond to lengthening. The mind and body are always communicating, and when the mind is busy their connection is weakened. What one did and what one has to do are thoughts that often cause a level of anxiety undetectable to a busy brain but are enough to interfere with the reflex arcs.

Stretching can act as a time out from the daily routine and unite the physical with the mental. Instead of the muscles reacting to the brain (stress), the brain should *interact with* the muscles when stretching. For instance, if a stretch becomes uncomfortable, one can back off, breath through it, or hold it anyway while gritting the teeth and hardly breathing (yes, you). This last technique usually adds more stress than it takes away. Instead, interact with the muscle by breathing smoothly and clearing the mind, this takes practice. Then it is possible to feel the muscle and each tightness surrounding it. Without reacting to the tightness the breath can be used to sooth the muscles and establish a new and improved length that wasn't possible with the old reflex arc, not to mention increase circulation and body awareness.

This doesn't have to be an enlightening experience, rather a timeout from the outside world and a union with the inside. This moment should be enjoyed; it's a great thing to be able to improve health just by breathing and paying attention to the body. *Without this "timeout" stretching is just another movement that can add stress to the body.*

This is of course an ideal way to stretch that is not always possible, but time should be taken to have ideal sessions whenever possible. Also remember that incorporating dynamic movements into a workout is a great way to stretch.

❖ In general, if stretching is not the mind's focus and enjoyable, then it will not fully benefit the body.

Stages of Stretching

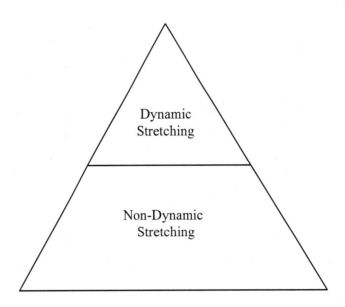

Stretch Progression Stage I
Non-Dynamic Isolated Stretching

Description

This stage is the foundation of stretching and is for beginners and advanced persons. Non-dynamic isolation stretches allow for the greatest lengthening of the muscle because only one muscle or small group of muscles will limit the stretch and little to no movement is used. They are also the safest because they keep the muscle in the most controlled environment (always supported by the floor, an object, or body part). In these ways non-dynamic stretching is just like isolated strength exercises; they are the safest, easiest to learn, produce the greatest results for individual muscles, but they don't tap into the potential of the neuromuscular system (control of balance and coordination).

Guidelines

- All beginners, even those without imbalances, should start with Stage I until they feel comfortable with the stretches.
- All stretches must be passive, self-myofascial release, active, isometric, or active assisted.
- Fascia and nerves are important to stretch during this stage in order to prepare the tissues for the complex movements of Stage II stretching.
- While improving major imbalances is the focus, all areas of the body should be stretched so that blood flow and mobility improve throughout.
- If there is a spine injury, spinal movement is often contraindicated and should be approved by a doctor.
- Most of the stretches should be performed while maintaining a neutral spine position.

Priorities

- Focus on correcting major imbalances.

- Stay within the limits of the tissues, overstretching can be worse than not stretching.
- Make stretching an integral part of the workout regimen, before and after exercise.

Variables

- Frequency   5-7x per week
- Intensity   Light to Moderate

Choosing Stretches

- Choose the technique (passive, self-myofascial release, active, isometric, or active assisted) that is most appropriate for the situation, i.e. no prolonged passive stretching before exercise.
- Focus on correcting major imbalances and reciprocal inhibitions with isolated movements, then move on to more general stretching.

Stretch Progression Stage II
Dynamic Integrative Stretching

Description

Dynamic flexibility is the key to injury prevention but seemingly impossible for some people to attain. This stage requires patience and practice to acquire the body awareness necessary to integrate multiple muscles into a stretched and coordinated position. This stage will prepare the body for any position it encounters by training the neuromuscular system to control complex movements which lengthen areas of the body to their functional limits.

Guidelines

- Some of the stretches should only be performed by athletes or those who need to put their body into extreme positions.
- The elderly or fragile should practice dynamic stretching, but only ones that are specific to their daily activities.
- Once a person has an injury, no matter what their skill, they should avoid Stage II stretches that involve the injury and practice simple flexibility in Stage I.
- Continue Stage I stretches to help prevent imbalances, up to seven days a week.

Priorities

- Stay within the control of the segmental stabilizer muscles.
- Utilize as many stretches as possible in order to coordinate, lengthen, and prepare the body in all different directions for slips and falls.
- Push the body to its limits of dynamic flexibility while staying within the limits of the neuromuscular system.

Variables

- Frequency 3-5x per week
- Intensity   Moderate to Difficult

Choosing Stretches

- Challenge the body with as many different positions as it can safely handle.

Chapter 5   Proprioception

Proprioception is often referred to as a sixth sense that creates our physical awareness by constantly communicating the body's position to the brain via receptors located throughout the body, even in fascia[30,31,32] and spinal ligaments.[29] It allows the body to regain balance during a slip or to touch the nose while the eyes are shut. It is mostly an unconscious system that functions along with the vestibular system (inner ear) to provide the sensory input needed to respond to our physical environment. Whether the body responds appropriately or not depends on the condition of these two systems along with the conditioning of the neuromuscular system.

The proprioceptive system has the ability to cause specific muscles to contract or relax through unconscious reflexes[18,19] and is the same system responsible for the stretch reflex described in chapter 4. For example, when stretching the hamstrings too far or too fast, muscle spindles will cause a reflex contraction of the hamstrings to control and resist the movement. It does this through feedback from three main receptor types[5,16,18,19,26]:

1. *Golgi Tendons* - monitor *tension* and rate of tension change. They are located in the tendons and cause an inhibitory effect on the stimulated muscle and facilitate its antagonist.[4,5,17,19,26] Golgi tendon reflexes will override excitatory inputs (muscle spindles) if sufficient tension is present.[18]

2. *Muscle Spindles* - monitor muscle *length* and rate of length change. They are located throughout the muscle and excite the stimulated muscle (create a contraction) and inhibit the antagonist.[5,18,19,26,28]

3. *Joint Receptors* - monitor joint *position*, pain, and pressure changes. They are located in and around the joint and ligaments and can inhibit or excite muscle contractions.[5,16,26]

Significance of Proprioception

If one was to lose most or all of their proprioception they would not be able to reach for a drink while talking to someone and still maintain eye contact with that person. They would have to constantly watch their hand (because the proprioceptive system isn't telling the brain where it is) and consciously move it towards the cup through the feedback of the eyes. Then do the same thing on the way up to the mouth. This is basic proprioception that most people have and don't need to train for but it shows the main principle of proprioception that is strived for, and that is being able to perform efficiently during complex movements without having to think about it.

For example, specific repetitive training can improve proprioceptive ability and teach the neuromuscular system how to properly jump, throw, and land while only having to think about who to throw it to, not how to do it. Or it can train the system to instantly and unconsciously react to slips and falls.

The proprioceptors are also part of the simplest reflex in the body, the stretch reflex. The main reason for the stretch reflex is to oppose passive stretching of the extensor muscles caused by the gravitational forces when standing upright[18,19]; a knee buckling for no apparent reason would be one example of the stretch reflex kicking in unconsciously to maintain alignment in the body. A similar example would be the head jerking upright when someone is sitting and falling asleep and their head falls forward.

With the exception of sleeping, the body is constantly utilizing proprioceptors for simple, complex, unconscious, and conscious movements. It is for this reason that Exercise Progression spends a lot of time developing this sixth sense in order to develop a more efficient neurological system to control the muscles.

Posture and Stability Effects on Proprioception

Good posture and stability are keys to efficient proprioception because they keep the body in the best position to resist gravity and place the muscles in their most effective position. Segmental stability must be achieved before advanced balance (reflex) or proprioception training begins, otherwise the body will find ways to compensate for segmental weaknesses by recruiting gross stabilizers. This will lead to segmental instability and eventually injury. It is common for athletes to be able to perform advanced levels of balance training using mostly their gross stabilizers;

this is due to great talent and poor training. These athletes often experience joint pain in the absence of any noticeable injury. Simple posture and stabilization exercises often correct the problem.

Movement Education and Proprioceptive Memory

The proprioceptive system has an unconscious memory of daily movements. It is this memory that allows the arm and hand to pick up a cup with the precise amount of tension needed so it doesn't jerk the cup and spill its contents. When learning a new movement or relearning one after an injury or surgery, a *conscious* effort must be made to eliminate faulty and protective compensation patterns by repeatedly practicing the proper movement and tension patterns. Once it is learned or "memorized" the proprioceptive and neuromuscular systems can operate on a more *unconscious* level by utilizing the memories of the proprioceptive system; shooting a basketball is a perfect example. Proprioception can also record specifically trained postures into a memorized sequence of appropriate muscle interactions which will achieve ideal functioning, such as finding a neutral spine (see pg. 81).

There is also a more conscious aspect of proprioception which allows one to pick up a box of unknown weight without falling over backwards. The key word here is *conscious,* because if a conscious effort is not made in an unknown situation, injuries can result due to an unconscious application of inappropriate memories that create too much or too little tension in the muscles. This conscious effort requires a state of heightened awareness similar to that needed when walking on a wet or slippery floor. Conscious proprioception during unknown circumstances is more difficult to apply because it never becomes automatic; it must be consciously applied every time.

The conscious or subconscious mind can also hinder efficient movement by analyzing normally unconscious situations and therefore interrupting proprioception. For example, an athlete who can normally make a free throw with their eyes closed can miss the same shot with their eyes open if the mind interferes by thinking about the consequences of the situation, i.e. a championship game with one second left and a tie score. The unconscious proprioceptive memory is disturbed by emotional feelings in the muscles. This is part of life and most often times the "clutch" athletes are able to focus on the task at hand without any distractions. So when you hear an athlete say "I was just concentrating on putting the ball in the basket", they're really saying "I was just trying to tune into my unconscious proprioceptive memories".

Proprioception Training

Many people do not have the ability to properly access their neurological system and recruit the specific muscles needed in order to strength train efficiently because they have been inactive for a prolonged time or have numerous compensations throughout the body. This is where balancing posture followed by proprioception training will 'wake up' the neuromuscular system and encourage better strength straining results.

The soles of the feet are the foundation for proprioception while standing, so there must be an emphasis on proper foot positioning. It is commonly called *"small (or short) foot"* and is helpful for increasing afferent input (neurological input to the brain), mostly from the sole.[4,41] The short foot position is accomplished by bringing the ball of the foot towards the heel, without curling the toes, which will raise the arch a little bit and place the entire body in a position that is well suited for coordination and balance. Of course overall posture must be aligned in order for the body to be properly placed over the feet. This takes practice and often requires repeating many times while sitting before it can be done standing.

Proprioception training occurs during any exercise, but specific reprogramming is often necessary to replace faulty motor patterns due to injury or bad habits. This involves proper techniques and PMAP repeated over and over until they become automatic. Proper training can condition the proprioceptive system to become more responsive to the length, tension, and position stimuli which are constantly stimulating the receptors. Proprioception can be negatively affected by injury, pain, or inactivity, thus post-injury and surgery training are essential for regaining balance, stability, and coordination. After surgery or serious injury it is often necessary to start with the foundation of proprioception training, which is termed proprioceptive neuromuscular facilitation (PNF). These techniques are mostly for the extremities; the spine will utilize more balance and reflex improving techniques, along with the PNF techniques. Proprioception training for specific body parts will utilize appropriate PNF techniques, while the reflex training will enhance priorioception for the entire body, especially the spine. Tai chi, yoga, and pilates are also excellent for challenging the proprioceptive system.

See Exercise Progression Vol. II for pictures and descriptions of the proprioception exercises.

PNF Technique Guidelines

PNF techniques were originally used for stroke victims or those with cerebral palsy[5], but are great for anyone who's relearning proper movement patterns or building strength, stability, and control of specific or general ROM's. These movements are at first assisted and then resisted by a practitioner and usually involves moving the shoulder or hip along with its extremity in a spiral and diagonal pattern. The proprioception involvement can be focused in the extremities, spine, or both depending on body position. For example, lying supine with both feet on the floor and moving the arm in a diagonal pattern will mostly challenge the arm and shoulder's proprioception, while lying supine and maintaining a bridged position and performing the same movement will include the core and spine.

Different PNF techniques can also be used to stretch a muscle and are explained further in the stretching chapter. The following are general guidelines for PNF strengthening techniques:

• Each pattern should be repeated against resistance 1-3 times for 10-15 reps of a complete cycle.
• Normal, uninterrupted breathing will be difficult at first, but should be a goal in order to avoid hyperventilating and enhance coordination and stability throughout the body.
• Extremity movement patterns are spiral (rotation) and diagonal, this increases muscle recruitment and decreases shearing and compression forces.[5]
• All movement patterns are fully explained to the participant and understood before starting.
• PNF techniques are used mostly to improve function in a rehabilitation setting and are not for everyone, but they can be used to improve certain non-injury dysfunctions.
• PNF techniques are not meant to replace a strengthening program, rather enhance it by being the foundation of coordination and stability.
• These techniques require experience and expertise to administer; this text is only informative and should not replace professional training.

PNF Movement Patterns

The following four patterns are considered the most efficient movements for increasing muscle fiber recruitment and are the basis for the PNF techniques.[5] Each description is only for one direction of the pattern; reverse the directions to complete one cycle or rep.

Upper Extremity Patterns

1. The client begins with their fist on the opposite shoulder and the forearm supinated. They then sweep the arm downward while internally rotating the shoulder, pronating the forearm, adducting the scapula, extending the wrist, and opening hand, ending in slight extension of the arm.
2. The client begins with a fist in the opposite pocket and the forearm pronated. Then they sweep the arm upward while supinating the forearm, externally rotating the shoulder, adducting the scapula, extending the wrist, and opening the hand, ending in a tray carrying position.

Lower Extremity Patterns

1. The client begins with their knee up towards the opposite shoulder, knee flexed, and ankle in dorsiflexion and inversion. Then the leg is moved down toward the table or floor while the knee is extended and the ankle in plantarflexion and eversion.
2. The client begins with their knee towards the same shoulder, hip slightly abducted and externally rotated, knee flexed, and ankle in dorsiflexion and inversion. The movement is the same as the previous pattern.

PNF Techniques

The following four PNF techniques are adapted from the American Academy of Health, Fitness, and Rehabilitation Professionals.[5] These techniques are used to assist a person through one or all of the appropriate patterns mentioned above. Always begin with the client in supine position, progress to sitting and standing if necessary or applicable. PNF techniques should not begin until weeks 5-8 of Stage III due to their open chain movements.

Rhythmic Initiation

The professional begins by passively moving the client through the explained pattern. Once the pattern is allowed by the body without resistance the client begins to assist the movement through the pattern. If the client can perform the pattern correctly and without pain, then resistance is added to the movement throughout the entire pattern. The resistance is in a direction that forces a concentric contraction in each direction, thus, agonists will work in one direction of the pattern, and then their antagonists will work in the other. This is different than the next technique where only the agonist will be resisted.

Combination of Isotonics

This technique uses all three types of contractions

(eccentric, concentric, and isometric) to increase strength and coordination of an agonist. The same procedures are used as in the technique above, except that the resistance is applied in the same direction throughout the movement, thereby affecting the same group of muscles on both directions of the pattern.

❖ Rhythmic Initiation and Combination of Isotonics are techniques that are helpful for those who have a hard time controlling a contraction or movement and need improved strength and coordination in a specific area. If there is a point in the pattern that causes pain, it is possible to still improve function by focusing on the non-painful zones. Special emphasis on specific points in the pattern can be used at anytime to improve function.

Isotonic Reversal

This technique utilizes alternating concentric contractions. A concentric contraction begins the movement and reverses direction at any point in the pattern. The goal is to shift smoothly from one direction to another and focus on areas with the most dysfunction.

Rhythmic Stabilization

Alternating isometric contractions are used on specific points in the pattern in order to improve joint stability.

PNF techniques are useful for assessing a person's ability to control movement without compensation or pain. For example, many times it is possible to perform certain exercises without pain because the body compensates, often with extremely small and difficult to notice patterns. These compensations are much easier to detect while applying a PNF technique than while observing an exercise because it is possible to feel and see the weakness as it occurs while the compensations simultaneously take place.

Spine Techniques

Proprioception training for the spine is different than other parts of the body because the spine doesn't move very much, if at all during the exercises compared to the extremities. The training can be very similar to PNF techniques but with *modified hip positions or* it can focus on *reflex (balance) exercises.* The spinal PNF techniques use the same patterns as mentioned above (upper and or lower body) but place the hips off the floor with the knees bent and feet flat. This challenges the spine's ability to maintain proper alignment while the extremities are moved, with or without resistance, and will establish new patterns of neuromuscular recruitment which increase stability and strength throughout the whole body. The reflex training is focused more on body awareness and improving reflexes and does not require a partner.

Reflex training utilizes unstable surfaces (balance disks, wobble boards, foam rolls, balls, etc.) to challenge the spine against gravity while the extremities move about to further test the spine's ability to maintain its proper alignment. D.A.M.'s and proper lifting techniques are also great for spinal proprioception training (see chapters 7 & 10) because they provide the opportunity for the neuromuscular (proprioception) system to practice and learn relevant tasks for each individual.

Summary

Every movement or exercise involves the proprioceptive system, so a key to improved performance and function is to *properly* stimulate the system to obtain a specific coordination. Some people even unknowingly take advantage of the system by pushing down on the center of the quadriceps muscle as they get up from a sitting position. This creates a slight stretching of the muscle that activates the muscle spindles, which are concentrated in the center of the muscle, and their stretch reflex, which facilitates a quadriceps contraction and thus helps the person stand upright.[18]

The saying "If you don't use it you lose it" definitely applies to proprioception. As we grow older or more sedentary our proprioceptive team "sits on the bench" more than it "plays" and thus becomes deconditioned and slow to react. This can be improved with specific training no matter how long it has been inactive or how old the person or injury is. Proprioceptive training is a necessity if the maximum benefits of exercising or rehabilitation are desired because it allows the muscles to fire on all cylinders. Proprioceptive training is also great for warming up the neuromuscular system prior to exercise.

If someone has abnormally poor proprioception and coordination it is useful to ask about their diet; B12 deficiencies are associated with a poor sense of balance and joint position awareness, clumsiness, and decreased reflexes to name a few of the many side affects.[128]

Guidelines for Proprioception/Reflex Training

- Manual therapy techniques can be applied directly to the golgi tendons and muscle spindles of the muscles that have proprioception deficiencies before reflex training starts.
- PMAP for hip abduction and extension, trunk flexion, and arm abduction should be had, along with the ability to find a neutral spine before starting proprioception training. In other words, Stage I of Exercise Progression should be completed.
- All movements are controlled and muscle contractions pain free.
- Bare feet are recommended whenever possible to enhance sensory input.
- Proprioceptive reflex training can be injurious if the exercise is too difficult because it will encourage compensation patterns from the dominant muscles and reflexes, the same ones that the training is trying to modify. Make sure that **stability is the focus rather than extreme acts of balance.**
- In order to properly activate the deep stabilizers without interference from the gross mobilizers there is a systematical progression in regards to body position that is as follows;

    1. Standing (closed chain)
    2. Seated (semi-closed chain)
    3. Lying or on all four's (open or semi-closed chain)
    4. Complex and functionally oriented towards a goal

    And:

    o Passive > active assisted > active unassisted > active resisted movements
    o Stable > unstable
    o Eyes open > eyes closed (not always appropriate)
    o All contractions utilized, (concentric, eccentric, and isometric)
    o Two > alternating > single (extremity)
    o Forward and backward > side to side > rotation > dynamic combinations

Stages of Proprioception

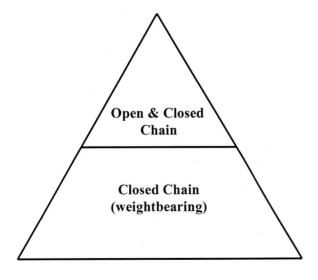

Stage I	**Closed Chain** **Reflex Training** • Fully or partially supported on unstable surfaces. • Unsupported on stable surfaces (standing on one leg on the floor).
Stage II	**Open & Closed Chain** **Reflex Training** • Fully, partially, or unsupported on unstable surfaces. **PNF Techniques** • Fully to partially supported

Proprioception Progression Stage I
Closed Chain Exercises

Description

The reflex exercises here are very simple and designed for those who are imbalanced and who do not have the ability to properly utilize their neuromuscular system at a basic level; this can include athletes who are normally advanced but due to imbalances utilize compensations for simple movement patterns. This stage is not meant to stand alone; it needs to be implemented with the other components of Exercise Progression in order to fully benefit the body. This stage should not be performed until Stage I of Exercise Progression has been completed.

Guidelines

- If compensations are noticed, modify or stop the exercises until they are corrected.
- If a specific exercise is painful or too difficult, move on for the time being to avoid compensations and focus on PMAP until ready.
- Perform proprioception exercises after a proper warm-up, and before a strength training workout.
- Repeat the same exercise over and over until it is performed efficiently, and then move on to a different one. This will improve the memory and efficiency of the reflexes.

Priorities

- Utilize the segmental and gross stabilizers with minimal assistance from the mobilizers by performing closed chain weightbearing balance exercises.
- Proper body alignment is essential, otherwise faulty movement patterns will result.
- Increase body awareness.

Variables

	Sets	Reps/Time	Intensity	Rest	X per wk	Duration
Reflex Exercises	1-3	2-4 min	Controlled up to max effort	20-30 sec or simply switch sides	5-7	4-8 weeks

Choosing Exercises

- Perform closed chain weightbearing exercises, i.e. standing on 1 leg on a stable surface or 2 legs on an unstable surface

Proprioception Progression Stage II
Open and Closed Chain Exercises

Description

The PNF techniques are used only for those who require special attention to an area or have decreased neuromuscular functioning. There is no limit to the reflex exercises in this stage as long the movements are controlled. Complex movements can mean simple reflex exercises while tossing a ball and catching it in the opposite hand, or inventing tasks that utilize balance and coordination which are appropriate for the individual performing the task.

Guidelines

- Apply all Stage I guidelines.
- Some of the exercises do require strength, so it is important not to overdo it and fatigue the stabilizing muscles prior to a strength workout.

Priorities

- Controlled movements first, ROM second.
- Focus on weaknesses, do not repeat exercises that are easy (the necessary reflexes are already possessed).

Variables

	Sets	Reps/Time	Intensity	Rest	X per wk	Duration
PNF Techniques	1-3	10-15	Controlled up to max effort	45-60 sec	2-5	6-8 weeks
Reflex Exercises	1-3	2-4 min	Controlled up to max effort	20-30 sec or simply switch sides	5-7	6-8 weeks

Choosing Exercises

- Choose as many different exercises as possible, including those from Stage I, in order to challenge the proprioception system in all of its capabilities.
- Once Stage III of Exercise Progression has been completed, proprioception exercises of all sorts should be used throughout the warm-up sessions of Stage IV.

Chapter 6 Strength Training

Strength training without the knowledge of how the body compensates or progresses during strength training is like eating without the knowledge of what is healthy food; both will eventually create problems that start off small but can end up causing irreversible damage. This chapter gives a brief description of strength training and a detailed description of the proper way to progress one's strength. The strength progressions at the end of this chapter are not meant to stand by themselves, they are part of a whole that can progress the body to any physical goal as long as the other components of Exercise Progression are also utilized. Strength training by itself without these complementary components (assessments, stretching, D.A.M.'s, cardio, and proprioception) can lead to the reinforcement of compensations and eventually deterioration of the tissues. Reading this entire manual is recommended for a complete understanding of these compensations and their influences.

Strength training can be done for many different reasons by using a variety of techniques, but to reap the maximum benefits one must:

- Begin with proper posture alignment, segmental stability, and core functioning so that the rest of the body can be trained to operate on a strong foundation.
- Utilize assessment findings to start with corrective exercises (including stretching and proprioception), and progress accordingly.
- Progress within the connective tissue's ability (muscle strengthens faster than connective tissue).
- Have proper rest and nutrition; exercise contributes to only one third of the results.
- Push past the comfort zone (tissues permitting).
- Focus on PMAP, see pg. 13.
- Fatigue the stabilizing muscles at the end of a workout so that they are able to stabilize throughout the main workout.
- Know the proper technique for each exercise.
- Know individual limitations.
- Warm-up the body's temperature and neuromuscular system (coordination) prior to working out.
- Incorporate stretching.
- Visualize the area being strengthened.
- Utilize proper breathing patterns.

Benefits of Strength Training

Health

➢ Increases bone density
➢ Improves balance and coordination
➢ Increases confidence and ability to do daily activities
➢ Manages stress
➢ Controls body weight and lean mass
➢ Rehabilitates and prevent injuries
➢ Improves posture and joint mechanics

Fitness

➢ Increases strength, speed, and endurance
➢ Improves balance and coordination
➢ Improves overall performance

Types of Muscular Contractions

1. Concentric
2. Eccentric
3. Isometric

Concentric

A concentric contraction involves the muscle fibers *shortening* to produce a force or movement. This is the most common type of contraction trained. Even though eccentric contractions (the lowering or deceleration phase) occur during most movements, they are rarely focused on. This neglect creates an imbalance of movement control that enhances acceleration strength (getting out of a chair or jumping), but ignores and thus reduces deceleration strength (getting into a chair or landing from a jump) and creates a body that is prone to injuries and compensations.

Eccentric

An eccentric contraction involves the muscles fibers *lengthening* to produce a force (often against the force of gravity) in order to decelerate a movement (sitting down into a chair or lowering a child into their car seat). Eccentric training is known to cause increased post-exercise soreness but is essential to functional balance. Weakness in eccentric strength is the cause of many injuries, especially in sports.

Isometric

Isometric contractions involve no muscle length changes at all, but can still create a powerful force within the muscle. These contractions are essential for maintaining proper posture and segmental stability throughout movement. It is important to breathe during isometric contractions in order to control blood pressure (BP), which can rise significantly during prolonged isometric contractions. Someone with hypertension should be tested for BP levels during an isometric contraction to see if it is safe for them to engage in this type of contraction. Always refer to their doctor for safe BP levels.

Specificity Training

At first, training should be slow enough to optimize control, balance, and utilization of the stabilization muscles, but once a solid foundation is established, i.e. Stages I-III of Exercise Progression, faster speeds can be practiced in order to prepare the body for real life situations.

If the body always trains slowly, then the neuromuscular system will be insufficient during sports or slips and falls. But if it is rarely trained slowly the body will not establish a strong foundation of stabilization strength.

The more an exercise resembles a specific activity (speed, movement, endurance, etc.), the greater its results will carry over into that activity. This is referred to as the *transfer-of-training effect*, and is based on the *SAID* (Specific Adaptation to Imposed Demands) principle, which states that the body will change in response to particular training and activities.[13]

Many sports (basketball, water polo, football, soccer, etc.) and manual labor jobs [construction worker, mom (laundry, vacuuming, dishes, groceries, and floor scrubbing, now that's a circuit!), warehouse worker, garbage man, fireman, police officer, etc.], utilize strength, power, and aerobic conditioning all at once or in cycles throughout the day and during practice and competition.

To gain the unique strength and stamina needed for each person it makes sense then to combine the three variables (strength, power, and aerobic conditioning) within a single workout in a way that mimics their environments. This is best done with circuit training. For example, 3-5 min of cardio immediately followed by 3-5 min of strength exercises and then 3-5 min of power exercises. These make up one circuit, with 3-4 circuits per workout being the norm. For more intense

training, 2-3 minute cycles can be used with higher levels of exertion.

Once an individual has completed Stage III of Exercise Progression they can train this way by utilizing the activity specific routines in Ch. 14, instead of the common half hour of cardio followed by a half hour of weights, or vice versa workouts. This will ensure that training results are tailored to the individual.

Adaptations to Exercise

It has been consistently shown[244-254] that the first 4-8 weeks of resistance training results in substantial neural adaptations as opposed to increases in muscle size. This reinforces the significance of balancing posture and eliminating compensations prior to intense strength training; these both allow the body to most efficiently utilize the initial neural adaptations.

When the body is regularly trained with the same movement patterns, it will adapt by getting stronger yet utilizing less motor units.[247,255-257] In other words, it evolves and becomes more efficient. This is ideal for sports and specific activities, but not for general exercising because it burns fewer calories and limits growth/strength potential by recruiting less motor units.

Therefore, an exercise program must be varied if the maximum benefits are to be achieved.

Muscle Growth

Muscles can atrophy, maintain strength, or gain strength. In order to optimize muscle growth:

1. The stimulus must be greater than the muscle's existing ability.
2. The stimulus must be varied and progressed.
3. The body must be balanced (no reciprocal or arthrokinetc inhibition, or synergistic dominance)

Growth Stimulating Variables

Box 6-1

• Intensity	• ROM
• Velocity	• Exercise Selection
• Volume (repetitions, sets)	• Exercise Order
• Rest	• Frequency
• Plane of Motion	• Proprioceptive Challenge

All of these variables should be mixed up about once a month to keep the body challenged and prevent overtraining or boredom.

Plane of Motion

There are three different planes of motion; all three are utilized in functional movements. If one plane is underdeveloped, that direction of movement will most likely lead to wear and tear or injury. A comprehensive exercise program needs to include and systematically progress each plane of motion.

The three planes of motion:

1. *Sagittal* – forward/backward
2. *Frontal* – side to side
3. *Transverse* – rotation

Adaptations to Specific Variables

It is known that training with specific variables will produce specific results. In order to obtain each specific adaptation, choose a weight that causes failure (cannot lift another rep without extreme effort or breaking form) at the given rep range listed in Table 6-1. Table 6-1 is based on widely accepted associations between variables and the adaptations they produce[13,267-269]; some modifications have been made (the addition of power/stamina and increased intensity level for endurance by 10%):

The variables are: sets, reps, intensity, rest, and tempo. Tempo numbers are in seconds and represent the *eccentric-isometric-concentric* phases of the contraction. Tempo numbers are only guidelines and can be interchanged to achieve combined adaptations or more specific goals. For instance, many athletes need quick speed (power) for more than five reps, thus the variables are changed to more endurance like levels but with more of a power tempo, which will vary depending on the goal. This allows for the development of longer lasting quickness (swimming, tennis, etc.). Strength and more intense power exercises are still needed to develop maximum power, but the combination are needed to achieve power with stamina.

The secret to achieving specific results comes from adhering to the appropriate variables in Table 6-1.

Table 6 – 1   Adaptation to Specific Variables

Adaptation	# of exs's	Sets	Reps	Load % of 1 rep max	Rest	Tempo	X/wk	
Max Strength	3-6	4-6	1-5	85-100%	3-5 min	3-1-1	3-5	**Strength Adaptations**
Strength	3-4	3-4	6-8	75-85%	45 sec- 5 min	3-1-1	3-5	
Hypertrophy	3-6	3	9-12	70-85%	45-90 sec	4-2-2	3-5	
Endurance	2-4	1-3	12-25	50-80%	1-3 min	3-2-1	3-4	
Stabilization	3-5	1-3	12-25	40-70%	0-1.5 min	Slow	3-5	
Power/Stamina	2-4	2-3	12-30	50-75%	3-5 min	Explosive	2-3	**Power Adaptations**
Explosive Strength 1x	2-5	3-5	1-2	80-90%	2-5 min	Explosive	2-3	
Explosive Strength mult.x	2-5	3-5	3-5	75-85%	2-5 min	Explosive	2-3	
Ballistics (upper body)	2-3	3-5	10-20	Variable	2-3 min	Explosive	2-3	
Ballistics (lower body)	2-3	3-5	1-3	30%	2-3 min	Explosive	2-3	
Plyometrics (upper body)	2-3	2-4	1-10	30-45%	2-5 min	Explosive	2-3	
Plyometrics (lower body)	2-3	2-3	1-10	0-45%*	2-5 min	Explosive	2-3	

* Only add weight to a lower body plyometric exercise if the individual is an elite athlete with no major injuries and is between the ages of 18-35ish.

The Variables

Power and Endurance

See below for descriptions.

Strength

If strength gains are desired for the *advanced* person, this type of training will promote it best.

Hypertrophy/Toning

This type of training produces growth and strength gains for the beginner but results will taper off once the person adapts to the weight being lifted. This is the ideal training for maintaining health and general strength.

Power/Stamina

This is the ultimate combination that athletes strive for, which is to be strong and explosive over a prolonged period of time and still maintain stability and technique.

Types of Strength

- Functional
- Endurance
- Transition
- Stabilization
- Maximum
- Relative
- Core
- Power
- Ideal

Functional Strength

The ability of the neuromuscular system to efficiently control and stabilize the body throughout static and dynamic movements by utilizing both the stabilizers and mobilizers. This includes concentric, eccentric, and isometric contractions, along with acceleration and deceleration in all planes of movement. Ideal or 100% functional strength is not as much strength as it is a combination of factors which is roughly;

- 20% Strength
- 40% Neuromuscular coordination
- 40% Proper posture and muscular balance

Stabilization Strength

➢ **Segmental Stabilization:** This is the most important type of stabilization and is part of the strength foundation for Exercise Progression. It involves small, one joint muscles that hold a joint in its most efficient position. The rotator cuff, small hip rotators, transverse abdominis, and deep paraspinal muscles are a few of the segmental stabilizers. These muscles often need special endurance exercises to keep up with the strength of the larger muscles.

➢ **Global Stabilization:** Global or gross stabilization comes from larger and more superficial muscles that stabilize across one joint. The external obliques, spinalis, and gluteus medius are global stabilizers.

❖ These two types of muscles are responsible for stabilizing the entire body throughout movement and static posture during predictable and non-intense situations. However, once a situation becomes unpredictable or intense, the mobilizers will co-activate in order to stabilize the body against buckling. See pg.'s 10-11 for details.

The strength goals for stabilizers are endurance and strength throughout the joint's functional ROM. Segmental strength must be the foundation of stabilization training, otherwise the gross stabilizers will be stabilizing a joint that is out of position.

CORE Strength

CORE strength is the sum of the *strength* of the CORE muscles and their *ability* to stabilize the lumbo-pelvic-hip region in its most efficient position throughout all types of movement. CORE strength is next to useless if it is activated at the wrong time or in the wrong order. See pg. 80 for proper activation techniques.

Endurance Strength

Endurance strength is the ability to generate and sustain forces over prolonged periods of time. These can be related to power events (tennis, wrestling, sprinting, etc.) or more normal activities (jogging, stay at home mom, massage therapist, etc.). Either way, endurance strength in the appropriate muscles is essential to avoiding injuries and maintaining posture.

Maximum Strength

The maximum force a muscle can generate in one attempt. This type of strength is also a key factor in the initiating phase of power.

Power

The combination of speed (how fast the muscle can contract) and force (strength) through distance equals power. Power has four phases of strength; 1) initiating, 2) speed (continuing), 3) transitioning (amortization), 4) deceleration phases, not necessarily in that order. All are essential to overall power efficiency.

$$\text{Power} = \frac{\text{Force x Distance}}{\text{Time}}$$

Maximum force production occurs when the speed of movement is slow (i.e. a 1 rep max lift) or zero (i.e. isometric).

On the other hand, as the speed of contraction increases, the force decreases. Therefore, a high velocity contraction results in a relatively low force production.

Somewhere between these two extremes is an optimal point for power output, and according to research, maximal power occurs at intermediate velocities when lifting moderate loads.[270,271] These loads are said to be about 30% of the 1 rep max.[13,270,272]

With that being said, there are four main techniques for developing power, and only one of them utilizes the "ideal" 30% load. Each of them has their place, but some, as you will read here, may be too advanced or demanding for the general population and those with major imbalances.

1. Heavy strength training
2. Explosive strength training
3. Ballistics
4. Plyometrics

Heavy Strength Training

Heavy strength or weight training influences the top ½ of the power equation by improving the peak force production.[273-275] This is essential for the initiating phase of power, i.e. starting from a stationary position.

This means that the greater a person's strength is the more explosive the initial phase can be and the greater their potential for power output is. However, this initial momentum requires the next phase, speed strength, to continue the movement into a powerful action. Therefore, heavy strength training has a limited but potent affect on power.

Because heavy strength training (70-100% 1 rep max) is associated with slowing down the rate of force production[276], individuals who already possess adequate strength should not focus on this type of training to improve their power. However, this is an ideal initial strategy for beginners who desire power and lack sufficient strength.

Explosive Strength Training

Once strength gains plateau, it is appropriate to begin more explosive methods of training. While 30% of the 1 rep max seems to be the optimal load for producing maximum power, it is difficult to control such a light resistance (weights, cables, etc.) at this high speed. These high speeds cause unwanted antagonistic contractions (trying to decelerate and stop the resistance before it is launched from the body) that minimize the adaptations for power.

In order to reduce the interference from the antagonists, heavier loads are recommended for explosive strength training, see Table 6-1. Also note in table 6-1 the increase in load and reduction in reps for "Explosive strength 1x", which refers to activities such as throwing, hitting, and other one time power exertions. This differs from the "explosive strength mult.x", which refers to sprinting, team sports, or any other activity requiring multiple power efforts in succession.

Note that the 30% 1 max rep recommendation is for free weights. High tech cable machines can be used for explosive strength training, but because of the different types of pulley systems, the actual weight lifted will always be a little different that what is indicated.

The goal with explosive strength training is quality over quantity, not training to exhaustion.

Ballistic

Ballistic actions use higher speeds and lower loads than the previous two methods and involve throwing objects and jumping with resistance, i.e. medicine balls and jumping squats holding dumbbells. Ballistic and plyometrics techniques reduce the activation of antagonistic muscles because the resistance is moved without restriction rather than decelerated and stopped. This allows for maximal adaptations for contraction velocity.

Generally, 30-35% of the 1 rep max is recommended[269], but some individuals, like a shot putter or Olympic lifter, will need higher loads for the throwing actions.

Reps are relatively high with certain ballistic throwing exercises due to the greater rest between reps, which comes from throwing and retrieving a medicine ball. Reps for the jumping exercises are relatively low due to the extreme demand on the joints. See the differences in Table 6-1.

The goals here are 1) to reach maximum acceleration at the instant the object is thrown or body is lifted and 2) throw or jump as far as possible.

Ballistics can be very dangerous for the uncoordinated and those with joint abnormalities. Even individuals with healthy joints should be aware of the extreme amount of pressure and force these techniques place on the ligaments and cartilage of joints, especially decelerating the jumping squats with weight.

Progress should always be gradual from unloaded to loaded and care taken to not perform these exercises if fatigue is present.

Plyometrics

Plyometrics consist of exercises that promote a maximum muscular force in the shortest amount of time.[267] The unique quality of plyometrics is the fact that the transition phase (as well as the three other phases of power) is utilized with every exercise.

For example, a ballistic jumping exercise will have a pause between the eccentric and concentric contractions, thus eliminating the transition phase. A plyometric jumping exercise will continue through the two different contractions without hesitating and thus utilize all four phases of power.

The transition phase is what allows plyometrics to be most sport specific type of exercise that results in the most sport-specific muscle memory. This does not mean that it is the best however; it is yet only another key component to developing power.

The secret behind the transition phase is the stored energy within the muscle and tendons caused by the "loading" or stretching of the eccentric contraction. The stretch reflexes of the stretched muscles will activate those muscles and contract them vigorously once the direction of movement is changed. The elastic energy that is created from the muscle and tendon stretch (i.e. the quadriceps during the down/eccentric phase of a squat jump) will cause the concentric contraction to be more powerful than that from a stationary position.[277,278]

For example, going continuously from standing, to squatting, and then immediately jumping up will produce a higher vertical jump than the same jump that was performed from standing, squatting, pause a few seconds, and then jumping.

Plyometrics can be upper body (medicine ball throws) or lower body (all types of jumping). The difference between ballistic and plyometric upper body exercises is that plyometrics will not pause like ballistic exercises after bringing the ball back into a ready position. Instead they (plyometric exercises) will utilize the transition phase by continuing the motion between eccentric and concentric.

An important differentiation needs to be understood when developing plyometric exercise programs. It is that that there are two main types of lower body plyometrics, high and low impact, and they each have their own place and guidelines.

High impact lower body plyometrics should be limited to 60 "impacts"/reps per workout and have ample rest (10:1 ratio) between each set and each workout (72 hours). For example, a set of high impact jumps (8-10 reps) that takes 30 seconds to complete should be followed by 10x 30 seconds (300 seconds = 5 min) of rest. This is obviously going to take a longer time than other types of workouts. That's ok. The goal here is fresh muscles so that quality dominates quantity. Muscle fatigue during explosive training will lead to injuries and bad habits.

Low impact lower body plyometric exercises can withstand a higher amount of reps per workout and even per set. For example, it is not uncommon to perform 10-20 zig-zag jumps or 1 legged hops at a time. These types of low impact exercises can total up to as high as 120 or 140 reps per workout.

Taking it a step further, most people will train with both types of high and low impact exercises in a single workout. A combination like this will require a blending of guidelines that resemble the following. Each combined workout should consist of *90-100 total reps (high and low impact)* per workout, with up to *60 of them being high impact.*

These guidelines are based on the author's experience and education, and because of limited research on the topic, there are no proven regulations for plyometrics, only opinions. Just remember that everyone responds to plyometrics differently depending on their experience, sport, time of year in their sport, history of injuries, skill and coordination levels, etc.

Below is a sample of a combined lower body plyometric workout in order to grasp the concept of how it is shaped and how important a proper warm-up is.

1. 15-30 min cardio warm-up
2. Dynamic stretching if necessary
3. 5-10 min dynamic exercise warm-up
4. 2-3 sets of low impact lower body plyometrics
5. Complete workout (2-3 sets of 2-3 exercises) for lower body, high impact plyometrics
6. 2-3 sets of low impact lower body plyometrics
7. Cool-down stretching

#'s 1-4 are basically a warm-up for the high impact plyometrics.

Now, with all of that knowledge of power exercises, which one is the best? None of them! One or a few of them are probably more important for each person depending on their weaknesses and specific activity they are training for. A combination of strength, agility, coordination, speed, and endurance are all necessary to reach optimal power potential.

In fact, power adaptations are maximized by utilizing heavy (85-100%) strength training and lighter (30%) power training.[13,235-243] It is recommended to perform these power exercises at 30-45% of 1 rep max or up to 10% of body weight.[13]

Transition Strength

Transition refers to the phase between an eccentric and concentric contraction, i.e. the changing of direction between deceleration (force reduction) and acceleration (force production). The ability to achieve stability in this phase comes from strong segmental and global stabilizers that are efficiently activated with the mobilizers; this is essential in preventing wear and tear and injuries, especially at high speeds.

Relative Strength

The maximum force an individual can produce in relation to their body weight.

Ideal Strength

Ideal strength is the maximum force a muscle can produce while maintaining the health of its surroundings. Understanding this type of strength is vital to rehabilitating injuries and achieving health.

If a muscle's strength has surpassed its related tendon and ligamentous strength (common with steroids or progressing too fast) or creates compensation patterns, it is not an ideal strength.

❖ *Ideal health functions through ideal strength.*

Exercise Options

Isolated Muscle Group Exercises
Utilizes as few muscles as possible to do a specific movement. Ideal for beginners, rehabilitation, balancing posture, and body building. These exercises are needed to establish proper individual muscle activation during simple movements Only then can integrated movements be done without compensations. Example: Bicep curl
Integrated/Dynamic Exercises
Utilizes the coordination of many muscles to perform complex movements or tasks that prepare the body for any goal (sports, daily activities, etc.). Unstable surfaces can be added to isolated exercises to make them an integrated exercise. Example: Squat with a row

Training Systems

- Single Set
- Multiple Set
- Super Set
- Pyramid Set
- Circuit Training
- Multiple Circuit Training
- Split-Routines

Single Set

Perform one set of each exercise. These routines are ideal for beginners.

Multiple Set

Perform multiple numbers of sets for each exercise. This is more appropriate for advanced individuals but can also be used by beginners.

Super Set

Perform a few different exercises in succession with no rest. The exercises should have a common goal. For example, antagonists can be worked in succession (chest and back), or the same muscle can be worked with a couple different exercises in succession.

Pyramid Set

Progress the weight with each set from heavy to light, or light to heavy. Progress from 1 or 12 reps to 12 or 1 reps respectively in a 3-6 set period.

Circuit Training

Perform a series of 3-5 exercises in a row with minimal to no rest. This is ideal for training the entire body in a short time as well as mimicking specific environments.

Sets and reps will vary greatly depending on the goal, with 3 sets of 8-12 reps and 2-3 min rest between circuits being the norm. Each set can be the same or different exercises.

Multiple Circuit Training

Perform 3-4 exercises in a row (1 circuit). Then rest 30 sec-1 min and perform a new circuit. Anywhere from 2-4 circuits can be used per multiple circuit, ideally with no two exercises the same. 1-2 multiple circuits can be performed per workout, with 2-5 min rest between them. Reps will vary with 8-12 being the norm. See Stage III for examples of how to create multiple circuits.

Split-Routine

Isolate different muscles on separate days. One to three muscles per day and up to five strength workouts per week is normal, depending on how everything is split up. Bodybuilders (or anyone with mainly hypertrophy goals) use this system because more work can be done by one muscle in a workout, which facilitates more growth in that one area. There are many different combos to use and it's hard to go wrong unless there's not enough rest between one muscle group's workouts; usually 72 hours between intense workouts of the same muscle group is needed for full recovery.

Stage Outlines

The following outlines give a general overview of the Exercise Progression strength philosophy. A more individual outline is presented for the low back on pg. 237.

Stages of Strength Training

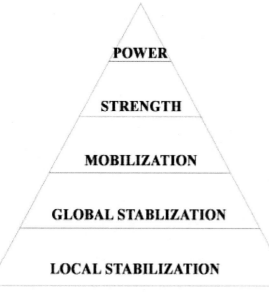

POWER

STRENGTH

MOBILIZATION

GLOBAL STABLIZATION

LOCAL STABILIZATION

Stage I	**Local Stabilization** • Corrective activation exercises • Utilize segmental stabilizers • Muscle control • Activate inhibited muscles
Stage II	**Global Stabilization** • Corrective isolation exercises • Engraining PMAP • Slow/endurance training • Closed chain/weightbearing • Integrated uniplanar exercises
Stage III	**Mobilization** • Corrective integration exercises • Closed and open chain exercises • Develop open chain stability • Integrated multiplanar exercises
Stage IV	**Strength** • Intense training • Advanced dynamic training
Stage V	**Power** • Explosive exercises • Training for extreme activity • Prepare all populations for quick movements, i.e. slips/falls

Strength Progression Stage I
Local Stabilization

Description

The foundation of strength and PMAP comes from segmental stability and the ability to recruit the smaller and more central muscles in the body. These muscles need to be specially trained while the gross movers need to be rested in order to momentarily take them out of the neuromuscular loop and establish new and improved recruitment patterns. Pain, bad posture, or bad habits will alter the sequence of muscle contractions for a given movement or posture and cause certain muscles to overwork while others weaken or tighten up. These patterns will lead to pain and injury if left unattended. To change these faulty patterns the body must start from ground zero, i.e. simple activation exercises, otherwise the larger and more dominant muscles will continue to move the body on an unstable skeleton. It is very difficult to properly perform complex tasks while in pain or imbalanced, even if it was once possible for the person in the past with a healthy body.

Once pain and major imbalances are greatly reduced or eliminated, the body can start to integrate multiple muscles into complex tasks (Stage III). If this principle is reversed it will further engrain the faulty patterns by constantly utilizing the wrong muscles. Training must start with the activation of important inhibited muscles, strengthening the segmental stabilizing muscles, and balancing overall posture no matter what area is the focus, then the areas of injury or interest can be fine tuned.

Without this fundamental stage the neuromuscular system will function with compensations that eventually wear down the joints and soft tissues. *Isolate, then integrate.*

Guidelines

- If there is a repetitive strain soft tissue injury, the acute stage of healing must be complete along with exercise clearance and advice from a doctor before starting this stage.
- If there is a traumatic soft tissue injury, the subacute stage of healing must be complete along with exercise clearance and advice from a doctor before starting this stage.
- Everyone should start with this stage. Advanced persons will progress faster, but only as fast as their imbalances and control, not skill or strength, permit.
- Keep exercises simple and movement minimal (isolate muscles).

Priorities (in order of importance)

- Establish PMAP by learning to activate specific postural and local stabilizing muscles (particularly multifidus and transverse abdominis).
- Focus on major imbalances and inhibited muscles.
- Incorporate into daily routine, do not limit to exercise program.

Variables:

- Duration   1-4 weeks (depends on health and ability)

	Sets	Reps/Time	Intensity	Tempo	Rest	X per wk
Workout	1-3	2-5 min	40-60%	Slow/Isometric	1 min	5-7

Choosing Exercises:

- Choose Stage I exercises that focus on correcting posture and inhibitions
- Simple, isolated, and uniplanar movements, if any movement

Strength Progression Stage II
Global Stabilization

Description

This stage introduces more integrative exercises while maintaining a corrective isolated approach. The focus here is weightbearing and closed chain exercises that utilize either the sagittal or frontal planes while emphasizing functional groups of stabilization muscles. This stage will strengthen both the local and global stabilization systems by gradually adding unstable surfaces and build the necessary recruitment patterns that stabilize the body for safe gross movement and more intense training.

Guidelines

- There are two 2-4 week programs that use the same or similar exercises but different surfaces (stable to unstable).
- If there is a repetitive strain soft tissue injury, the acute stage of healing must be complete, Exercise Progression Stage I must be completed, and exercise clearance and advice from a doctor must be had before starting this stage.
- If there is a traumatic soft tissue injury, the subacute stage of healing must be complete, Exercise Progression Stage I must be completed, and exercise clearance and advice from a doctor must be had before starting this stage.
- Circuit training can be utilized to increase stamina and maximize time.
- If post exercise soreness greatly reduces daily functioning or remains longer than 72 hours, the intensity should be lowered.
- Progress from bilateral to unilateral where appropriate.
- Continue developing the same principles as Stage I (corrective, stabilizing, and muscle control) while incorporating weightbearing exercises into integrated uniplanar exercises (squat with a shoulder press).

Priorities

- Establish PMAP and maintain proper spinal alignment throughout integrated uniplanar closed chain exercises.
- Strengthen all types of muscle contractions (concentric, eccentric, and isometric) in order to control body weight in upright positions, i.e. sitting to standing, standing to sitting, etc.
- Correct major imbalances and compensations in order to prepare the body for dynamic strength exercises.
- Find an intensity level that promotes growth, not damage.

Variables:

- Duration   4-8 weeks (depending on ability)

	Sets	Reps/Time	Intensity	Tempo	Rest	X per wk
Workout	3-5	15-25 reps or 1-3 min	50-75%	Slow/Isometric	45-60 sec	3-5

Choosing Exercises:

- Choose from Stage II exercises
- Utilize integrated (multiple muscles) uniplanar exercises that focus on weightbearing stabilization
- Add unstable surfaces to appropriate exercises to increase joint stabilization, core recruitment, proprioceptive efficiency, and functional strength
- Focus on lengthening (eccentric) and holding (isometric) contractions, especially body weight

Strength Progression Stage III
Mobilization Exercises

Description

The purpose of this stage is to utilize the gross movers (large muscles) while maintaining local and global stability. Many different things will be going on during this stage, such as; open chain exercises for the mobilizers, closed chain exercises to further develop the stabilizers and incorporate the mobilizers, and for the first time in the strength progression, multiplanar movements and segmental spinal movement. This is the final corrective stage before intense exercise begins, therefore all types of movement and coordination must be introduced here (with little to moderate resistance) in order to prepare the body for dynamic action.

Guidelines

- There are two 3-4 week programs that use the same or similar exercises but different surfaces (stable to unstable).
- Circuit or multiple circuit training is utilized to increase stamina and maximize time.
- Open chain movements should have already been introduced in the stretching component of the early stages, and thus they will begin here in the strength training against resistance as long as proper spinal alignment and PMAP can be controlled.
- Incorporate Stage II exercises into multiplanar movements (add rotation).
- Incorporate segmental spinal movement, i.e. curl-ups, bent knee dead lifts, etc.
- Practice open and closed chain exercises with extremity movements while maintaining a stable spine.

Priorities

- Ability to move extremities while maintaining a stable or neutral spine.
- Establish PMAP throughout integrated multiplanar (dynamic) movements against light to moderate resistance.
- Achieve strength and stability in complex multiplanar movements with all types of muscle contractions (eccentric, isometric, and concentric).
- Incorporate more advanced proprioception and strength exercises.
- Learn to activate each major muscle throughout its functional ROM with proper segmental stabilization.
- Increase intensity, duration, and tempo to meet individual needs (with the exception of explosive movements).

Variables:

- Duration   6-8 weeks

	Sets	Reps	Intensity	Tempo	Rest	X per wk
Open & Closed Chain	2-3 or within a multiple circuit	Exercise dependent	50-75%	Slow/Moderate	Training system dependent, i.e. circuit or multiple sets	3-5x

Choosing Exercises:

- Choose from Stage III exercises, open and closed chain, add unstable surfaces to appropriate exercises
- Isolated multiplanar exercises (abdominal crunch or back extension with a twist)
- Integrated multiplanar exercises (squat with a one arm row into a twist or push-ups with a twist)

Strength Progression Stage IV
Strength Exercises

Description

Now that all major imbalances have been controlled, intense strength training and complex movements can be practiced without compensation. This stage will begin to emphasize the intensity and specificity of any sports or activity specific actions. For those who need extreme strength, this is the stage too focus on. For those who need strength and speed, i.e. power, Stage V should be focused on, but only after completing at least 4 weeks of Stage IV.

Guidelines

- There are two 4 week programs that follow the same principles and progress each exercise to its potential, ideally each exercise is mastered before moving on to others.
- Weeks 1-4 are regular tempo and weeks 5-8 progress to explosive concentric contractions.
- All major imbalances and pain must be corrected before starting this stage.
- High intensity strength training is optional during this stage and is not for everyone.
- Circuit training can be utilized to increase stamina and imitate real life situations.
- Plyometrics are optional in weeks 5-8 (body weight only and no transition phase, i.e. pause between concentric and eccentric).

Priorities

- Achieve strength and stability in movements that are relevant for each individual.
- Achieve ideal strength and stability throughout complex high resistance movements.
- Increase intensity, duration, and tempo to meet individual needs and prepare for Stage V.

Variables:

- Duration   4-8 weeks
- Frequency   3-5x week total   (depends on how muscle groups are spaced out)

	Sets	Reps	Intensity	Tempo	Rest	X per wk
Endurance	2-3	12-25	60-80%	varies	30-60 sec	3-5
Hypertrophy	3-4	9-12	70-75%	varies	45-90 sec	3-5
Strength	3-4	6-8	75-85%	varies	2-3 min	3-5
Max Strength	3-5	1-5	85-100%	varies	3-5 min	3-5
Plyometrics	3-5	8-15	85-100%	explosive	2-5 min	1-3

➢ Varies signifies goal dependent

Choosing Exercises:

- Same or similar to Stage III strength exercises but much more intense
- Any type of training system can be implemented (circuit training, split-routine, etc.)
- Integrated multiplanar exercises with intensities that are specific to the individuals goals
- Add unstable surfaces to appropriate exercises
- Plyometric exercises in weeks 5-8 can utilize any activity specific movements that the person needs as long as no resistance is used and there is a pause between eccentric and concentric contractions
- After the first 4 weeks, the second 4 week program can be implemented *or* a Stage II routine can be used to rest the body until it is ready for the second Stage IV program or Stage V

Strength Progression Stage V
Power Exercises

Description

With a solid foundation of strength, speed, and coordination established, explosive movements with resistance and whatever else one can think of (be careful) can be trained in this stage. This is the most explosive and activity specific stage. Athletes are not the only ones who need power. Power training can prepare the neuromuscular system to quickly jump out of harm's way or simply start a lawn mower (the older models of course). Lifting heavy loads (85-100%) and light loads (30%) as fast and as controllably possible is necessary to enhance results.[13,235-243]

Guidelines

- CORE conditioning is the combination of intense cardio followed by CORE exercises that train the CORE to function during exhausting situations (for athletes or extremists only).
- There are two 4 week programs with three main types of exercise, see Ch. 14 for examples:
- Weeks 1-4   1. Total Body   2. Strength & Power Pairs   3. CORE Conditioning
- Weeks 5-8   1. Total Body   2. Transition Power   3. CORE Conditioning
- Power training for weeks 1-4 focuses on the speed of contraction for one contraction phase at a time, meaning that there is a brief pause between the concentric and eccentric contractions, i.e. no transition phase. A strength exercise of similar biomechanics is also utilized immediately before the power exercise in order to promote the strength component of power and maximal neuromuscular recruitment.
- Power training for weeks 5-8 focuses on: 1) the transition phase of power (the changing of direction and stability strength between eccentric and concentric contractions) 2) the speed of this transition 3) the ability to maintain this power and stability throughout an activity specific action of predetermined time, i.e. stamina power can last up to 1 min or 30 reps. Stamina power is optional and not as intense as strength power.
- Training the elderly to their limits of ROM, velocity, and strength will prepare them for trips and falls (little to no weight is needed with this population).

Priorities

- Achieve ideal strength and stability throughout explosive movements.
- Strengthen the CORE to withstand extreme activity.
- Mimic sport or job with explosive exercises.
- Maintain strength gains from Stage IV with total body exercises.
- Increase intensity, duration, and tempo to meet individual needs.

Variables

- Duration   8 weeks
- Frequency   3-5x week total (depends on how muscle groups are spaced out)

	Sets	Reps	Intensity	Tempo	Rest	X per wk
Hypertrophy	3	9-12	70-75%	varies	45-90 sec	3-5
Strength	3-4	6-8	75-85%	varies	2-3 min	3-5
Max Strength	4-6	1-5	85-100%	varies	3-5 min	3-5
Power	4-8	1-10	85-100%	explosive	3-5 min	1-2
Power/Stamina	2-3	12-30	75-85%	explosive	2-5 min	1-2
CORE Conditioning	varies	varies	75-90%	varies	2-3 min	1-2

➤ Varies signifies goal dependent

Choosing Exercises:

- Choose from Stage IV strength exercises for the total body section
- Power exercises can focus on power, or both power and stamina depending on the person's goals
- **<u>Weeks 1-4</u>** To develop power, use a strength, toning, or max strength exercise immediately followed by an explosive exercise of similar movement (power pairs); explode concentrically and eccentrically but utilize a brief pause between the concentric and eccentric phase in order to eliminate the transition phase and build a foundation of stability for each contraction phase; try to imitate sport or significant activities
- **<u>Weeks 5-8</u>** To develop power/stamina, use exercises that can be safely controlled through the transition phase of the exercise at high speeds and that mimic significant activities performed by the individual (squatting up and down as fast as controllably possible with no stopping, jumping is optional)
- CORE conditioning circuits should include any form of cardio, preferably the type that the individual utilizes the most in sports, along with exercises that challenge all aspects of the CORE (side bending, rotation, lower abs, upper abs, and lower back)
- Depending on the goal, different combinations (times per week) of the three main exercises (total body, power, and CORE conditioning) are possible during one week, see Ch. 14 for different combinations of exercise routines
- Use 5-10% of body weight for power exercises, or little to no weight for special populations
- Athletes like a shot putter will use heavier weight and fewer reps than the norm

Chapter 7   Daily Activity Modifications (D.A.M.'s)

D.A.M.'s are used to teach the body more efficient ways of performing daily movements and decrease the amount of wear and tear the body is subjected to each day. They are for people who are injured or in pain, or who are interested in improving their daily functioning and improving compensation patterns. The goal with these exercises is not reps or duration; it is learning how to do the movements correctly and then applying them throughout day. This way a separate workout isn't needed for them, they become part of life. Occasional practice in the gym is needed to reinforce proper techniques, but too much practice will wear the body down for when these movements really need to be performed.

Unlike a proper workout, real life doesn't usually involve a warm-up before having to lift something (kids, furniture, etc.) or other complex movements. Unfortunately these activities are best done when the body is warm and after the movement pattern has been repeated a few times to ensure proper form. So the question often times is this; would you rather risk feeling silly by squatting up and down a couple of times in order to warm-up before lifting something? Or would you rather risk being immobilized by pain for the next week because of improper lifting techniques?

D.A.M.'s are necessary because exercises don't transfer their effects over to real life situations as well as practicing the real life situations do. D.A.M.'s are an exception to the progression philosophy of saving the more complex exercises for the later stages because these activities often have to be performed daily. Therefore, the earlier the proper techniques are learned, the sooner the body will break from bad habits and have the ability to function efficiently. D.A.M.'s are ideal for low back pain sufferers because these people often fall into a cycle of bad movement patterns that are a result of the pain. These bad movements reinforce the pain, thus adding to the cycle. Once the movements and activities are improved, daily functioning and pain also improve.

D.A.M.'s are only performed in Stages I and II, after that they should be incorporated into the daily routine, although they can and should be practiced every so often in the gym to ensure proper form and adherence.

See Exercise Progression Vol. II for pictures and descriptions of the D.A.M.'s.

The Daily Activity Movements

1. *Kneeling on knees* (like a quad stretch without leaning back, good for being on the ground)
2. Kneeling on tip toes (*washing hands in river* - reaching things on bottom shelf - picking things up off the floor – etc.)
3. *Putting on shoes and clothes/scrubbing feet* (1 leg balancing and other techniques)
4. *Vacuuming*
5. Standing *overhead reach*
6. Rolling over and *getting in and out of bed or off the floor*
7. *Sitting flexion*
8. *Standing twist*, no weight
9. *Standing lateral bend*, no weight
10. *Golf pick-up* (pencil)
11. Modified *Golf/Soap pick-up in shower* (one leg squat/touch toes/other hand supported on wall)
12. *Opening doors* (push-pull at lumbar level)
13. *Momentum lifting* (medicine ball on table)
14. *Getting out of and into chairs*
15. *Mini squat* with hands on abdominals and low back
16. Box pick-up off floor
17. Using *knees against trunk* of car (groceries) or front of wash machine for leverage during lifting
18. *Backwards door close kick* (glute squeeze w/leg swing/push)
19. *Standing Posture Hold* (tense stomach and stand tall/squeeze gmax/activate lumbar erectors/ground through feet/push heels out/etc.)
20. Standing Tip Toe *Garage Door close*/straight arm lat pull
21. Squat w/one arm on knee and other arm picking up a light weight (*toilet seat pick-up*/down)
22. *Garbage toss* without weight, progress to tubing/cable
23. *Lawn mower start* without resistance, progress to light tubing and then "bent-over dumbbell row w/twist"
24. *Long hair management* (combing over a chair, etc., i.e. not standing and stooping)
25. *Squat w/object fall and catch* (speed work)
26. *Shoveling*

27. *Stepovers* (standing and stepping over different heights until hips have to hike) forward/backward/sideways/with a twist
28. *Squat with ball pick up*
29. Cooking or *leaning over counter*

30. *Floor Scrub* on knees like ab/wheel exs
31. *Laundry unloading* (med ball pick-up from hip-high object (table, tall chair, etc., then twisting throw-push to person (i.e. into the dryer or laundry basket)
32. Rotating step-overs (over a chair or corner of bed)

D.A.M.'s Progression Stage I

Description

There is only one stage for D.A.M.'s, and it can be done at anytime and in conjunction with any other Exercise Progression component. For someone who trains others, it is important to spend a good amount of time teaching the proper techniques, especially to those who are injured or in pain, if proper muscle activation patterns and pain improvement are goals.

Guidelines

- Only focus on the activities that are difficult or applicable to the person (not everyone needs to know how to shovel, but if time permits it is useful to learn).
- Little to no weight should be used for the lifting techniques until proper form is established, especially for those in pain or who are injured.
- The D.A.M.'s mentioned above only scrape the surface of possible activities in need of modification; use your imagination and detailed assessment of the individual to create as specific a DAM as possible.

Priorities

- Learn proper techniques of appropriate activities and apply them on a daily basis.
- Realize that one activity done wrong once a day is enough to 'pick at the scab' of an injury and keep it from healing.
- Have fun and spend enough time with this stage because it can dramatically improve a person's lifestyle by making a daily activity easier and pain free.

Variables

- Duration   Anytime
- Intensity   Light to Moderate
- Frequency As often as necessary to learn the movement

Workout

- Reps and sets are not as much a factor as time spent, which should be at least 10 min for those who need it.
- The tempo should be at whatever speed is most useful for the task.

Choosing Exercises

- Choose activities that 1) normally cause pain 2) are done repeatedly wrong on a daily basis and therefore reinforce faulty muscle recruitment patterns 3) are the most relevant for each individual.

Chapter 8   Warm-up and Cool-down

Warm-up

Warming up the body for strengthening exercises or strenuous activity is similar to warming up a car before it is driven. If the car is going for a mellow drive around town, then it needs little warming up and can even warm up while driving around town. But if the car is going to perform at a high level, it must be driven around for awhile to prepare the engine and tires for serious action.

The body requires the same type of attention before performing. If an exercise or activity about to be done is fairly simple (a few muscles moving in one plane) than the warm-up can be as simple as repeating that motion for a few sets with a lighter weight. But, if the workout is going to involve *complex or explosive* movements, then the warm-up needs to consist of complex actions that warm up the body's core temperature and neuromuscular system (coordination and balance). Warm-up stretching can also be used to improve specific inhibitions that might impede the workout. Some of the benefits of warming up are:

- Decreased post activity soreness and stiffness.
- Increased coordination and neuromuscular ability, and therefore increased strength and performance.
- Decreased chance of injury.
- Improving reciprocal inhibitions that can decrease performance.

Notice that the main theme of warming up is movement, not stretching. Prolonged static stretching can reduce strength and power before working out.[21/22/23] Flexibility is of course needed to avoid injuries, but should not be the primary focus of warm-up, see stretching before exercise pg. 39.

Time can be a major factor limiting a warm-up routine. This can be remedied by turning the warm-up into a mini workout. Exercise Progression utilizes a warm-up routine that is challenging yet safe. It can actually be considered working out, but with a different purpose; to prepare the body for more intense training. This way it doesn't seem like such a waste of time for those who don't want to be bothered with a warm-up.

A typical warm-up should include the following components in the following order:

1. At least 5-10 minutes of aerobic activity that increases core temperature and blood flow to the appropriate areas (jumping jacks, jumping rope, shooting a basketball, cardio machines, etc.).
2. Specific active stretches that improve major imbalances and inhibitions which might affect the workout.
3. 5-10 minutes of proprioception training (this is optional, mostly for those who lack coordination).
4. A group of exercises and or dynamic stretches that prepare the body for action.

In general, it is only necessary to warm-up the area that is going to be used. For instance, an upper body workout should utilize an arm ergometer or shooting a basketball rather than riding the bicycle for warm-up. But if the upper body workout is going to include dynamic or explosive movements, then a more complete total body warm-up should be performed.

The warm-ups presented in Stage IV of Ch. 14 are for a total body workout because the intensity and complexity of a Stage IV workout requires advanced utilization of the body's neuromuscular system.

Warm-up

Warm-up Progression Stages I-IV

Description

Each stage uses the same principles but the warm-up exercises will have a higher degree of difficulty for each progressing stage. There are many different ways to warm up the body; the warm-up exercises in the appendix have worked best for the author as a warm-up routine. It is encouraged to create an individual warm-up regimen utilizing the principles described in this chapter.

Guidelines

- o Stage I of Exercise Progression is so simple that it does not require a warm-up routine.
- o Stages II and III utilize 1) cardio 2) corrective stretching 3) proprioception for a warm-up routine.
- o Stage IV utilizes 1) cardio 2) a circuit combining 7-10 warm-up exercises (see below) and stretches that challenge the neuromuscular system in a way that prepares the body for that particular workout.
- o Body weight (push-ups, squats, supermans, etc.) and unstable surface exercises are ideal for warming up.
- o For Stage IV, pick 7-10 exercises and cycle through them like a circuit 1-3 times, with the appropriate rest in-between sets and circuits, see Ch. 14 Stage IV for an example of a general warm-up.

Priorities

- o Get a little sweat going.
- o Prepare the body for whatever activity it is about to perform.
- o Incorporate warm-ups into *every* strengthening workout.

Variables

	Sets	Reps	Intensity	Exercise Rest	Circuit Rest	# of Exercises
Workout	1-3	10-15	40-70%	5-10 sec	30-90sec	7-10

Choosing Exercises

- o Choose exercises and stretches from the appropriate stage.
- o Choose exercises and stretches that warm up the body in all of the planes of movement that will be challenged in the workout.

Cool-down

The need to cool down isn't so much a performance or injury issue, rather a health and comfort choice. Cooling down helps to clear the body of lactic acid that builds up during intense exercise, as well as prevents blood from pooling in the larger muscles when intense exercise is stopped immediately. Depending on how intense the workout is will determine the duration of the cool-down. *Generally a cool-down should be at least 5-10 minutes of easy activity*, i.e. walking, biking, light swimming, etc., *followed by stretching of the major muscle groups,* which is at least another 5-10 minutes. See appendix for an example of a cool-down stretch routine.

A post-workout stretching session is ideal because the muscles are already warm and it will help restore the muscles to their normal resting length. Cool-down stretching and easy activity are the muscle's reward for working hard. They also help rejuvenate the muscle so that it is best prepared to work hard again soon.

How to Fit in a Warm-up and Cool-Down

The dilemma now is how to find time to fit a warm-up and cool-down into an hour or half hour workout; of course if there is no time limit then there is no dilemma. The following is one example of a proper *one hour strength training workout* for Stage III.

1. Aerobic warm-up (bike, basketball, walking, etc.): 5-10 minutes
2. Corrective active stretching: 5-10 minutes
3. Proprioception: 5-10 minutes
4. Strengthening workout : 25-35 min
5. Aerobic warm-down (bike, walking, light swimming, etc.): 5-10 minutes
6. Stretching cool-down: 5-10 min

❖ #'s 1-3 are warm-up, # 4 is the main workout, and #'s 5-6 are cool-down.

The following is one example of a proper *one hour strength training workout* for Stage IV:

1. Aerobic warm-up (bike, basketball, walking, etc.): 5-10 minutes
2. Dynamic stretches and exercises that are activity specific and prepare the body for the following workout: 5-10 minutes
3. Strengthening workout: 25-35 min
4. Aerobic cool-down (bike, walking, light swimming, etc.): 5-10 minutes
5. Stretching cool-down: 5-10 min

❖ #'s 1-2 are warm-up, # 3 is the main workout, and #'s 4-5 are cool-down.

Sometimes only a half hour is available to workout. This limits the intensity and complexity of the workout because of insufficient time to warm up and cool down. Therefore, simpler and less intense workouts are recommended when only short periods of time are available.

The following is one example of a proper *half hour strength training workout:*

1. Aerobic activity: 5-10 minutes, **Or**
   5-10 minutes practicing each exercises before it is performed in the workout, but with less weight.
   2-3 sets of 10-20 reps
2. Strengthening workout (simple movements, can include proprioception training): 20 minutes
3. Easy aerobic activity or stretching utilizing the muscles just worked: 5 minutes

❖ # 1 is warm-up, # 2 is the main workout, & # 3 is warm-down.
❖ A more in depth stretching routine should be performed later that day.

Chapter 9   Corrective Actions Guidelines

This chapter describes the basic philosophies of corrective strategies for the various phases of injury and different categories of assessment. See Ch. 13 for details on the specific corrections of the low back.

Figuring out where to start with a corrective exercise program can be overwhelming due to the abundance of assessment findings. A priority list is helpful for creating a progressive exercise program that focuses on health, function, and overall strength. The following list is in order of priority.

1. Find any red flags and refer to a specialist.
2. Pain is often a sign of injury, improper mechanics, or trigger point involvement and its origin should be identified before starting an exercise program. Refer to a specialist whenever necessary.
3. Neurological involvement must be identified as nerve root or peripheral entrapment origin. Nerve root problems require referral to a specialist while peripheral nerve entrapments can often be relieved by appropriate manual therapy or stretching techniques.
4. Joint dysfunctions must be identified as structural or muscular. Structural abnormalities should be corrected with manual therapy before any advanced exercising, while muscular involvement requires that the appropriate muscles be stretched and strengthened, and PMAP practiced.
5. Follow the priorities (#'s 1-7) listed in Stage I of Exercise Progression in Chapter 14.

Corrective Action Categories

Asymptomatic	Palpation
Repetitive Strain	ROM
Posture/Gait	Muscle Testing
Neurological	Functional Tests
Structural	Traumatic Injuries

❖ *Asymptomatic Population*

Start with Stage I of the low back progressions. If major imbalances are present, then specific corrections should be added to the general progression.

❖ *Repetitive Strain*

The following guidelines are for the different stages of repetitive strain and should only be advised by a licensed practitioner and will vary with individual cases. Each section is in the proper order of application from top to bottom.

Acute (2-3 days avg., up to 1 wk)[41]

- PRICE (protection, rest, ice, compression, elevation)
- Anti-inflammatories
- Manual therapy (focus on improving blood and lymph flow)
- Light stretching if tolerable
- Daily activity modifications (ergonomics, poor posture, faulty biomechanics, and detrimental habits)
- Educate with handouts

Subacute (6-8 wks avg., up to 16 wks)[41]

- Physical therapy (if necessary)
- Manual therapy (chiropractic adjustments and soft tissue mobilization) as needed
- Exercise clearance from doctor or physical therapist
- Create a specific exercise program utilizing the methods in this manual and advice from doctor.

Chronic (until pain free and function is restored)

- Refer to a specialist if daily functioning is severely impaired, medication is habitually used for relief, psychological factors seem prevalent, or a reason for the pain cannot be found.
- Manual therapy (chiropractic adjustments and soft tissue mobilization) as needed.
- Modify any detrimental habits or faulty patterns of movement.
- Utilize chronic pain forms and other educational handouts when appropriate.
- Create a specific Exercise Progression program by utilizing the methods in Stage I; a home exercise program is essential to improving symptoms.
- If symptoms persist, evaluation by a pain specialist is recommended.

Posture

- Improve ergonomics
- Teach awareness of ideal posture positions for the work place, home, car, etc.
- Activate weak postural muscles with specific exercises.
- Stretch tight areas that are dominant and create postural stress.
- Apply manual therapy to restricted areas.
- Teach the principle that proper posture will not become *permanent* in most cases because of the environment we live in; instead it must be constantly achieved through awareness.

Gait

Results from gait and posture analysis give incite on where major imbalances lie and which neuromuscular and biomechanical dysfunctions are probable. See the low back corrective actions section for specific corrections.

Neurological

Failure of the neurological tests does not assure neurological involvement, because there are tissues other than nerves that can mimic failure of the tests (trigger points, facet joints, etc.). Start by correcting (using manual therapy) any abnormalities found in the supplementary tests and then retest the nerve roots. If the test is still positive it points towards neurological involvement (or inadequate treatment) and referral to a specialist is recommended. If the retest is negative then non-neurological factors might be the cause of weakness/paralysis, *or* the body's adaptive systems may be overloaded from the manual therapy and cause a false negative test. Therefore it is best to test again after at least one day of non-treatment. If the weakness/paralysis is still improved one day later, then one can assume that the treatment was appropriate.

If a person with diagnosed neurological dysfunction is cleared for treatment, care should be taken during manual and exercise therapy due to the hypersensitivity of healing nerve tissue. The exercise or manual therapy treatment should follow the doctor's guidelines.

These guidelines can be helpful for the following conditions:

Weakness/paralysis

1. PNF techniques[2]
2. Isolated muscle contractions[2]
3. Electrical stimulation[2]
4. Balance influential postures throughout the body.

One or all of the above can be utilized, with PNF techniques seeming to be the most effective due to its complex neurological organization demands. A home program and good posture are also essential to recovery.

Pain/inflammation along a nerve path

1. Manual therapy along the entire path to release adhesions and yet sooth the nerve.
2. Gentle stretching of the nerve may be useful in moderation.
3. Local strengthening exercises are contraindicated until inflammation is much improved, but general fitness (walking and movement of the uninvolved tissues) can be helpful.
4. Balance influential postures throughout the body.
5. Ice the inflamed areas, do not heat.

Structural

Positive tests only give hints of joint dysfunction and can sometimes be mimicked by other tissue traumas (trigger points, ligament strains, etc.). Start by correcting (using manual therapy) any abnormalities found in the supplementary tests and then retest the joints. If the joint test is still positive then a joint dysfunction is likely present and a referral to a specialist is recommended to learn the extent of the dysfunction. Once cleared for exercise or manual therapy, treatment should follow the doctor's guidelines.

Palpation

Inflammation or swelling contraindicates any exercise without a doctor's release.

Tenderness should be compared with other test results to discern regular from abnormal tenderness.

Any adhesions or trigger points which are found that impair crucial functioning should be relieved with an appropriate manual therapy before any complex or intense exercise is performed. Simple stretching is not always sufficient to remove TP's or adhesions.

Soft tissues that feel dry and rigid will need to progress slowly because of the greater chance of injury and decreased rate of blood flow within the tissues. Extra water and massage is often helpful.

When interconnecting areas of the body are restricted together or the skin feels stuck to the underlying tissues, restricted myofascia is usually present and requires special stretching of the appropriate fascial lines.

It should be noted that tight or rigid areas can sometimes be the result of a protective mechanism for an underlying problem and therefore should not be the focus of manipulation or manual therapy. Instead, an understanding of why the movement or tissue is restricted should be had before trying to improve mobility. For instance, someone with a lateral disc herniation can have unilateral muscle guarding that protects the nerve from being pinched, releasing that tightness would only encourage pinching of the nerve.

If the palpation skills are possessed then the energetic condition of the body can be interpreted, which is reflective of the intensity of activity required to best improve the health of the individual. For instance, a frail or ill person emits an obvious low energy vibration that is easily overwhelmed by average exercise and therapy intensities. Obvious cases such as this can be seen with the naked eye but the more subtle ones require touching the body and feeling its pulse and overall energy.

ROM

Limitations in ROM only give clues about which muscles to stretch, they don't necessarily mean that the muscle failing the test is the cause of the limitation. For example, a failed hamstring test could be influenced by short hip flexors tilting the pelvis anteriorly, which creates the illusion of short hamstrings. In this case the test would be corrected by stretching the hip flexors, not the hamstrings. Improving ROM deficiencies is safe only if the antagonists of the short muscles can stabilize the joint(s) in the new position. Hypermobility is a common cause of instability and is described on pg. 41 in ROM and Weakness.

The end-feel of ROM tests is the most important factor in determining the cause of limitation. A leathery 'give' at the limited range signifies soft tissue restrictions, while an abrupt and solid stop of movement points to a structural blockage or adhesions from scar tissue. A restricted leathery 'give' will respond well to stretching, structural limitations often require mobilization, and scar tissue adhesions within the joint are permanent after about 14 weeks[6] unless surgical intervention is used.

If pain accompanies a ROM test, then all other assessment categories need to be compared in order to find the cause of pain. It should be noted at what ROM the pain is present and worst.

Muscle Testing

As with the ROM testing, failed or weak tests do not verify that the muscle being tested is responsible for the dysfunction, they only show that function is altered. Results must be compared with the other assessments to find the true source of the problem. Correcting any altered firing patterns is a priority, see Ch. 13 for individual corrections. Strengthening or "waking up" inhibited muscles can be done with specific activation techniques.

A weak muscle test can be the result of reciprocal or arthrokinetic inhibition, poor mechanics from faulty posture, pain, or many other factors. Muscle testing is performed after the ROM and posture assessments in order to confirm any of the above mentioned factors as well as fine tune the overall picture created from the relatively passive assessment performed up to this point.

Functional Tests

Failed or deficient functional test results are improved by incorporating the tests into the workout regimen and correcting any correlating tests or imbalances. Functional restoration is a priority *after* correcting major imbalances and faulty movement patterns, unless the functional tests can be done without compensating, or immediate function is more important than symptom control and long term function.

When working with athletes or manual labor workers it is important to find the functional weaknesses that relate to their activity and explain to them how balanced muscles are able to work more efficiently and thus function for longer periods of time, which protects against fatigue injuries. This explanation can encourage dedication to correcting the imbalances and shed light on the reasons for their dysfunction or pain.

Traumatic Injuries

The following guidelines are purely educational for the unlicensed professional. They are meant to shed light on what someone should go through before they arrive for post-rehabilitation work. If someone is in Stage I or II of recovery and presents themselves to a personal trainer before seeking the help of a doctor, they should be immediately referred for physical therapy and not trained until they are released to the fitness professional.

Soft Tissue Injury Response

All of the following time frames are depending on the

severity of the injury and are a compilation of findings from Slosberg[75], Colby and Kisner[6], and Liebenson.[41]

0 - 30 minutes	Initial trauma and tissue deformation
0 - 36 hours	Coagulation/blood clotting
2nd hour - 2nd week	Inflammation response
2nd day - 6th week	Repairing and healing
3rd week – 12 months	Maturation and remodeling

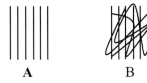

A   B

Fig. 9-1   Scar tissue formation. A shows regular, linear tissue fibers. B shows the random configuration of scar tissue that grows to make the tissue stronger in all directions. This is great for strength but bad for vascularity and flexibility.

Soft Tissue Injury Response

Phases:

1. Acute or *Inflammatory* (lasts 12-96 hours) Swelling, redness, warmth, and pain are common symptoms. Very vulnerable

2. Subacute or *repair* and *healing* (lasts 1-2 weeks average and up to 6 weeks) Scar tissue is forming and inflammation is decreasing. Vulnerable

3. Chronic or *maturation and remodeling* (Starts at about the 3rd week and lasts 3-14 weeks average and up to 12 months post injury) Injuries that never properly healed or keep getting re-injured are often stuck in this phase. *Inflammation is gone* and scar tissue is growing thicker and realigning to the stresses placed on it.[6] The first 8-10 weeks scar tissue is remodeling it can be manipulated using cross friction massage with the muscle in the shortened position to form a more flexible scar, but after 14 weeks the scar tissue is mostly unchangeable without surgical intervention.[6] If cross friction or deep tissue massage is applied too intensely or before the repair and healing phase is complete (1-3 weeks post-injury), the tissues will break down even more and thus increase scar tissue formation and healing time. Semi-vulnerable

Re-injury during any of these phases leads to increased scar tissue and prolonged healing time. Re-injury can occur from returning to activities too soon or from too intense of an activity (overstretching is common)

during the healing process. It is imperative to educate about the healing process to those who are injured if progress is to be made with a post-rehabilitation exercise program.

Traumatic Injury Rehabilitation Guidelines

The following guidelines for phases one and two are from Kisner and Colby.[6]

Phase 1. *(physical therapy)* – Acute

- Medication is sometimes required for pain and inflammation.
- Resistance and stretching exercises are contraindicated for the inflamed tissues.
- Gentle massage, passive movements, PRICE treatment, and modalities promote healing best during this phase.
- Move as much as tolerable.
- Active ROM at the site of injury is often contraindicated, but there are exceptions.
- D.A.M.'s are generally necessary.
- Sometimes a low back disorder is such that any exertion aggravates the condition, this situation is ideal for the McKenzie[79] methods or simply finding positions that help the pain and then repeating them throughout the day, as well as avoiding movements or positions that cause pain. This tactic should also be used in the subacute stage.

Phase 2. *(physical therapy)* - Subacute

- Controlled ROM and intensity are crucial to the progression of tissue growth.
- Active exercise within the pain-free ROM.
- PNF techniques should be utilized to progress from passive, to active-assisted, to active-unassisted, and then to active resisted ROM.[5]
- Concentrate on exercises and stretches that balance tension around the injured area and correct influential postures.
- Submaximal isometric exercises are ideal to start with because they teach muscle control.
- Progress to all painless angles and take care to not overstretch the injured site during the contractions or tears can occur.
- Low intensity resistance exercises for the injured tissues can begin once the isometric contractions can be done with a pain level less than four.[5]
- Utilize closed chain exercises and progress to open chain depending on the injury and focus on eccentric contractions once the tissues can tolerate it.

- Mild stretching is recommended for the injured tissues.
- Pain and swelling should decrease during this stage. Great skill is required to distinguish between normal exercise discomfort, which can seem like pain to someone who is very deconditioned, and pain as a result of destructive exercising.
- In general, if pain is accompanied with swelling or lasts longer than a couple of hours at the site of injury, the exercises need to be less intense, modified, or completely changed.
- Pain should not be experienced while exercising.
- Gentle cross-friction massage can be applied at the latter part of this stage if tolerated by the tissues.
- Modalities, mobilization, and other manual techniques are often useful at this stage.

Phase 3. *(Exercise Progression)* - Chronic

- Continue to progress all the components above to meet the physical needs of the individual.
- Utilize Exercise Progression assessments to figure out what stage the individual should begin training at and which corrections and exercises are needed.
- Increase intensity of cross-friction massage.
- Swelling is a sign of too much or the wrong type of exercise.

Chapter 10   Program Design for Low Back Disorders (LBD's)

Exercise Post-Rehabilitation for LBD's

Exercise has yet to help acute low back pain (LBP) with any consistency, but is more promising for chronic LBP[80], the latter of which is a primary focus in this manual.

Up to 85% of disabling LBD cases have no true pathoanatomical diagnosis[37,81], this means that most of the time the practitioner doesn't know what they are trying to correct. This is one reason that many low back rehabilitation attempts fail. Another reason is that the low back is often treated as if it is its own entity, snuggly hidden away from the rest of the body, with the consequences of forward head posture and rounded shoulders going unnoticed.

In reality, *the lumbar spine is a shock absorber for many misalignments throughout the body*, and often times posture correcting exercises that don't directly involve the low back will reduce pain and allow proper healing of an injury without the popular but invasive lumbar exercises; these exercises can increase scar tissue formation and magnify symptoms.

Knowing which exercises cause the most compressive forces on the lumbar spine is a key to low back rehabilitation. This is very important with disc herniations and other motion segment maladies, especially since *exercise is no more proven to help LBP than the body's natural healing process.*

The low back is different from any other body part because it requires balancing the cervical, thoracic, and lumbar spine with the lower and upper extremities. For example: If the legs or arms are too weak to lift a box, then the low back has to compensate with increased flexion and or increased contractile force, which translates to greater intra-discal pressure and chance of disc protrusions. Therefore the *weakest parts of the body must be identified* and corrected to ensure a long lasting recovery, even the seemingly unrelated rotator cuff muscles.

The spinal erectors do not always need to be the primary target of exercise, in fact, they are usually facilitated while the abdominals are inhibited and in need of strengthening. Many upper and lower extremity exercises will indirectly strengthen the spine if a neutral posture is maintained throughout the different movements. This is ideal for those who have to limit their lumbar ROM and compressive forces due to instability, herniations, or acute pain.

Care should be taken when recommending isolated lumbar spine and abdominal exercises because they tend to place the moment force directly on the low back, thus encouraging injury or re-injury.

While stabilization training seems to be a popular way to rehabilitate the spine, it is too often done without first balancing the muscle tension and activation patterns throughout the body, which is fundamental for stability. What good is practicing stabilization exercises if the muscles are not *balanced* and functioning in harmony?

For example, learning to activate the abdominals first isn't very beneficial if one side or layer is much stronger than the other; it could actually promote spinal instability.

In order to affect the spine's stability, the body's joint protection mechanisms must be efficient. They are assessed two ways[138]; 1) testing the activation of the muscular corset, and 2) testing the ability to attain normal spinal curves.

The testing of spinal position is unnecessary if the individual is unable to properly activate the abdominal corset (even if they could find a decent spine position, they would be utilizing the wrong muscles). In this case, the activation patterns are learned first, followed by the practicing of proper spinal position.

A corrective exercise program that equalizes tension throughout the kinetic chain and teaches PMAP for the CORE muscles should be the foundation and initial stage of rehabilitation or post-rehabilitation of the low back. That being said, *spinal stabilization training is essential to low back rehabilitation* and should be incorporated as soon as the body is ready. *Isolate, and then integrate.*

Spinal Stabilization Training

There are three stages of spinal stabilization training and they make up the first three stages in Exercise Progression. Spinal stabilization is necessary as a first step for most people, LBP or not, because of the cumulative effects of deloading.

Deloading (reduction of weightbearing and sensory input regarding gravity, i.e. sitting or swimming) tends to cause the stabilizing muscles in the body to atrophy and lose function.[138]

Spinal stability must not get confused with balance or total body stability training. Spinal stability is closely related to its overall and symmetric segmental stiffness; exercises that challenge the body on one leg or with balance devices are testing overall kinetic chain stability and balance, not spine stability.[37] The spinal stabilization system consists of three components;[45] (Box 10-1).

One muscular miscue or damaged ligament can cause enough instability to promote injury if the load is enough. In order to prevent injury due to spinal instability there must be extreme muscle activity.[46]

Box 10-1

Components of Spinal Stabilization Training
   1. Active (muscles)
   2. Passive (osteoligamentous)
   3. Controlling (neurological)

This is where a balance of muscle tension, appropriate coordination, and speed of contractions are essential in maintaining stability. The co-contraction of the abdominals is also essential to spinal stabilization.

Once passive stiffness is lacking due to structural or ligament injury, active stiffness from muscular balance and coordination becomes the only hope for stability. Active stiffness must be retrained after injuries because of the disturbed motor patterns associated with pain and trauma.

Spinal stability requires different muscles and tissues to "take up the slack" with every change of position. It also requires different amounts of tension that are directly related to the task at hand. This takes a lot of practice to permanently groove the patterns into the conscious and eventually subconscious neurological system as well as erase any pain and injury induced patterns.

Some of the more important stabilizing muscles are the multifidus, transverse abdominus, internal oblique, diaphragm, pelvic floor muscles, latissimus dorsi, and the quadratus luborum, see pg. 15 for details about the CORE muscles..

There are three main stages to spinal stability training, see box 10-2; these three stages progressively incorporate the three stages of motor control learning, which are[47];

1. Kinaesthetic awareness
2. Conscious control
3. Subconscious control

Stage one of spinal stabilization training introduces new and improved simple neuromuscular patterns that can be quite difficult for the beginner or those in pain to feel or gain kinaesthetic awareness of.

These populations must be supervised closely at first in order to detect any compensation, such as the abdomen "puffing out" instead of tightening or the superficial spinal erectors arching the low back instead of the multifidi activating with no resulting movement in the spine.

The practitioner or individual should place their hands on the back and abdomen or use additional feedback methods to ensure proper muscular coordination and positioning.

Postural alignment during these exercises should be viewed form the side *and* anteriorly or posteriorly whenever possible, otherwise it is easy to overlook any right vs. left iliac crest and 12th rib height discrepancies if only the common side observation is used.

Without a foundation of corrective, isolated, and segmental exercises, stabilization training is essentially building a strong house (global muscles) on a weak foundation (segmental muscles and the joints) that will always be limited by structural and neuromuscular imbalances.

It is obvious when someone has a nice house with a weak foundation by looking at an accomplished athlete with low back problems. They can often perform very difficult stabilization exercises with ease but only by utilizing the mobilizing muscles; this is due to muscular imbalances and poor training and eventually leads to wear and tear followed by pain and injuries.

Therefore, total body or advanced stabilization exercises should be introduced after posture is more balanced, segmental strength is gained, and PMAP is learned. *Isolate, and then integrate.*

Stage two focuses on engraining the newly learned activation patterns into the neuromuscular system and progressively incorporating the global stabilization system into weightbearing movements.

While speed is a priority in stabilization contractions, it cannot be trained for until the appropriate positions are learned and practiced at a slower pace. Then speed can be the focus by using labile surfaces and other techniques. Endurance is also essential to stabilization and is most often best trained by performing the exercises until exhaustion while maintaining proper alignment.

A great way to safely train to exhaustion is to perform the most difficult exercise possible for as long as possible and then immediately switch to an easier stabilization exercise that is similar until proper form is no longer possible. This is continued down the line of exercises until the person is exhausted. Training of this sort is called "peeling back", and according to Craig Liebenson[41],

"Finding the patient's limit and peeling back is the art of spinal stabilization."

Spinal stabilization training should work up to at least 30 minutes of exercises that challenge the various positions possible by the spine if lasting and functional results are desired. Repetitions are not the goal, fatigue is, and thus time is a better gauge for improvement and keeping track of performance.

Stage III involves the entire muscular system with an emphasis on open chain movements and the development of the larger muscles in non-weightbearing positions. Exercises from Stages I and II are incorporated as well in order to fully integrate both systems.

The Abdominal Wall and Spinal Stability

As described in Ch. 11, there are four muscles in the abdominal wall that each creates unique forces on the lumbar spine when activated. Research[37] has shown that activation of the external and internal obliques along with the transverse abdominis produces superior spine stability compared to other activation patterns while in an upright position. *This pattern of activation is done by sucking in and tightening the stomach at the same time, not simply sucking it in or pushing it out. If done properly, activating the stomach will result in little to no change in the position of the abdomen[37], i.e. pushing out, sucking in, or bulging laterally [weak transverse abdominis (T.A.)].*

A weak or inhibited T.A. along with an overactive rectus abdominis (R.A.) is very common and leads to a decreased stabilization ability by the CORE. The point at which lumbopelvic stability ceases can be seen or felt and has been described as the *stabilization threshold.*[212] It is noticeable as a stomach protrusion, which signifies that the T.A. is inactive and therefore stability is minimal. This occurs from either too much load, i.e. during a squat the abdomen only protrudes at the end ROM or from too much weight, or the muscle is simply inhibited. In the former case, corrective actions would be to practice the squats only in the positions and weight ranges that stability can be maintained and then slowly progress. The latter situation calls for Stage I training for PMAP of the CORE.

It is important to note that PMAP for T.A. needs to be trained in various positions because the ability to utilize the T.A. and CORE muscles does not

Box 10-2

Stages of Spinal Stabilization Training

Stage I   Activation of Local Stabilizers

• Learn individual muscle activation patterns (especially multifidus, gluteus maximus, and transverse abdominis) and integrate them into awareness of proper static posture, progress from 1) lying 2) sitting 3) standing; *do not advance to Stage II until proper form can be held in all three positions for 10x 10 seconds.*

• Simple and isolated strengthening exercises are focused on segmental muscles that balance postural stresses (only if a neutral spine can be maintained) in the body to effectively pull the spine into a more even stiffness, in other words, enhance stability.

• In general, utilize *active* stretches for the hip flexors, pectorals, and upper abdominals to strengthen the gluteus maximus, scapula adductors, and thoracic extensors respectively.

Stage II   Integration of Global Stabilizers

• Incorporate the PMAP learned in Stage I into closed chain weightbearing (compression) exercises, i.e. squats and lunges, overhead press, etc.

• Engrain proper form with daily repetitions.

• Posture correcting exercises are still used.

Stage III   Integration of Mobilizers

• Utilize more functional open and closed chain exercises at higher speeds to involve the mobilizers.

• Posture correcting exercises are still used.

Each stage coincides with Stages 1-3 of Exercise Progression. See chapter 14 for more details and how to progress each stage.

automatically transfer from position to position. In other words, someone who can properly activate their T.A. and CORE during a squat does not always have that ability during a lunge.

When training for spinal stability it needs to be emphasized that there are different optimal activation patterns of the abdominal wall depending on the position of the spine and body. For instance, while standing, squatting, or sitting upright, the best combination seems to be the tightening method mentioned above, but with a flexed lumbar spine the best activation pattern seems to be contracting the transverse abdominis first (sucking in the abdomen) followed by a tightening of the abdominal wall. This focuses on the transverse abdominis and therefore its ability to resist the injurious anterior shear forces caused by forward flexion.

McGill[37] makes an important incite to the overuse of abdominal 'hollowing' or sucking in of the stomach for spinal stability training. This technique is known to activate the transverse abdominis, which is desirable in some situations as mentioned above, but is only one of the important stabilizing muscles of the abdominal wall. And as research[37] has shown, stability is greatest when the oblique abdominals are also activated. See pg. 84 for discussion on proper breathing techniques to increase stabilization affects (IAP).

Neutral Position

This position is ideal for optimal healing of lumbar injuries because it *provides the best support against gravity and is a foundation for stability*. Finding it is as easy as 1-2-3. Meaning, whether sitting, standing, or lying, it can be found by tilting the pelvis upward to twelve o'clock, then downward to six o'clock, and finally placing it somewhere in-between the two at the most stable spot. Then, if there are any pelvic abnormalities and pain allows, assume the corrective pelvis position, see pg. 209. Sometimes this last position can be too much for an acute LBD, but once ready, this position can solidify the spine's stability.

The neutral position is usually described as the most comfortable position for someone with LBP, but this can be misleading for those with a non-serious musculoskeletal based pain or dysfunction because they will lean and function (often undetected) towards tightness and facilitation and away from weakness to find comfort, this is not stable.

In this case, training inhibited muscles and learning PMAP needs to be applied *first* in order to have the *ability* to find stability, otherwise faulty recruitment patterns will be practiced. If the pain is serious (pinched nerve, inflamed joint, etc.), then a position of comfort is best practiced to protect the tissues until the injury is past the acute or painful stage.

This is not a universal position; it is unique to the individual's structural makeup and will even change throughout the healing or strengthening process as the spine strengthens into balance. For some, finding it is a relatively easy task, but for others who lack body awareness or have muscular inhibitions from pain interference it is quit difficult.

A lot of time and coaching are needed to learn this position prior to exercising or stretching. The neutral position should be introduced as a new best friend to those with motion segment disorders and serious lumbar pathologies. *It should be emphasized as the position of choice for most activities and exercises until healing and PMAP are satisfactory.*

While this position is the safest position for injured tissues, training the spine in only this position will leave it vulnerable to situations that challenge the posterior ligamentous system, such as sports, accidents, and falls. Therefore kyphotic (more flexed) positions must be strengthened and coordinated to achieve dynamic strength in the spine and its passive tissues. Only an experienced practitioner will know when the spine is able to withstand such training.

See the proper lifting techniques section on pg. 83 for details on techniques. It takes endurance strength from CORE muscles to maintain this position for a prolonged time, so home practice is essential.

Safety Zone

This refers to the ROM that the lumbar spine can move in all directions without pain or injury while maintaining a stable position; it is also called the "functional range". It must be practiced until it becomes automatic. This zone can grow larger with increasing strength and flexibility, but proper healing time is also vital in the decision to increase the zone.

The safety zone and neutral position are integral pieces of a low back program, without them the best of exercises can be injurious. Constant practice of these positions can lead to muscular stability for hypermobile joints, but the stability only lasts as long as the muscles do so endurance training is essential.

Great patience is needed during the building of stability to restrain from cracking one's own joints and slowly build up a stable environment.

Guidelines for Back Extension Exercises

People with low back pain tend to have trigger points in overactive erector spinae and inhibited thoracic extensor and multifidus muscles. These trigger points correspond with the Law of Facilitation, as well as findings from Travell and Simmons[7] that state "trigger points can refer inhibition or excitation to functionally related muscles, especially if the targeted muscles also have trigger points".

This means that training the erector spinae in the absence of thoracic extension can further promote the inhibition of the thoracic extensors and create numerous imbalances in regards to spinal movements. For this reason, thoracic extension will be a large part of all back extension training in this manual. See chapter 11 for more details on erector spinae and thoracic extensor functions.

Keep in mind, as mentioned in the spinal stabilization section, there are two stages of stabilization exercises to learn before the larger gross movers (erector spinae) should be trained. This is very different then the common training regimen that entails erector spinae strengthening at the beginning.

The following guidelines describe mostly open chain exercises that require a foundation of closed chain segmental stabilization strength to maintain proper alignment during the movements.

Positions

The pay offs for segmental or isolated contractions of the spine extensors are that inhibited areas can be activated and facilitated areas neutralized, as well as reduced total compression force on the spine. This can be done by (in order from least to highest amount of lumbar stress) utilizing;

1. Isolated thoracic extensions
2. Opposite arm and leg reaches (quadruped)
3. Double leg raises or torso extension
4. Both arms and legs reaching (superman)

The opposite arm and leg reach quadruped produces about one half of the spinal compression compared to the commonly used back extension machines that utilize both sides at one time.[37]

A common mistake for those with LBD or general health needs is training the erectors in a standing bent over position and holding heavy weight. While this technique strengthens the muscles maximally, it also stresses the posterior spine elements maximally.[58] The erector spinae have been shown to be most active while standing and flexed at the hips about ninety degrees.[99]

This position also places the maximum strain on the lumbosacral junctions compared to a bent knee squat[100], little or no weight should be repetitively lifted in this position.

Strategies

Extension exercises or movements are ideally done after flexion exercises (sit-ups) in order to protect the intervertebral disc[117], i.e. counterbalancing the posterior migration of the nucleus caused by flexion with anterior migration caused by extension.

Endurance is the goal over strength. *Endurance training of the back extensors is known to be crucial in preventing recurrent low back pain[97], as well as preventing first time occurrences.[98]* Studies have shown that *people with LBP have the same strength as the control group but significantly less endurance strength.[138]*

Five to ten second isometric holds followed by slow repetitions are great for strengthening the spinal erectors. Natural to faster speed repetitions are also needed to train the back for sudden movements and other activities, but they should not be the foundation of spinal strength. Lifting at high speeds can more than double the compression force on the spine.[129]

There are four main quadrants to back extension, upper left and right, and lower left and right. The more quadrants that are used during an exercise the greater the compressive load is on the spine. Therefore, segmental extensor contractions like the opposite arm and leg extensions, which utilize two quadrants, place smaller compressive loads on the spine than the double arm and leg "superman's", which utilize all four quadrants.

Relatively heavy extension exercises that isolate the erector spinae should be avoided for the average person because it is unnecessary and involves high compression forces. However, heavier squat like lifting techniques are more beneficial because they have a functional carryover that proves to prevent injuries during manual labor, (see proper lifting techniques below).

Hyperextending past neutral should also be avoided for most people, especially repeatedly, because of the higher compressive loads and non-functional results associated with it; an athlete who needs hyperextension is an exception.

Fig. 10-1 Hyperextension of lumbar the spine

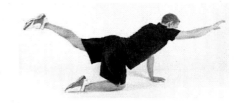

Athletes are often the exception and require exercises with greater loads and thus higher risks of injury. Very often this population needs explosive movements with rotation and or extension and flexion against resistance.

Wear and tear can be minimized by maintaining a safe ROM, enough recovery time in between workouts, and proper technique throughout the movements.

Stretching the Low Back

It has been shown that *increased spine ROM can increase the chance of future back problems[104,105]*, but keeping the spine relatively flexible is advisable, in fact, those with limited spinal mobility have higher than normal peak bending moments on the lumbar spine while those with more supple spines have lower than normal measurements.[134]

In other words, a more flexible spine, to a certain extent, leads to less spinal stress, although this does not mean that stretching an injured spine will improve the injury, by then it is too late, at least until the tissues are healed and ready.

Focused stretching of the lumbar spine is not desirable during low back post-rehabilitation unless the pathology is strictly muscular and tolerable to elongation stress. Stretching other areas of the body in order to balance tension and correct posture should be the focus of low back stretching during post-rehabilitation.

Those who have LBD should be educated about this because this population frequently tries to stretch their way out of pain by flexing and twisting the spine.

In general, stretching most parts of the body should be done with a neutral spine, especially with a low back injury.

Proprioception for the Low Back

Retraining the proprioceptive system of the spine after an injury or due to lack of conditioning is essential because it helps harmonize all the intersegmental movements of the vertabrae via the deep paraspinal muscles, LDF, and ligaments along the spine.

Manual therapy directly on these structures is ideal for fast recovery and proper alignment. See chapter 5 for more on proprioception training.

Proper Lifting Techniques

Because we walk less and sit more than ever before our legs and passive spine system (muscles, fascia, and ligaments) have become deconditioned along with an increase in spinal flexion. Bad habits and postures have predisposed the spine to problems that require preventative actions if health is a goal.

We must learn when and how to lift even the lightest of weights, as well as keep the spine in good enough condition to accomplish individual needs. For many people, proper technique must be learned and practiced as much as unlearning the bad habits of lifting. There are a number of different lifting techniques, and depending on the spine's condition and what's being lifted, some are better than others.

The golden rule in low back care for lifting is *moderation with variation*. Any one position is bad if it's held for a long time, repeated frequently, or too much weight is present. Proper lifting techniques are

just like proper sitting postures in that no one is best and *variations are needed to distribute the stresses* to different tissues instead of constantly loading the same areas.

The more lifting techniques a person knows the more options they have for protecting their low back before, during, and after it is injured.

Biomechanics

The degree of curvature in the lumbar spine during a lift is very important for the average person and most important for those with injuries. There is a 'danger zone' or 'critical point' in lifting that comes when the activated erector muscles relax and transfer the load to the passive system of the ligaments, fascia, and relaxed muscles (which were just previously contracted).

The range when the load is transferred from passive to active tissues or vice versa (the danger zone) depends on the weight of the load and is as follows;[109]

- *Heavy loads* – at about 25-35° of flexion the spinal erector muscles relax and the posterior passive system takes over the load.
- *Light loads* – at about 50-60° of flexion the spinal erector muscles relax and the posterior passive system takes over the load.

The danger zones are also in effect on the way back up from a lift, i.e. the muscles take over for the ligaments at the same range. These parts of a lift must be executed with great skill, otherwise the slightest bit of un-coordination can create failure and injury in the spine. The tensing of the T.A. and LDF is essential during this point of the lift in order to resist anterior shear forces.

It is commonly stated that the erector spinae muscles become relaxed or myoelectrically silent at a certain degree of flexion and then transfer the load to the passive system. Unfortunately it is not commonly mentioned that the muscles themselves become part of the passive system once they are relaxed. McGill and Kippers[110] demonstrated that the lumbar extensor muscles produce a substantial elastic force by way of stretch tension during full spine flexion. This is important if extreme muscle tension or stretch stress needs to be avoided.

A common error in lifting is to adhere to the lumbo-pelvic rhythm that is noted to involve only lumbar flexion for the first 60 degrees of torso flexion followed by flexion about the hips for the rest of the movement. According to McGill[37], "we have *never* measured this strict sequence in anyone. In fact, Olympic weightlifters attempt to do the opposite – they lock the lumbar spine close to the neutral position and rotate almost entirely about the hips."

This reinforces the findings which show that a moderately flexed[107] or neutral spine[108] is stronger than a fully flexed spine.

Choosing a Lifting Posture

Depending on the situation, *a kyphotic or lordotic* lifting posture will be best. A kyphotic posture can cause full lumbar flexion which will put more stress on the posterior disc, posterior ligamentous system, and posterior connective tissues, therefore resulting in more ligament sprains, fascia strains, and disc damage during a lift.

A lordotic posture is more stable because it locks the facet joints into place by using the erector muscles and thus does not allow dangerous shearing forces. It also tightens the strong anterior longitudinal ligament. This posture mainly uses muscle contractions for support and thus results in more muscle strains. A strain is preferable to a sprain because it heals faster and isn't likely to cause permanent instability at the involved joint like a sprain does.

Fig. 10-2 *Lifting techniques*

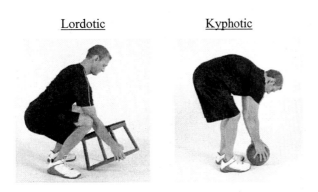

Lordotic   Kyphotic

When dealing with disc herniations or other intervertebral disc pathologies it is helpful to know that an applied compression force of 500N can be reduced by 40% in the nucleus when in a position of 4 degrees of extension, compared to a neutral position; this is due to the load bearing qualities of the adjacent vertebrae's neural arches.[135] Conversely, the pressure in the nucleus increases 100% in full flexion.[80]

Therefore, in general, someone with lumbar instability or injury is better off not flexing the spine much, if at all, and adopting a more lordotic posture, particularly when lifting, until health is attained. On the other hand, a relatively healthy spine should use both kyphotic and lordotic lifting postures to build overall

strength because if a kyphotic posture is rarely used then the ligamentous system will atrophy and not be strong enough to support the body during awkward situations (slips, falls, sudden movements, etc.). But, if a kyphotic technique is used frequently or at the wrong times it can create permanent damage in the lumbar spine.

See chapter 7 for descriptions on the many different lifting techniques.

Intra-Abdominal Pressure (IAP)

Increased IAP increases abdominal muscle activity, intradiscal pressure, and spine compression.[111,112]

Increased IAP causes an increase in low back EMG activity.[113]

IAP adds stability to the low back and protects against "buckling".[37]

Conscious elevation of IAP should only be done by those lifting extreme weights and is not appropriate in most rehabilitation programs.

For intense lifting it is important to take a full diaphragmatic breath in order to develop sufficient IAP.

The elevation of IAP should come naturally once proper lifting techniques are learned and should be in proportion to the load being lifted.

Lifting Guidelines

Always keep spine memory (pg. 94) in mind when lifting an object after a prolonged time of resting or sitting.

Choose a lifting technique by how much and often the weight needs to be lifted, as well as the condition of the spine.

Determine if and how much IAP is appropriate.

When lifting heavier loads, utilize the stability created from the pressurized abdominal cavity by slowly letting out the breath through tight lips as the load is lifted[212] (this will make an audible sound similar to loud blowing). If the breath is let out all at once, then so is stability, just watch a professional weight lifter and notice the sounds they make and when they make them.

Even with proper form repetitive lifting will eventually wear down the body. If lifting must be excessively repeated on a daily basis, a smarter lift should be used, i.e. a forklift, objects or devices that create leverage, two people, a pulley system, etc.

Mix up the techniques whenever appropriate to avoid repetitive overload and encourage uniform strengthening of the tissues.

Always try to align the body so the weight lifted is directly in front and close to the body, don't reach or twist unless it's unavoidable

Always tighten the abdominal muscles first and in proportion to the load being lifted in order to support the spine. If the abdominals activate too early, too late, too much, or too little, then the resultant stabilization force will be inadequate.[45,194]

Avoid lifting asymmetrical loads i.e. heavier on one side.

Lifting with a stomach full of food can be dangerous because of insufficient abdominal bracing.

Lifting with straight legs leaves less room for error because the spine's tolerance for compression is much greater than for shear forces[37], it also doesn't allow the gluteus maximus muscle to engage and contribute to the extension force and taughtness of the LDF.[50]

Co-contraction of the abdominals is agreed to increase stability of the trunk, unfortunately it also increases spinal compression by up to 45% during lifting techniques.[136] This explains why even proper lifting techniques can be painful for those with a herniated disc.

The proper lifting technique depends on:
1. The individual's capabilities
2. Type of injury
3. Object to be lifted

See Box 13-1 for contraindications for specific situations and injuries.

Summary

The past is a definitive clue to the spine's present situation. Once it has been seriously injured it will forever require special care, and odds are that LBP will reoccur randomly or regularly. The best form of special care is preventative maintenance in the form of corrective exercise, posture awareness, and knowledge of mechanical dos and don'ts.

Low back care comes down to a few things; good mechanics, endurance and stability in the CORE muscles, and a variety in lifestyle with moderation being the key. Without one the others are lacking. For example:

• Sitting in a chair with proper lumbar support and posture or working in a warehouse with perfect lifting technique for twenty years will still degenerate the spine because it is stressing the same tissues the same way over and over again. Solution: Use different sitting postures with frequent standing and walking breaks. Use different lifting techniques wherever possible and use objects or devices for leverage.

• Working a job that requires physical labor for a few hours but the muscles only have the endurance to last for one hour due to inadequate training and nutrition will cause failure and injury to the joints and muscles. Solution: Appropriate training and nutrition.

• Sitting at a desk or driving for an extended time then having to stand up and immediately pick up a heavy object can cause disc protrusions because of the increase pressure in the disc from sitting and instability from lax ligaments. Solution: Stand up and extend the spine and walk around for a few minutes.

Unfortunately many jobs demand these types of situations so it is the spine's fate to suffer from accelerated degeneration until management empathizes with the needs of the body. Until then, the best way to combat the stresses of daily living is by understanding how the spine works and incorporating healthful ways whenever and wherever possible.

Chapter 11   Anatomy & Injury Mechanisms of the Low Back

Understanding the low back starts with the knowledge of its structure, function, and then mechanisms of injury. This chapter deals with structure, function, and the injury mechanisms plus other helpful hints regarding the low back and exercise.

The muscles and structures described in this chapter are, in the author's opinion, the most essential to identifying the causes of and designing exercise and treatment programs for LBD.

Motion Segments of the Spine

The spine can be broken down into five sections; 1) cervical 2) thoracic 3) lumbar 4) sacral 5) coccyx, each with their own tendencies and structural variations. Within these sections there are segments that are intimately related by movement and function; the lumbar and cervical regions are also directly related to one another regarding movement or lack there of. The joining segments are called the functional spinal unit (FSU) and three joint complex (3-Jt. complex), see fig.'s 11-1, 11-2, and Box 11-1.

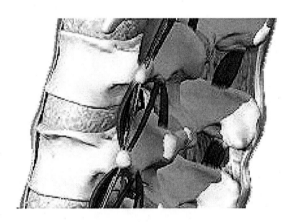

Fig. 11-2   The functional spinal unit (FSU) consists of 1) two adjacent vertebrae 2) disc in between 3) all of the connecting ligaments 4) connecting soft tissue and muscles. The FSU, along with the 3-Jt complex, paint a detailed picture of a person's history and show essential dysfunctions that occur during movement.

The FSU, also known as the motion segment, consists of two adjacent vertebrae with the disc in-between, ligaments, and soft tissue that connect them.[40] The 3-Jt. complex consists of the disc and two facet joints.[40] An injury in any of the units, i.e. nucleus, annulus, endplates, facets, ligaments, or soft tissue of one FSU will influence nearby joint mechanics and eventually spread its effects over an entire spinal region.[40,92] How each is affected is explained in detail in the following sections and in the injury mechanisms section on pg. 92.

The Intervertebral Disc

- Nucleus
- Annulus Fibrosis

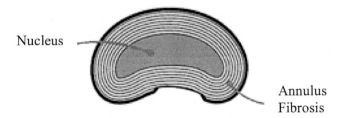

Nucleus

Annulus Fibrosis

Fig. 11-3   The disc consists of a phlegm-like nucleus surrounded by the dynamic fibrous layers of the annulus. Seen from the top.

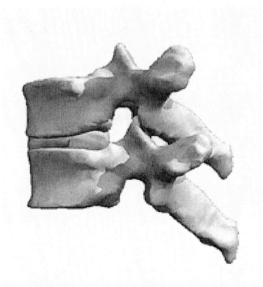

Fig. 11-1   The 3-Jt complex consists of two adjacent vertebrae and the disc in-between.

Degenerative Phases of the 3-Joint Complex

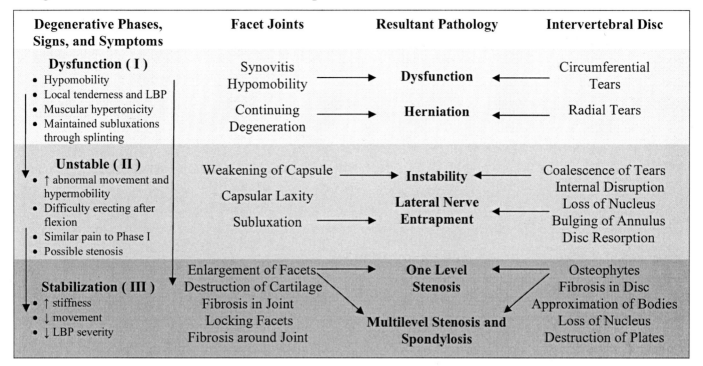

Degenerative Phases, Signs, and Symptoms	Facet Joints	Resultant Pathology	Intervertebral Disc
Dysfunction (I) • Hypomobility • Local tenderness and LBP • Muscular hypertonicity • Maintained subluxations through splinting	Synovitis Hypomobility Continuing Degeneration	**Dysfunction** **Herniation**	Circumferential Tears Radial Tears
Unstable (II) • ↑ abnormal movement and hypermobility • Difficulty erecting after flexion • Similar pain to Phase I • Possible stenosis	Weakening of Capsule Capsular Laxity Subluxation	**Instability** **Lateral Nerve Entrapment**	Coalescence of Tears Internal Disruption Loss of Nucleus Bulging of Annulus Disc Resorption
Stabilization (III) • ↑ stiffness • ↓ movement • ↓ LBP severity	Enlargement of Facets Destruction of Cartilage Fibrosis in Joint Locking Facets Fibrosis around Joint	**One Level Stenosis** **Multilevel Stenosis and Spondylosis**	Osteophytes Fibrosis in Disc Approximation of Bodies Loss of Nucleus Destruction of Plates

Box 11-1. This box contains the degenerative changes of the 3-joint complex and the relationship between the facet joints and discs. The two arrows on the left pointing down signify the progression of degeneration. The single longer arrow also represents a progression of degeneration which involves skipping directly to Phase III from Phase I, although it is not quite understood why Phase II is not experienced. It is also possible to go back to Phase I from phase II if proper healing takes place. Modified from Kirkaldy-Willis.[213]

The disc has two main parts, a center, or nucleus, and a layered circumference called the annulus fibrosis. The disc shares the duty of resisting forces placed on the spine with the vertebral endplates, facet joints, ligaments, and conjoining soft tissues. The *discs are not the primary shock absorbers of the spine*, rather the vertebrae and end plates are[37,39], it is because the vertebrae are filled with blood and bone marrow that they are likely to act as shock absorbers.[84]

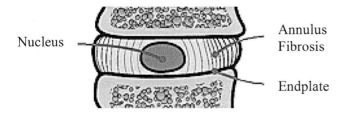

Fig. 11-4 Although it appears like the disc would be a primary shock absorber, it is mostly involved with resisting bending and twisting forces.

Nucleus

The nucleus is gel like and surrounded side to side by

the annulus and top to bottom by the vertebral bodies and their end-plates. It sits in the posterior center of the disc and acts like a marble between two planes (the vertebrae), meaning it shifts slightly when the vertebrae are moving[89]; this is how it oozes out and compresses the spinal cord or its nerves if the annulus is deformed enough. This leaking of the nucleus reduces disc height and resilience which alters the mechanics of the motion segments and thus accelerates degeneration throughout the FSU.

During flexion the nucleus slides posteriorly[37,40,89] while the annulus bulges anteriorly[40], the former is the most common direction for the nucleus to herniate. In general, the younger the nucleus the more liquid and pressure it contains, making it more vulnerable to herniations and heavy lifting[40,80,84], likewise, the amount of nucleus fluid decreases with age and or degeneration.[80]

Fluids and nutrition pass to and from the disc via the vertebral end plates[37,39,40,84] and segmental branches of the aorta, which are attached to the annulus[80,84], until adulthood where the nucleus has no blood or nerve supply.[40] At this point only the outer part of the disc can heal from injuries.

Prolonged inactivity is detrimental to the influx of

nutrients to the disc.[39,40,84] When referring to the nucleus, Buckwalter[86] states that "no other musculoskeletal soft tissue structure undergoes more dramatic alterations with age".

Annulus Fibrosis
(Fig.'s 11-3, 11-4, &11-5)

The annulus fibrosis is made up of approximately 15-25 distinct layers called lamella, with the number of layers varying depending on the spine level, circumferential location, and age of the individuall.[87] Only every other lamella can resist torsion (twisting) in a given direction due to their fiber arrangement, the other half are made to resist in the opposite direction.[37,39,40,84]

The annular fibers elongate in response to shear, rotation, compression, and flexion-extension; rotation forces cause more elongation than compression, flexion-extension, or both combined, but maximum elongation results from combining compression, rotation, and shear.[39]

Annular fibers are similar to ligaments in the sense that they will become permanently elongated if excessive tension is placed on them[39] and they connect adjacent vertebrae while restricting their excessive motion.[4] According to Cailliet[39], "The annular fibers are the key to the integrity of the intervertebral disc", they are also extremely vulnerable to axial rotation[40], with the innermost fibers usually tearing first because they are shorter.[39]

The annulus degenerates from recurrent strains that initially cause a number of small circumferential tears which weaken the disc and facilitate repetitive injury, eventually growing larger and merging together to form radial tears that reach the nucleus; once radial tears are present, relatively minor traumas can cause a localized disc herniation.[84] Bogduk and Twomey[82] hypothesized the possibility of an annular sprain in the outer layers (when placed under excessive torsion) that is similar to an ankle sprain of the ligaments.

The outer annulus communicates with pain receptors[80,137] and receives blood from the segmental arteries[80,84,137], so any damage to the outer annulus can cause pain and retard the healing process of the disc. The nucleus and annulus function as a unit, as do the facet joints and disc of a 3-Jt. complex, therefore dysfunction in one will lead to the breakdown of the other.

The following are a few deformations that can occur to the nucleus and annulus fibrosis, based on descriptions by Pate.[170] These terms are often misused and confused, but the focus here should be the different results and consequences of disc injury, not the name of each problem.

Disc Bulge – radial tears in annulus allow increased disc volume (centrally or laterally)

Disc Herniation or Protrusion – nuclear matter protrudes into the radial tears displacing surrounding structures, i.e. nerves, but does not escape the annulus (subligamentous)

Extruded Disc – a non-contained disc that has herniated past the posterior longitudinal ligament (transligamentous)

Sequestered Disc – a progressed extrusion, the herniated disc material no longer is connected to the disc, it can now migrate within the canal and become a free fragment

Fig. 11-5 Disc Pathologies – Discs can bulge or protrude in any direction, including posteriolaterally (A.), up into the end plates (B.),and posteriorly (C.). B. requires a fracturing or eroding of the end plates, as opposed to tears in the annulus like A. and C.

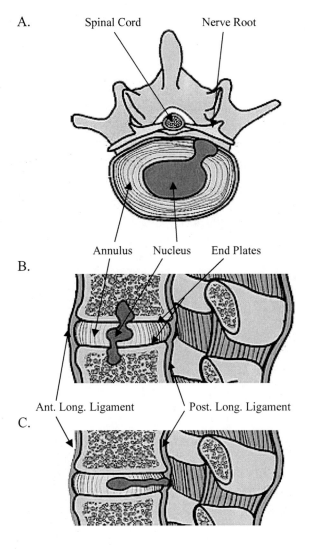

A.   Spinal Cord   Nerve Root

Annulus   Nucleus   End Plates
B.

Ant. Long. Ligament   Post. Long. Ligament
C.

The Facet Joints

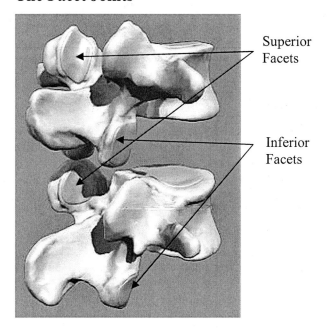

Fig. 11-6 There are two superior and inferior facets per vertebrae. All of which are responsible for resisting torsion and providing proprioceptive feedback to spinal stabilization reflexes.

The facets are posterior articulations (synovial joints) of the vertebrae that connect the adjacent vertebrae above and below and contain a meniscuslike structure that according to Cailliet[39] is "well innervated with proprioceptive nerve endings and nocioceptor fibers thus they function for position sense and as a site of pain". Facet pain can actually be referred into the lateral hip and buttocks, as well as into the anterior upper thigh.[93] The pain referred is most often downward, and hardly ever upward.[44]

Facet joints are extremely important in resisting torsion (about 40% of total torsional resistance) and shear forces (although not much resistance is given to posterior shear forces[40]), as well as approximately 25% of an axial compression load.[84]

The facet is the first structure to incur a twisting (torsion) failure due to its mechanical barrier to rotation, which is well before the elastic limit of the disc.[83] This mechanical barrier is much better at resisting torsion in the upper lumbar vertebrae than in the lower, which are better suited for resisting the anterior shear forces that concentrate in this area, especially L5-S1.[40]

L4-L5 is the main region affected by rotational strains because of their facet configuration and the strongly reinforced L5-S1 joint via ligaments and bone[84], thereby leaving the L4-L5 segment hypermobile in comparison. While they can resist torsion forces in an upright position, the facet joints separate during flexion and thus pass on the duties of resisting excessive rotation forces to the posterior annular fibers.[39]

The function and health of the facet joints and intervertebral disc are strongly connected, dysfunction in one leads to dysfunction in the other, in fact, Kirkaldy-Willis[84] states that "nearly every case of disc herniation is accompanied by a pathologic lesion in the facet joints" while Farfan[91] suggests that gross injuries of the facet joints do not occur when the intervertebral disc is normal.

Other relationships are mentioned by Cailliet[39] that propose facet dysfunctions can create hypermobility which leads to increased degeneration in the 3-Jt. complex, spondylolisthesis, and annular tears.

The Ligaments

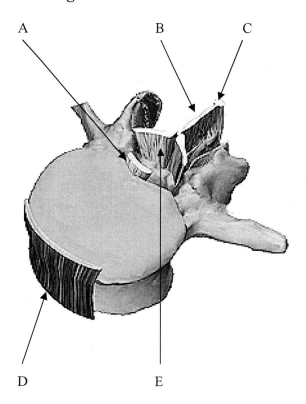

Fig. 11-7 Top view of a vertebrae with ligaments cut and exposed.

The following ligaments are the most influential to the low back. See Fig. 11-8 for the sacro-iliac, tuberous, and spinous ligaments.

- Anterior longitudinal (D)
- Posterior longitudinal (A)
- Ligamentum Flavum (E)
- Intertransverse
- Interspinous (B)
- Supraspinous (C)
- Iliolumbar
- Sacroiliac
- Sacrotuberous
- Sacrospinous

Fig. 11-8 - Sacral Ligaments

A. Posterior superficial view. B. Posterior deep view C. Anterior view

A.   *B.*

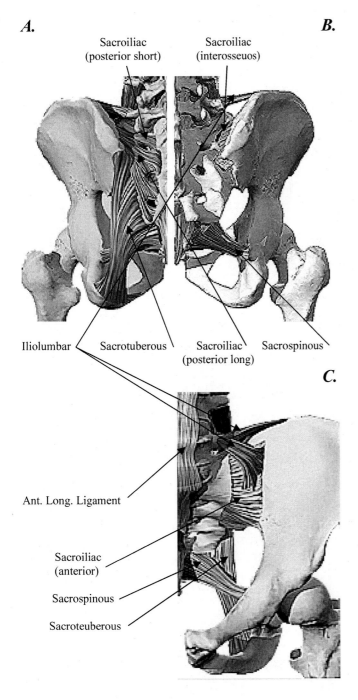

Sacroiliac (posterior short)   Sacroiliac (interosseuos)

Iliolumbar   Sacrotuberous   Sacroiliac (posterior long)   Sacrospinous

C.

Ant. Long. Ligament

Sacroiliac (anterior)

Sacrospinous

Sacroteuberous

original structure.[40]

Repetitive loading can cause fatigue and failure to the ligaments[84], which will most likely cause injuries elsewhere in the 3-Jt. complex, but the ligaments seem to be injured themselves more by traumatic events when the spine is at its end ROM as opposed to regular daily errors in movement.[37]

Spinal ligaments are thought to have proprioreceptive functions[88], and due to the longer healing time of ligaments (see appendix) could be a reason for prolonged recovery of spine coordination after certain injuries.

Anterior Longitudinal Ligament (ALL)

Attachments

A wide, strong band of fibers that traverses along the anterior surface of the vertebral bodies from the 2nd cervical vertebrae to the sacrum. It consists of multiple layers of fibers, with the most superficial being the longest and spanning 4-5 vertebrae, the middle layer 2-3 vertebrae, and the deepest layer only 2 vertebrae.

Functions

• Resists excessive extension forces
• Serves as attachment site for tendinous fibers of the crura of the diaphragm (L1-L3)

Posterior Longitudinal Ligament (PLL)

Attachments

A wide, strong band of fibers situated within the spinal canal that traverses along the posterior surface of the vertebral bodies from the 2nd cervical vertebrae to the sacrum. It consists of two layers of fibers, with the most superficial spanning 3-4 vertebrae and the deep layer only 2 vertebrae.

Functions

• Resists excessive flexion forces
• Is the last barrier between herniated disc material and the spinal cord

Ligamentum Flavum

Attachments

Posterior to the spinal cord, this highly elastic ligament connects adjacent vertebral laminae and makes up the anterior capsule of the facet joint.

The spinal ligaments allow movement in the joint until they reach the end of their elastic range, which corresponds with the end ROM of the spine, where they immediately resist the force of injurious situations. Ligaments regain their normal length when stretched within their limit, but excessive stretching will cause some permanent deformation, called plastic deformation, leaving it longer and weaker than the

Functions

- Resists excessive flexion forces
- The elasticity allows the ligament to contribute tension upon returning to an upright position from one that was flexed
- Acts as a lateral barrier to matter that could otherwise penetrate the spinal cord

Intertransverse Ligament

Attachments

Connects one transverse process to the next.

Functions

- Resists excessive flexion forces
- They act more like a connective tissue membrane that separates the lumbar anterior muscles from the posterior

Interspinous Ligament

Attachments

Oblique fibers that connect adjacent vertebral spinous processes and merges with the supraspinous ligament.

Functions

- Resists posterior shear of superior vertebrae
- Creates anterior shear forces in full flexion due to its obliquity
- Controls rotation of vertebrae during flexion, thereby helping the facet joints maintain proper alignment
- Provide proprioceptive feedback

Supraspinous Ligament

Attachments

Vertical fibers that connect the tips of adjacent spinous processes.

Functions

- Resists excessive flexion forces
- Provide proprioceptive feedback

Iliolumbar Ligament

Attachments

Bands of fibers crossing directly in front of the S.I. joint and connecting each transverse process of L5 to the ipsilateral ilium; some fibers arise from Q.L. fascia and the anterior sacroiliac ligament.

Functions

- Is more muscle tissue in infants, then ligamentous as an adult, and eventually degenerates into fatty tissue later in life
- Resist anterior migration of L5 over the sacrum
- Stabilizes L5 on the sacrum against virtually all motions; the lumbosacral joint is an area of concentrated stress in the spine because it is at the foundation, which is evident by the large size of the L5 transverse processes
- Can refer pain to anterior medial thigh and inguinal area[38]

Sacroiliac Ligaments

Attachments

- Interosseous (strongest)
- Posterior (short/long)
- Anterior

There are three distinct fiber arrangements of the sacroiliac ligament(s). Included are deep and superficial layers with anterior and posterior connections. Many of the sacral nerves are held within the sacroiliac ligaments, which connect all around the sacrum and nearby ilium. Anteriorly and posteriorly, some fibers merge with the LDF and surrounding myofascia.

Laterally they are continuous with the sacrotuberous ligament and medially with the posterior lamina of the thoracolumbar fascia.

Functions

- Stabilize the S.I. joint (all)
- Resists (very strongly) downward motion of the sacrum with respect to the ilium (long posterior fibers)
- Resists anterior motion of the top of the sacrum (short posterior fibers)
- It is the main connection between the ilium and sacrum (interosseuos fibers)

Sacrotuberous Ligament

Attachments

Lateral band – Spans from PSIS to ischial tuberosity

Medial Band – From the coccygeal vertebrae to the ischial tuberosity

Central Band – Connect the lateral band to the lateral sacral crest

Superior Band – From the PSIS to the coccygeal vertebrae

The saccrotuberous ligament also blends together with the biceps femoris and sacral fascia, making it a part of the superficial back and spiral myofascial line.

Functions

- Stabilizes sacrum against excessive nutation (superior border of sacrum rotates anteriorly)
- Is a major anchor point for the posterior myofascial system involved with resisting forward flexion forces
- Can refer pain down the entire posterior leg, lower buttocks, heel, and lateral thigh[38]

Sacrospinous Ligament

Attachments

Blending medially with and lying directly beneath the sacrotuberous ligament, it is attached to the anterior portion of the lower sacrum and upper section of the coccygeal area. From there it converges onto the ischial spine.

The sacrospinous ligament also lies directly posterior to the coccygeus muscle and can cause referred pain patterns down into posterior buttocks and leg.[4]

Functions

- Assist the sacrotuberous ligament

Low Back Injury Mechanisms

If you haven't had low back pain (LBP) before, just wait a while and you probably will. Most of the general population (60-80%) will experience LBP at least once in their life[41] and many will have no idea what caused it, including their doctors. Unfortunately, up to 85% of low back disorders (LBD) are of unknown etiology.[37,81]

Around 85-95% of the LBP population will recover within 6 weeks, although recurrences are common, while the non-improved individuals (5-15%) are unresponsive to treatment and maintain their disability[41], ultimately being labeled as chronic. It is not too far-fetched to label many LBP sufferers as acute-chronic if the incidence of recurrence is taken into account, which is often as high as 70-75%[232,233], along with the fact that numerous LBP specialists have concluded that the best predictor of future LBP is a history of LBP.[226-231]

The point to make here is that it is often helpful to see the big picture (chronic) instead of viewing repetitive acute episodes as simply "acute".

What starts the pain is often a mystery, one reason is because it can take a couple of days after an injury to a disc for it to maximally swell and cause pain.[37] Sometimes it's from too much yard or house work, too much sitting or standing, too much or too little activity, or sometimes it just appears upon waking up.

How could this happen? Nothing unusual occurred, no accidents or traumatic injuries, and yet it is impossible to bend over and tie shoe laces the next day. This is how it can happen.

There are certain patterns of movement and posture that the spine should follow in order to function properly, and for some reason the body doesn't always intuitively know these ways, or due to pain and limitations has compensated with unhealthy habits.

Like any part of the body, the spine is susceptible to genetic and developmental misfortunes that can cause many difficulties, some of which are very similar to the consequences of bad posture, incorrect movements, repetitive use, and age.

Usually problems are not caused by one incident[84], although the start of pain can sometimes be traced back to one event, it is rather the accumulation of factors over time (Table 11-1) that lead to the breakdown of tissues until that unfortunate day when failure occurs somewhere in the joint and pain is finally perceived. *Pain is very tricky in that it is usually the last symptom to come but the first to go, so great care needs be taken after an injury is pain free because it still needs time to heal.*

Movement

The single most dangerous position for the lumbar spine comes when it is fully flexed, from here a combination of factors will increase its vulnerability, such as rotation, lateral flexion, repetitious bending, quick movements, being startled, and adding compression loads.

Repeatedly flexing the spine with minimal *or* substantial compression loads consistently produced disc herniations in a spine model[37] while lifting and rotating to one side is agreed to increase spinal compression[80] and the bending moment on the lumbar spine (up to 30%)[119] compared to straight forward lifting. It has also been shown that lifting quickly or while startled will increase spinal compression by 60%[129] and 30-70%[130] respectively.

TABLE 11-1. Detrimental Factors and their Consequences

Factors	Consequences
1. Aging	1. Less fluid in disc leaves less space between vertebrae and a greater chance of nerve compression[80] 2. Decreased blood flow and healing ability[40] 3. Increased scar tissue and joint stiffness, and thus increased chance of re-injury
2. Prolonged bed rest (greater than 8 hours)	1. Swollen discs from increased fluid[85] 2. Increased pressure and stress on three joint complex[85] 3. Three joint complex is vulnerable to activity soon after rising[85]
3. Prolonged Sitting with Vibration (truck driver)	1. Similar to regular sitting but more severe 2. Higher rates of LBD[215,218] 3. Swollen discs are likely 4. Deconditioning of weightbearing muscles due to inactivity
4. Cumulative hyperextension and full flexion patterns (gymnast)	1. Facet joint injury and degeneration 2. Pars injury and fractures, eventually spondylolisthesis[37] 3. Eventually leads to disc disease
5. Repetitive heavy lifting with large trunk motions for many years (warehouse worker)	1. Accelerated arthritic changes in the three joint complex 2. Increased risk of degenerative joint and disc disease 3. Stenosis[217]
6. Repeatedly bending or twisting the spine (even with minimal load)	1. Higher rates of LBD[37,219-223] 2. Intervertebral disc injury[37]
7. Bending to pick up an object while fully flexing the spine and twisting and side bending	1. Increased intradiscal pressure 2. Posterior disc herniation[224,225] 3. Posterolateral annual tears 4. Posterior spine ligament and connective tissue sprains
8. Repetitive exposure to unchanging work	1. Higher rates of LBP[216] 2. Intervertebral disc injury[217]
9. Prolonged standing or crouching while bending forward (roofer or gardener)	1. Excessive loading of the passive tissues due to muscle lengthening and inactivity 2. Increased laxity in passive tissues and soft tissue strains[37] 3. Decreased stability in three joint complex[37] 4. Laxity/instability remains for quite sometime[37] 5. Increased shear forces on vertebrae[37] 6. Increased posterior disc stress[37] 7. Progressive decrease in passive tissue strength[37] 8. Increased chance of disc herniation[37]
10. Prolonged Sitting (slouching w/out a Lumbar Support)	1. Increased intradiscal pressure compared to standing[214] 2. Increased posterior disc stress[37] 3. Increased laxity in passive tissues for a while after sitting[37] 4. Decreased stability in three joint complex after sitting[37] 5. Increased chance of disc herniation[215] 6. Deconditioning of weightbearing muscles due to inactivity

McGill[37] has shown that when bending forward, full lumbar flexion produces similar compressive forces to a more neutral spine (3145N and 3490N respectively), but the shear forces, which are more dangerous, were more than three times higher in the fully flexed position (954N vs. 269N).

This large difference is explained by the unrestricted *anterior* shear forces in the flexed position and the *posterior* shear forces created by the muscles and fascia during the neutral position that oppose the anterior shear force produced by the weight of the torso hanging over the hips.

In addition to the above risks, disc-bending stresses are estimated to increase by 300% and ligament stresses in the neural arch by 80% in the morning compared to later in the day due to the increased fluid in the disc from lying down[85], which therefore creates a greater risk of injury to the disc from forward bending stretches or lifting movements at that time of day. However, most of the effects of the increased water content are minimized after one hour.[131,132]

Torsion

Twisting imposes approximately four times the compression on the spine as an equal torque of flexion and extension, making it more vulnerable to rotation than flexion and extension.[37] When the spinal segments are challenged with torsional forces in the laboratory, fissures are produced in the annulus in the same posteriolateral location that is a common site for disc heriations; these fissures may or may not be in conjunction with nuclear matter leaking into them.[84]

Compression

Excessive compression on a neutral spine is known to fracture vertebral endplates before tearing annular fibers or herniating discs.[37,39,40,84] Without a major trauma it seems impossible for the nucleus to leak out of a healthy annulus fibrosis; instead of one incident it takes many to break down the three joint complex and cause problems (Table 11-1).

Heavy lifting at a young age can cause Schmorl's nodes which damage the vertebral end plates and start an early degeneration process.[40]

Shear

Shear is the horizontal translation between the disc and vertebrae which is always present in the natural lordosis of the lumbar spine and increases as flexion increases. It is resisted by the annulus and facets joints[39,40], as well as the posterior spinous ligaments[39], spinal erectors (when activated to form a neutral lordosis[37]), and lumbar dorsal fascia (when activated through the transverse abdominus and internal oblique[40]). The psoas muscle can actually increase anterior shear forces when it is activated, this is not good.

The spine has a much lower tolerance for shear forces than for compression forces[37], and thus it is easier to succumb to shear injuries than compression injuries, especially in fully flexed positions. Studies show that injuries sustained from high load anterior shear forces are in the form of pars and facet fractures which lead to spondylolisthesis, while lower load forces result in unidentifiable soft tissue damage.[94,95,96]

Fatigue

Fatigue plays a large roll in spine injuries by causing improper motion segment mechanics once muscular and intervertebral disc or ligament strength fail. The annulus itself can fail when fully flexing the spine repeatedly or for a prolonged time thereby weakening the 3-Jt. complex and leading to herniations.[37]

Ligaments will also fail from repetitive loading[84] and cause instability throughout the FSU which can lead to damage almost anywhere in the FSU depending on the activity. Multiple injuries to the 3-Jt. complex will build up scar tissue that stiffens the joint and alter FSU mechanics, leaving it vulnerable to re-injury and further degeneration.

Spine Memory

Different positions create different lengths, tensions, and pressures in the tissues of the spine. Time is needed for the ligament tensions and disc pressures to stabilize and return to normal after prolonged positions are changed.

When the spine is flexed the nucleus will migrate posteriorly in the annulus[37,40,89], thus creating a dangerous lifting posture if not allowed to slide back into proper position with some standing or extension exercises. Twenty minutes of sitting in a slouched position, fully flexed, resulted in a loss of intervertebral joint stiffness by fifty percent two minutes post slouching, some laxity was still present after thirty minutes of rest.[90]

Another study showed that just five minutes of sitting or standing in a flexed position (simulated in-vitro) reduced the ability of the intervertebral ligaments to protect the disc when bending by 40%.[133] This is important when dealing with truck drivers, athletes on the bench, gardeners, etc.

The Muscles

The muscles listed in this chapter are those which are most commonly involved with a LBD. Some, such as the adductors and gastrocsoleus complex have many more functions regarding other areas of the body, but because the focus here is on the low back, their descriptions will be limited to low back related facts.

Other influential muscles, such as the ones implicated in an upper crossed syndrome, will not be mentioned here because they are already adequately touched on (as far as the low back is concerned) in chapters 12 and 13.

Influential Muscles of LBD

These muscles or areas are the most essential for understanding LBD's.

- Abdominals
- Iliopsoas
- Hip adductors
- Posterior myofascia
- Latissimus dorsi
- Q.L.
- Paraspinal muscles
- Gluteus maximus
- Piriformis
- TFL/IT band
- Gluteus medius and minimus
- Hamstrings
- Gastrocsoleus complex

Note that in this chapter some innervations are followed by a number in parenthesis, (#), this indicates that the muscle is *sometimes* innervated by the segment in parenthesis, depending on which reference is used.

Muscle Abbreviations

A.L. - adductor longus
A.M. - adductor magnus
B.F. – biceps femoris
E.O. – external oblique
Gmax -gluteus maximus
Gmed – gluteus medius
Gmin – gluteus minimus
G.N. - gastrocnemius
I.C.L. – iliocostalis lumbothoracis
I.L. – iliacus
I.O. – internal oblique
I.V.M. – intervertebral muscles
Lats – latissimus dorsi
LDF – lumbar dorsal fascia

L.L. – longissimus lumbothoracis
L.T. – longissimus thoracis
M.H. – medial hamstrings
Mult - multifidus
Pect – pectineus
Piri - piriformis
P.S. – psoas
Q.L. – quadratus lumborum
R.A. – rectus abdominis
Sol – soleus
T.A. – transverse abdominis
TFL – tensor fascia lata

See glossary for other less used abbreviations. These are of course what work best for the author. It is recommended to use whichever abbreviations are easy to remember for each professional. They are a must for assessment note taking.

Origin/Insertion

The term *origin* denotes an area where the muscle attaches that is mostly stationary during a contraction, while *insertion* refers to the attachment site that moves towards the origin during a concentric contraction of the muscle. These points of reference can sometimes be switched to create a different movement, for example, with the pelvis fixed (the origin), a rectus abdominis contraction will cause the trunk to flex about the pelvis (a sit-up), but with the trunk fixed it will cause the pelvis to flex towards the trunk (a reverse crunch).

When describing muscle actions in this chapter, the letters I/O (insertion/origin) will describe actions that do not result from the most common origin-insertion type movement.

Functional and Dysfunctional Groups

Every major muscle has a group of muscles that is functionally and dysfunctionally related to it. The functional group is related solely by function while the dysfunctional group is similar but related by function, referred pain patterns, and the ability to cause compensation in the muscle, no matter how distant its location is.

When considering a muscle's individual involvement in a kinetic chain dysfunction, both of these groups should be assessed for primary or secondary involvement in order to find the root of the problem and encourage its complete recovery.

Corrective Actions

The corrective actions following each muscle are the most common and useful, there are of course exceptions. Sometimes an acute situation can be corrected by simply eliminating the contributing bad habits, but other times (chronic cases, severe imbalances, etc.) specific exercises that aim to balance the kinetic chain are necessary.

The lists of muscle, fascia, and ligament attachments, innervations, functional groups, and functions throughout this chapter are a compilation from various authors, all of whom have made brilliant contributions and incites about the human body and function that are the foundation of this chapter.

Thank you; Travell and Simmons[7,8], Stuart McGill[37], Kendall and McCreary[49], Richardson C A,

Hodges P, and Hides J[138], Chaitow and DeLany[4], Vasilyeva and Lewit[55], Hislop and Montgomery[53], Bogduk[137], Thomas Myers[63], and Henry Gray[54] for your influence on this chapter.

Pain Patterns

The following pain patterns can be broken down into even more exact areas of referral, but have been adapted as follows.

The muscular referred pain patterns are as described by Travell and Simmons[7,8] and caused by trigger points.

The facets referred pain is described by McCall, Park, and Obrien[93], and ligament pain by Vleeming et al[38]

Sciatica is the referred pain pattern from an irritated or "pinched" sciatic nerve, as described by Cox.[234]

History → Program Design

General Symptoms → Program Design

Pain Patterns → Program Design

Physical Assessment → Program Design

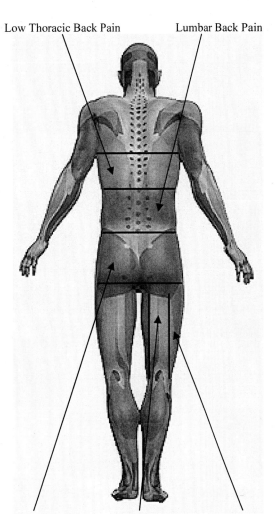

Low Thoracic Back Pain   Lumbar Back Pain

Sacral & Buttock Pain   Posterior Thigh Pain   Lateral Thigh Pain

Low Thoracic Back Pain

- Iliocostalis thoracis
- Multifidus
- Serratus posterior inferior
- Rectus abdomins
- Intercostals
- Latissimus dorsi
- Iliopsoas
- Local pathology

Sacral & Buttock Pain

- Longissimus lumbothoracis
- Multifidus
- Iliocostalis lumbothoracis
- Gluteus medius
- Gluteus mimumus
- Gluteus maximus
- Q.L.
- Piriformis
- Soleus

Posterior Thigh Pain

- Hamstrings
- Gluteus minimus
- Piriformis
- Obturator internus
- Sacrotuberous ligament
- Sacrospinous ligament
- Local pathology

Lumbar Back Pain

- Longissimus lumbothoracis
- Multifidus
- Rectus abdomins
- Iliocostalis lumbothoracis
- Iliocostalis thoracis
- Gluteus medius
- Iliopsoas
- Local pathology

- Obturator internus
- Semimembranosus
- Semitendinosus
- Rectus abdominis
- Pelvic floor muscles
- Sacrotuberous ligament
- Sacrospinous ligament
- Lumbar facet pathology
- Sciatica
- Local pathology

Lateral Thigh Pain

- Gluteus mimumus
- Gluteus maximus
- Vastus lateralis
- Piriformis
- Q.L.
- TFL
- Sacrotuberous ligament
- Sciatica
- Local pathology

Anatomy Groups for the Low Back

Lumbar Stabilizers	INDIRECTLY
1. Erector spinae	Dorsal rami of spinal nerves
2. External oblique	T5-T12
3. Rectus abdominis	T5-T12
4. Gluteus maximus	L5-S2
5. Pelvic floor muscles	S2-S4

Lumbar Stabilizers	DIRECTLY
1. Diaphragm	C4 (phrenic)
2. Deep paraspinals	Segmental spinal nerves
3. Latissimus dorsi	Thoracodorsal nerve, C6-C8
4. Psoas major posterior fascices	L1-L4
5. Transverse abdominis	T7-L1
6. Internal oblique	T7-L1
7. Q.L. medial fibers	T12-L3 (L4)

➢ The spinal ligaments and natural pressure from the disc also help to stabilize the low back

Posterior Shear Force	LUMBAR SPINE
1. Erector spinae fascicles	Dorsal rami of spinal nerves
2. Latissimus dorsi	Thoracodorsal nerve, C6-C8
3. Internal oblique	T7-L1
4. Transvers abdominis	T7-L1
5. Multifidus	Segmental spinal nerves

Force Closure of S.I. Joint	STANDING
1. Transverse abdominis	T7-L1
2. Piriformis	L5-S2
3. Coccygeus muscles	L5-S5

Force Closure of S.I. Joint	DURING GAIT
1. Latissimus dorsi	Thoracodorsal nerve, C6-C8
2. Transverse abdominis	T7-L1
3. Gluteus maximus (P)	L5-S2
4. Biceps femoris	L5-S3
5. Erector spinae	Dorsal rami of spinal nerves

The Abdominal Muscles

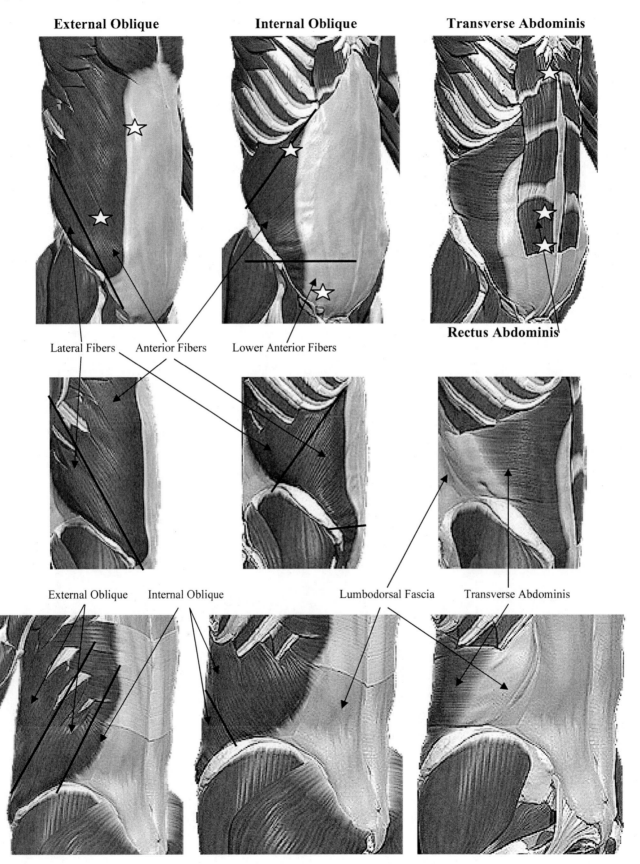

External Oblique

Internal Oblique

Transverse Abdominis

Rectus Abdominis

Lateral Fibers   Anterior Fibers   Lower Anterior Fibers

External Oblique   Internal Oblique   Lumbodorsal Fascia   Transverse Abdominis

Layers of the Abdominal Wall
1. Superficial – Rectus Abdominis (R.A.) 2. 2nd Layer – External Oblique (E.O.) 3. 3rd Layer – Internal Oblique (I.O.) 4. Deep – Transverse Abdominis (T.A.)

The abdominals connect the anterior torso to the posterior and are built to stabilize the spine against small and large forces from all directions as well as mobilize it about the pelvis during flexion, rotation, and side bending. Any movement in the body that places stress on the spine should be *initiated* with an appropriate abdominal contraction that is in proportion to the force required to stabilize the spine. This is an ideal recruitment pattern that has been seen in many tests which observe the CORE muscles in response to random and organized movements.

As described in chapter one, the transverse abdominis and posterior fibers of the internal oblique are part of an inner unit that the CNS activates prior to predictable imposed demands on the spine, while the rest of the abdominals are activated soon after to provide a more global stabilizing effect. Each layer has unique duties and is required to activate in harmony with the others in order to efficiently stabilize and mobilize the spine.

For instance, if during push-ups or squats the rectus abdominins is first to activate, then the abdominal cavity will not be properly pressurized and stability will be poor. However, if only the transverse abdominis contracted during a heavy lift, the spine would buckle.

It is essential for low back health to learn how to contract the abdominals for a variety of daily activities. This can be a long and arduous process if compensation patterns have been engrained into the neuromuscular system via chronic pain or poor posture, but it is still possible through practice and education.

Although not mentioned below, all of the abdominal muscles contribute to supporting and compressing the abdominal contents and assisting in respiration, especially forced respiration.

Rectus Abdominis

Muscle Type – Hyperactive/Mobilizer

Attachments

Origin – Pubic symphysis and crest of pubis

Insertion – Costal cartilages of ribs 5-7 and the xyphoid process

Innervation – T5-T12 intercostal nerves

Functions

Unilaterally

• Assists in side bending the trunk to the same side and controlling side bending away

Bilaterally

• Flexes the trunk over the pelvis (i.e. a sit-up)
• Flexes the pelvis towards the trunk while posteriorly rotating the pelvis. i.e. reverse crunch with a fixed trunk – mostly lower fibers (I/O)
• Controls spinal extension, especially in sudden movements that involve hyper-extension, i.e. sports
• Co-activates to stabilize the spine against sudden or intense movements, not against lighter loads; unless there are faulty recruitment patterns

External Oblique Anterior Fibers

Muscle Type – Hypoactive/Global Stabilizer and Mobilizer

Attachments

Origin – A flat, wide aponeurosis ending at the linea alba along its entirety of the anterior abdominal wall

Insertion – Anterior surfaces of ribs 4 or 5-8 and serratus anterior origin/fascia

Innervation – T5-T12 intercostal nerves – both fiber types (lateral and anterior)

Functions

Unilaterally

• Rotates the trunk, bringing ipsilateral shoulder forward
• Brings contralateral hip towards opposite shoulder, i.e. reverse crunch with a twist - fixed trunk (I/O)
• Controls spinal extension with rotation backwards or simply rotation backwards, i.e. if a quarterback makes a quick throw, the E.O. decelerates the torso rotation backwards and then accelerates it forward while the opposite E.O. simultaneously decelerates the trunk rotation of the throw

* Virtually all unilateral E.O. anterior fiber functions are in conjunction with the anterior fibers of the contralateral I.O.

Bilaterally

- Flex the trunk over the pelvis (sit-up)
- Flex the pelvis towards the trunk while posteriorly rotating the pelvis. i.e. reverse crunch with a fixed trunk (I/O)
- Control spinal extension
- Support and compresses the abdominal cavity contents

External Oblique Lateral Fibers

Muscle Type – Hypoactive/Global Stabilizer and Mobilizer

Attachments

Origin – Inguinal ligament and outer border of anterior 1/2 of iliac crest

Insertion – Edges of the serratus anterior and latissimus dorsi myofascia, and anterior surfaces of ribs 9-12

Functions

Unilaterally

- Side bends spine to same side
- Controls side bending away
- Assists anterior fibers with rotation
- Hikes ipsilateral pelvis (I/O)

* Virtually all unilateral E.O. lateral fiber side bending functions are in conjunction with the lateral fibers of the ipsialateral I.O. and often times the Q.L.

Bilaterally

- Assist anterior fibers with flexing the trunk over the pelvis (sit-up)
- Assist anterior fibers with flexing the pelvis towards the trunk while posteriorly rotating the pelvis. i.e. reverse crunch with a fixed trunk (I/O)

Internal Oblique Lower Anterior Fibers

Muscle Type – Hypoactive/Global Stabilizer

Attachments

Origin – Shares tendonous insertion with T.A. into the pubic crest, medial aspect of pectineal line, and aponeurosis of the linea alba

Insertion – Lateral 1/2 - 2/3 of inguinal ligament, and iliac crest closely surrounding the ASIS

Innervation – T7-T12 intercostal nerves and ilioinguinal and ilio hypogastric nerves (L1) – all fiber types (lateral and anterior)

Functions

Bilaterally

- Pull ipsilateral hip anterior, as in a forward pelvis posture

Internal Oblique Upper Anterior Fibers

Muscle Type – Hypoactive/Global Stabilizer and Mobilizer

Attachments

Origin – Aponeurosis of the linea alba and the cartilage of ribs 7-9 via the deep aponeurosis

Insertion – Anterior 1/3 of middle lip of iliac crest

Functions

Unilaterally

- Rotates the trunk, bringing contralateral shoulder forward
- Brings ipsialateral hip towards opposite shoulder, i.e. reverse crunch with a twist - fixed trunk (I/O)
- Assists in controlling side bending away while in a flexed position (lunging for ball in tennis)
- Assists in controlling contralateral trunk extension with rotation backwards or simply contralateral rotation backwards (initial phase of tennis serve or throwing a ball)

* Virtually all unilateral I.O. upper anterior fiber functions are in conjunction with the lateral fibers of the contralateral E.O.

Bilaterally

- Flex the trunk over the pelvis (sit-up)
- Bring the pelvis towards the trunk while posteriorly rotating the pelvis. i.e. reverse crunch with a fixed trunk (I/O)

Internal Oblique Lateral Fibers

Muscle Type – Hypoactive/Global Stabilizer and Mobilizer

Attachments

Origin – Central 1/3 of middle lip of iliac crest and the LDF

Insertion – Inferior borders of ribs 10-12

Functions

Unilaterally

- Side bend the trunk to the same side
- Hikes ipsilateral pelvis (I/O)
- Controls side bending away
- Assists anterior fibers with rotation

* Virtually all unilateral I.O. lateral fiber side bending functions are in conjunction with the lateral fibers of the ipsilateral E.O. and often the Q.L.

Bilaterally

- Flex the trunk over the pelvis (sit-up)
- Exert a posterior shear force on the thoracolumbar spine via the LDF

Transverse Abdominis

Muscle Type – Hypoactive/Global Stabilizer

Attachments

Origin – Linea alba, common tendon of T.A. and I.O., pubic crest, and pectin of pubis

Insertion – Inner surfaces of rib cartilages 6-12, diaphragm, LDF, anterior ¾ of inner lip of iliac crest, and lateral 1/3 if inguinal ligament

Innervation – T7-T12 intercostal nerves and ilioinguinal and ilio hypogastric nerves (L1)

Functions

Bilaterally

- Initial activator of the abdominal wall and works with the pelvic floor muscles and diaphragm to charge the abdominal cavity by increasing IAP and tensing the LDF and linea alba in order to stabilize the lumbar spine and trunk
- Exert a posterior shear force on the thoracolumbar spine via the LDF
- Contribute to force closure of the S.I. joint
- Major stabilizer of the low back

Functional Groups

Lateral Bending – external and internal abdominal obliques, latissimus dorsi, psoas, erector spinae, rectus abdominus, and the rotatores

Trunk flexion – rectus abdominis, oblique abdominals, iliacus, and psoas major and minor

Lumbar Extension – longissimus and iliocostalis lumbothoracis muscles, longissimus and iliocostalis lumbar fascicles, latissimus dorsi, serratus posterior inferior, psoas (standing upright), Q.L., and to a small degree the multifidi, rotatores and serratus posterior (although these smaller muscles are more for fine tuning stabilization movements), the hamstrings and gluteus maximus are involved with indirectly extending the lumbar spine

Lumbar rotation – primarily the abdominal obliques, and to a lesser degree the posas, multifidi, and rotatores

Lumbar Flexion – Rectus abdominis, oblique abdominals, and psoas major and minor

Anterior Tilting of Pelvis – iliocostalis and longissimus lumbothoracic, rectus femoris, psoas, iliacus, sartorius, and other hip flexors to a small degree

Posterior Tilting of Pelvis – Rectus abdominis, external oblique, hamstrings, gluteus maximus, piriformis, and other hip extensors to a small degree

Thoracic rotation – primarily the intercostals and abdominal obliques, and to a lesser degree the multifidus, rotatores, semispinalis thoracis, longissimus and iliocostalis lumbothoracis, and serratus posterior inferior

Contribute directly to stabilizing the lumbar spine – spinal ligaments, disc pressure, diaphragm, deep intervertebral muscles, posterior fascicles of psoas, medial fibers of Q.L., and the latissimus dorsi, internal oblique, and transverse abdominis muscles via the LDF

Contribute indirectly to stabilizing the lumbar spine - pelvic floor muscles, rectus abdominis, external oblique, and the erector spinae

Exert posterior shear forces on lumbar spine – iliocostalis and longissimus fascicles, latissimus dorsi, internal oblique, and transverse abdominis (the last three act via the LDF)

Exert anterior shear forces on lumbar spine – gravity forces on a flexed spine, and possibly activation from a facilitated psoas when the spine is flexed (antagonists)

Force closure of S.I. joint during gait – T.A., latissimus dorsi, erector spinae, gluteus maximus, and biceps femoris

Force closure of S.I. joint during static weightbearing – T.A., piriformis, and the ishipcoccygeas muscles

Increases intra-abdominal pressure (IAP) – diaphragm, abdominal muscles, and pelvic floor muscles
Myofascial Lines – (R.A.) superficial front and front functional lines - (E.O./I.O.) spiral and lateral lines

Dysfunctional Group

All the above mentioned.

Descriptions

Rectus Abdominis

The R.A. is enclosed in a sheath that is the tendonous extensions of the T.A. and oblique muscles.[28] This vertical muscle is commonly overworked from improper sit-ups. It is also chronically shortened in its upper fibers and lengthened in its lower fibers from a slouching and hyperlordotic posture (upper and lower cross syndrome).

Many people believe that the R.A. cannot be functionally separated into upper and lower fibers. Lehman and McGill[199] concluded that there is no such distinction and that the muscle could be effectively trained with only one exercise; however, McGill[37] later concluded that some individuals may be able to preferentially activate the two divisions.

Unfortunately, the former conclusion was based on a study that had the following faults and is continually feeding the debate with erroneous conclusions;

1. Only 11 subjects were tested, all of which were athletes or physically active, three of these routinely performed sit-ups at least three times a week prior to the study; although not mentioned, it is likely that the other eight athletes also frequently performed improper sit-ups.
2. It is likely that all or most of the subjects routinely performed abdominal exercises that engrained faulty recruitment patterns into the lumbo-pelvic stabilizing system, just like most other athletes; this was evident as the subject shown in the study's demos for the exercises displayed obvious faulty recruitment of the neck flexors.
3. All of the tests involved upper body flexion, some in conjunction with lower body resistance, but there was no isolated lower body stabilization or movement

exercises; this is when the lower abdominals should activate greater than the upper fibers!

Fortunately, the need for studies to prove results is not always necessary when personal experience can be observed. The differentiation of the lower and upper fibers can actually be felt if the proper exercises are performed, see for yourself.

Try the lower abdominal exercises (chapters 12-14) in exclusion of any other exercise one day, then notice where you feel sore the next day. If done correctly you will feel sore only in the lower part of the abdomen, this of course includes the lower portions of the obliques. If the upper and lower portions of R.A. are inseparable, then why doesn't the upper portion become sore?

More food for thought on this topic is found when observing poor posture, i.e. excessive thoracic kyphosis and lumbar hyperlordosis. It is obvious in this posture that the R.A. can be lengthened below (and probably inhibited) and shortened above (and probably overactive).

With this in mind it is interesting to compare the multiple segmental innervations of the R.A. and oblique abdominals and the many different functions of the obliques depending on which fibers are activated. It makes sense that the R.A. could also have this differentiation of fiber activation if the body needed it.

For example, an athlete extending backwards to catch a pass should activate the upper fibers of the R.A. to eccentrically decelerate trunk extension, while the lower fibers isometrically maintain a neutral lordosis.

It is this author's belief that by utilizing corrective exercise it is not only possible, it is probable and necessary for those with LBD to be able to preferentially recruit the two portions, and that at least two different exercises are required to completely strengthen the R.A.

Because the R.A. is a mobilizer, its duties are reserved for more intense or sudden actions so that it can co-activate with the other abdominals and mobilizers to prevent the spine from buckling. *Three significant errors are commonly made when training this muscle;* 1) it is most often strengthened while lying on the floor, thus utilizing a less than natural ROM 2) performing 100's to even thousands of repetitions per week is normal for an athlete or fitness addict 3) the head position is often pushed forward, like a chicken, instead of flexing with the rest of the spine.

The results of these poor training habits lead to inefficient and inappropriate activation patterns of the R.A. and subsequent instability in the low back.

For instance, training on the floor and performing sit-up type exercises neglects an essential strength component of the R.A., which is deceleration or stabilization of the spine while hyperextended, and then repositioning thereafter to a neutral or flexed position. This is a common posture of injuries in sports or slips and falls. Executing 100's of repetitions per week of the traditional sit-up type exercise is often times detrimental because it encourages the R.A. to become the dominant abdominal muscle, even in low load situations. This results in spinal stability coming in the form of a slightly flexed spine, improperly pressurized abdomen cavity, and posteriorly rotated pelvis; obviously this is not ideal.

The inner unit should stabilize first and hold the spine in neutral for low load conditions.[138] Finally, if the head is pushed forward each time it will encourage the mobilizers of the neck, mainly the sternocleidomastoid, to stabilize the neck in a vulnerable position whenever sudden or intense action is required, not to mention the daily aches and pains it causes in the neck and shoulders from the poor posture it creates.

Causes of R.A. Tightness

- Poor posture, i.e. slouching
- Excessive or poor technique abdominal exercises
- Prolonged cough, i.e. bronchitis, flu, etc.
- Soft tissue injuries occurring to the abdomen, usually in a hyper-extended trunk or hip posture
- Forward head posture
- Referred pain from the oblique abdominals, T.A., iliocostalis lumbothoracis, multifidi, or pyramidalis
- Emotional or visceral stress can affect the entire abdominal wall with TP formation[7,200,201]
- Hyper-kyphosis of the thoracic spine
- Improper breathing patterns
- Abdominal viscera problems, stemming from either organ pathology (indigestion, abdominal pain, etc.) or referred pain from the associated spinal nerves
- Hyper-activity in the upper fibers (due to shortening from slouched posture, rounded shoulders, excessive sit-ups, etc.) and inhibition in the lower fibers (due to lengthening from hyper-lordosis, facilitated hip flexors, etc.)

Effects of R.A. Chronic Tightness

- Depression of the rib cage and improper breathing techniques, both lead to the development of tension and trigger points in the respiratory neck muscles

- TP's in the R.A. can refer pain and tension to the low and mid back and the S.I. joints, as well as mimic appendicitis[7]
- Creates tension throughout the entire anterior superficial myofascia system
- Improper breathing patterns
- Over-activity in this muscle, or upper portion of the muscle, and a resultant instability in the thoracolumbar spine during low and high load tasks; mainly due to inhibition and delayed reaction patterns in the inner unit (T.A., diaphragm, etc.) caused by the hyperactive R.A.
- Bent over posture and resultant low back stress
- Weak lower fibers cause a protruding abdomen
- Pain with extension due to TP's in the R.A.
- Leaning to one side posture – unilateral

Individual Assessments

ROM (standing trunk extension), posture (bent forward at the hips), PMAP for 1) spinal flexion (sit-up test) 2) squats 3) lunges 4) push-pull exercise, and strength testing (sit-up against resistance and endurance tests) assessments and corrective actions are described in Chapters 12 and 13.

Corrective Actions

1. Improve any pain, faulty postures or breathing patterns, and bad habits (excessive/improper sit-ups).
2. Stretch and or apply manual therapy to any a) adhesions in the abdominal myofascia and b) short or overactive neck flexors, erector spinae muscles, Q.L., sternalis muscle, hip adductors, hip flexors, and any other influential muscles.
3. Learn how to properly activate the inner CORE unit, see pg. 80.
4. Utilize at least two different exercises in order to strengthen the upper and lower fibers, although the upper fibers are usually overactive and require stretching first, i.e. balancing posture in step 1.
5. Perform sit-backs (reverse sit-up, progress to a weighted ball caught overhead) to encourage the development of eccentric/deceleration strength.
6. Utilize training of the upper fibers in a hyper-extended position, i.e. lying on a ball or standing overhead medicine ball catches/throws.

External and Internal Obliques

Unlike the R.A., the E.O. and I.O. are great stabilizers *and* mobilzers. They usually function as one (contralaterally with rotation and ipsilaterally with side bending), even though they have separate functions(see above), most of which have to do with rotating or stabilizing the trunk. These are the trunk muscles predominantly used during swinging or throwing activities.

Imbalances between the right and left sides of each muscle as well as the same side E.O. and I.O. are common, especially in athletes or people whose daily routine involves rotation or bending to a dominant side. For example, a grocery clerk who continually swipes (torso rotation) items the same direction every time or a computer worker who sits rotated to one side is vulnerable to strength imbalances between the obliques.

These types of imbalances lead to postural faults that create spinal rotation and reduced stability throughout the spine. Therefore, it is essential to find out which side is dominant before simply adding oblique exercises into a fitness or post-rehabilitative routine. To find out which side is dominant two tests or observations are helpful;

1. Manual muscle testing
2. Posture (look for any torso rotation or bending)

If a side or muscle is found to be dominant, follow the corrective actions below.

Causes of E.O. and I.O. Weakness

- Dominant contralateral oblique is creating imbalance of strength between sides
- Sedentary lifestyle
- Hyperlordosis
- Sway back posture, mostly affects E.O., especially its lower anterior fibers
- Referred pain from R.A., multifidi, iliiocostalis lumbothoracis, or abdominal organs

Effects of E.O. and I.O. Chronic Weakness

- Rotated or side bending trunk posture, often times creating a functional scoliosis with the thoracic spine deviating towards the weak E.O. and the lumbar spine towards the weak contralateral I.O.[49]
- Sway back posture, mostly E.O. and especially its lower anterior fibers
- Decreased spinal stability, especially against torsion forces, therefore increasing the load and chance of injury to multifidus and other intervertebral muscles during twisting moments
- Decreased ability to posteriorly tilt pelvis or flex trunk
- Hyperlordosis
- Decreases respiratory efficiency and abdominal viscera support[49]

Individual Assessments

ROM (sitting or standing trunk rotation), posture (torso and pelvic rotation, iliac crest and rib cage levels, and scoliosis), PMAP during side flexion test, and strength testing (sit-up against resistance and endurance tests) assessments and corrective actions are described in Chapters 12 and 13.

Corrective Actions

1. Improve any pain, faulty postures or breathing patterns, and bad habits (sitting at desk or on couch with torso rotated).
2. Stretch and or apply manual therapy to any a) adhesions in the abdominal myofascia b) short or overactive neck flexors, erector spinae muscles, Q.L., sternalis muscle, hip adductors, hip flexors, and any other influential muscles.
3. Learn how to properly activate the inner CORE unit, see pg. 80.
4. Perform at least three times as many strength exercises for the weak muscle or side as the dominant side.
5. Once the obliques are balanced, utilize functional movement patterns, such as wood chop motions or old fashioned pull start lawn mower movements.

Transverse Abdominis

Along with the deep multifidus, the T.A. is the most important muscle for improving and preventing LBP. As mentioned in chapter 1, the T.A. is an integral part of the inner unit in which the CNS utilizes a feedforward neuromuscular system to stabilize the spine prior to the involvement of the intermediate and outer unit muscle groups during predictable imposed demands.

The T.A. is the main muscle involved with creating posterior shear forces via the LDF, and is the only muscle that can effectively do so regardless of the spine's position. This posterior shear force could be considered the most important factor in combating the injurious stresses caused by flexion of the lumbar spine; a neutral or lordotic spine position is another essential factor, but it cannot be maintained properly without the activation of T.A.

Although the T.A. doesn't produce much movement, the body utilizes the T.A. (as well as the other muscles of the inner unit) for just about every movement, and during repetitive movements or continuous actions the body utilizes it in a tonic or constant manner.[172,182] For instance, when running, the T.A. should be constantly activated at a low level in order to maintain stability throughout the entire body.

Ask any experienced runner about this and they will concur; if they don't, teach them how to activate the CORE and then have them try them how to activate it, odds are their speed and stamina will improve quite drastically.

Unfortunately, the T.A. is easily inhibited by factors such as inactivity, pain[175], intestinal disorders, etc. In our sedentary society it is necessary to be conscious of proper abdominal activation that should otherwise come naturally to a more active population.

Causes of T.A. Weakness

- LBP
- Poor posture
- Improper or excessive sit-up techniques
- Sedentary lifestyle
- Abdominal pains
- C-section surgery for child birth

Effects of T.A. Chronic Weakness

- Instability in the spine and pelvis, especially in the lumbar spine and S.I. joints
- Inefficient movement patterns throughout the entire body
- A lateral and anterior bulge of the abdomen during CORE activation
- Encourages protrusion of the anterior abdomen and subsequent increase in lumbar lordosis[49]
- Inability to pull the belly-button in towards the spine
- Improper breathing patterns
- Faulty PMAP during curl-up and forward flexion tests
- Facilitates weakness in the rest of the CORE muscles

Individual Assessments

Posture (protruding abdomen), PMAP of CORE during various movements, i.e. sit-up, squat, etc. (an anterior and lateral bulge during any of these tests indicates a T.A. weakness), and strength testing (should be able to squat to 90°, lunge so back knee touches floor, and

bend forward fully while maintaining proper CORE activation, i.e. stomach remains tense and does not protrude anteriorly or laterally) assessments and corrective actions are described in Chapters 12 and 13.

Corrective Actions

1. Improve any pain, faulty postures or breathing patterns, and bad habits (excessive/improper sit-ups).
2. Stretch and or apply manual therapy to any a) adhesions in the abdominal myofascia   b) short or overactive neck flexors, erector spinae muscles, Q.L., sternalis muscle, hip adductors, hip flexors, and any other influential muscles.
3. Learn how to properly activate the T.A. (suck in the lower abdomen while a) lying b) sitting c) on hands and knees d) standing.
4. Learn how to properly activate the inner unit as a whole, see pg. 80.
5. Incorporate these activation patterns into a) simple tasks b) simple tasks + resistance c) complex tasks d) complex tasks + resistance e) all the above at high speeds.

Abdominal Training

As a whole, the abdominals should be trained to stabilize the body throughout all relevant functional tasks. Therefore, unless someone needs to get up from a lying position 100's of times a day, 100's of sit-ups are unnecessary and probably even detrimental to the spine.

Strength training for the abdominals should consist of workouts that utilize resistance and 2-4 sets of 10-15 reps* for 1-2 of the muscles. Meaning that all of the abdominals should not be trained every day. It is best to focus on 1 or 2 abdominal muscles per session so that over training does not occur.

Because the lower abdominal exercises are usually the most difficult and stressful on the low back, it is a good idea to do them at the beginning of the abdominal workout to avoid straining the low back. Endurance training for the abdominals should come from circuit training which utilizes CORE exercises alternated with other functional exercises, not 100's of sit-ups.

*During the early stages of training there are cases where more reps or time are required to learn PMAP.

Iliopsoas

"The Deep Root of LBP"

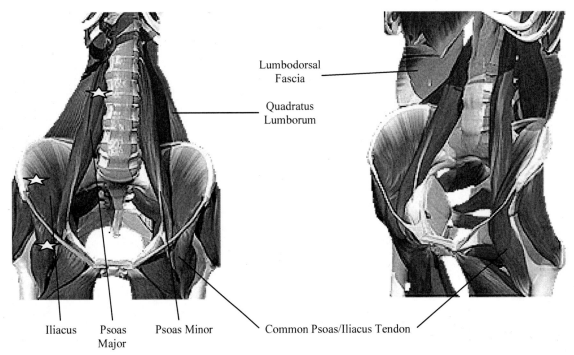

Lumbodorsal Fascia

Quadratus Lumborum

Iliacus   Psoas Major   Psoas Minor   Common Psoas/Iliacus Tendon

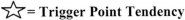 = **Trigger Point Tendency**

Psoas Major

Muscle Type – Hyperactive/Mobilizer

Attachments

Origin – Lateral aspects of vertebral bodies T12-L5 and to their intervertebral discs and medial half of the anterior inferior portions of the lumbar transverse processes

Insertion – Iliacus muscle/iliopsoas tendon and ending on the lesser trochanter

Innervation - Lumbar plexus, L2-L3, (L1/L4)

Functions

Unilaterally

- Flexes the thigh at the hip
- Assists lateral bending and flexing of lumbar spine to same side (I/O)
- Assists lateral rotation and abduction of thigh
- Compresses lumbar vertebrae on same side

Bilaterally

- Flex both thighs at the hips

- Exert substantial compression loads on the lumbar spine
- Assist trunk and lumbar flexion (I/O)
- Assist extension of the lumbar spine by increasing lordisis while standing with a normal lumbar lordisis (I/O)
- Play a major role in maintaining upright posture (sitting and standing)
- Anteriorly tilt the pelvis
- Can create nutation of the sacrum by pulling down and forward on L4-L5

Iliacus

Muscle Type – Undetermined

Attachments

Origin – upper two-thirds of the inner iliac fossa, internal lip of the iliac crest, lateral aspect of sacrum, and anterior portion of the iliolumbar and sacroiliac ligaments.

Insertion – psoas tendon, anterior lesser trochanter, and nearby femur.

Innervation – Femoral nerve, L2-L3, (L1/L4)

Functions

- Flexes the thigh at the hip, most effective after 30°
- Anteriorly tilts the pelvis
- Assists in abduction of thigh
- Assists lateral rotation of thigh
- Assists trunk flexion (sit-up)

Psoas Minor

Muscle Type – Hyperactive

Attachments

Origin – Anterolateral portion of T12, L1 and or L2, and the corresponding intervertebral disc(s).

Insertion – Superior ramus of the pubis, iliopectineal eminence, and iliac fascia.

Innervation - Lumbar plexus, L1-L2

Functions

- Assists psoas in extending normal lordosis
- Assists in lumbar flexion (bilaterally)
- Elevates the ipsilateral anterior pelvis
- Assists in lumbar flexion with a lateral component (unilaterally)

Functional Groups

Hip Flexion – psoas major, iliacus, pectineus, rectus femoris, sartorius, TFL, gracilis, and hip adductors

Hip Extension – gluteus maximus, hamstrings, and posterior adductor magnus (antagonists)

Myofascial Lines – deep front line

Dysfunctional Group

Includes all muscles in the functional group as well as the; diaphragm, Q.L., contralateral psoas, and the deep six lateral rotators of the hip. Because of their close relationship, this dysfunctional group is the same for the iliacus.

Description

The term iliopsoas refers to the collaboration of the posas major, psoas minor, and iliacus muscles, not one muscle. These muscles are similar in location and function but their small differences create important effects on the kinetic chain and lumbar spine.

The psoas major is the most often talked about muscle of this group because of its effects on lumbar vertebral shearing and compression forces on L5-S1[195] as well as its associations with many vital structures, i.e. colon, kidney, lymph nodes, aortas, diaphragm, lumbar plexus, femoral nerve, and more. Unless otherwise noted, the term psoas here refers to the psoas major.

The psoas minor muscle is difficult to assess because it is absent bilaterally in roughly 50% of the population[8] and has insignificant functional roles, but its tendon can be a palpable taught cord in some individuals which indicates its need for treatment. The iliacus is sometimes forgotten about in LBD because it is mostly connected with hip dysfunctions. But, LBD and hip dysfunctions are often related and the iliacus and psoas major are commonly dysfunctional together, along with the Q.L., due to their intimate myofascial connections. These factors alone make the iliacus muscle a key link in low back health.

The psoas major is the most influential postural muscle in the body[121] and can have a dominating effect on the entire kinetic chain when both the right and left sides are chronically short by causing hyperlordosis in the lumbar spine, muscle and vertebral compensations throughout the whole spine, and chain reactions throughout the rest of the body.

The psoas is an important muscle in low back post-rehabilitation because it is the link between the low back and legs, and it functions similarly to the abdominal muscles, but with two key distinctions;

1. The psoas *tilt the pelvis anteriorly* vs. the abdominals tilt the hips posteriorly.
2. The psoas cause *anterior shearing forces on the lumbar vertebrae*[37] vs. the internal obliques and transverse abdominis create a posterior shearing or extension force via the lumbardorsal fascia[40].

Along with their innate tendency to become overactive, psoas dysfunction is encouraged by prolonged sitting, bicycle riding, and other popular bent over hip flexion activities that cause the psoas to shorten and dominate the neuromuscular recruitment patterns during sit-ups and hip or trunk flexion.

This dominance is detrimental to the low back because of the resultant *high lumbar compression forces*[37] *and increased loading of the intervertebral discs*[122] the psoas create, not to mention the inhibition it causes in the abdominals that forces the paraspinal muscles to absorb forces they are not equipped for during daily and physical activities, especially rotation forces.

The balance between the iliopsoas, abdominals, hamstrings, gluteus maximus, and erector spinae muscles is crucial for maintaining a low level of lumbar compression and high level of functional efficiency.

Low back care is tricky because one goal is to strengthen the abdominals, but if the psoas are too tight they dominate most of the neuromuscular activity during sit-ups and other abdominal exercises which therefore limits any strength gained by the abdominals, as well as adds substantial stress to the low back.

There have been attempts to inhibit the psoas during sit-ups by pressing the heels into the floor (activating the hamstrings to create reciprocal inhibition in the hip flexors), but McGill et all[72] showed that this technique actually increased psoas involvement in order to stabilize the extensor hip moment caused by the hamstrings.

A similar technique of plantar flexing the feet during curl-ups is also likely to have a similar effect. Methods for strengthening the abdominals are presented in Chapter 13.

While the psoas plays a questionable role in rotation of the thigh, the rotation does seem to be important when stretching it. *The optimal stretch position for the psoas should include extension and medial rotation of the thigh while avoiding abduction*[8], but optimal stretching of the entire iliopsoas complex and its fascia requires a few different stretches, such as the Q.L., lats, lateral abdomen, and by reaching the ipsilateral arm upward.

Causes of Psoas Major Tightness

- Prolonged sitting, especially when the knees are higher than the hips and the thigh is externally rotated (driving), or the spine is held erect without back support
- Prolonged cycling or uphill walking
- Too many sit-ups, especially with the feet anchored
- Improper breathing patterns[4]
- Scoliosis convex towards the shorter psoas[49]
- Frequent walking or running on treadmill; the leg is thrown into extension by the momentum of the treadmill, thus relieving the gluteus maximus of that duty and forcing the psoas to decelerate the leg, as well as already having to accelerate it.
- Weak abdominals, especially the lower fibers
- Weak gluteus maximus
- Lumbar vertebrae or nerve disorder
- Sacroiliac joint dysfunction
- Pronated feet
- Wearing high heel shoes often
- Kidney, digestive system, or colon dysfunction

Effects of Psoas Major Chronic Tightness

- Inhibits the lower abdominals, gluteus maximus, and the deep lumbar paraspinal muslces
- Synergistic dominance during hip and back extension by the superficial erector spinae and hamstrings (due to compensations for the inhibition of the deep paraspinal and gluteus maximus muscles)
- Decreased hip extension
- LBP during push-ups
- LBP and inability to keep the lumbar spine flat against the floor during the lower abdominal testing
- Bent over posture (to same side as tightness if only one side is tight) with difficulty straightening up
- Hyperlordosis of the lumbar spine and subsequent shortening of the lumbar erectors
- Overloads and strains the hamstrings
- Sacroiliac and or facet joint syndrome
- Can perpetuate TP's in muscles as distant as the posterior cervical muscles[8]
- In conjunction with an ipsilateral Q.L. tightness can cause false leg length discrepancies.
- Pronated foot or feet
- Lumbar vertebral dysfunctions
- Scoliosis *convex* towards the shorter psoas[49]
- Facilitated psoas muscles can inhibit the lower abdominals and create a flexion-extension imbalance that causes anterior tilting of the pelvis whenever the lumbar erectors are activated (the lower abdominals do not counteract the lumbar erector's force), commonly seen in squats as the buttocks protrudes excessively.

Individual Assessments

ROM (supine leg hanging off table), posture (lumbar lordosis, scoliosis, ASIS height, femur rotation, and pevic tilt), and muscle testing (supine straight leg flexion against resistance) assessments and corrective actions are described in Chapters 12 and 13.

Corrective Actions

1. Improve any pain, faulty postures, and bad habits.
2. Stretch and or apply manual therapy to the psoas, hip flexors, anterior and lateral abdominals, Q.L., hip adductors, lumbar erectors, and any other relevant area.
3. Strengthen/activate the gluteus maximus.
4. Learn how to activate the lower abdominals without the psoas taking over, see chapter 13.
5. Balance tension between the left and right psoas muscles with strengthening and stretching exercises.

The Hip Adductors

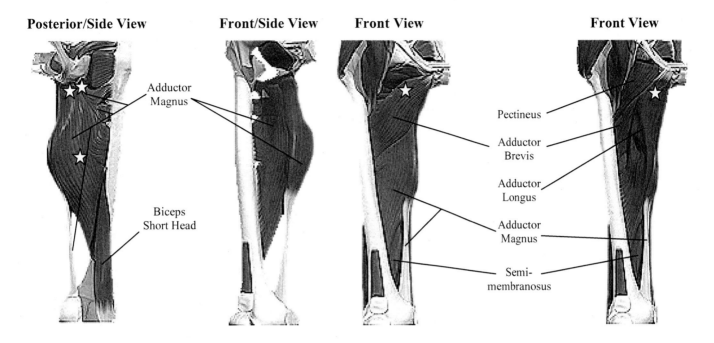

Posterior/Side View   **Front/Side View**   **Front View**   **Front View**

Adductor Magnus

Biceps Short Head

Pectineus

Adductor Brevis

Adductor Longus

Adductor Magnus

Semi-membranosus

☆ = **Trigger Point Tendency**

Pectineus

Muscle Type – Undetermined/Global Stabilizer

Attachments

Origin – Crest of the superior ramus of the pubic bone, lying deep and below the inguinal ligament and lateral to its attachment at the pubic tubercle

Insertion – Medial posterior portion of the femur, between the lesser trochanter and linea aspera (pectineal line)

Innervation – Obturator and femoral nerves (L2-L4)

Adductor Longus

Muscle Type – Hyperactive/Global Stabilizer and Mobilzer

Attachments

Origin – Small point between the symphysis pubis and obturator foramen, sometimes fusing with pectineus

Insertion – Medial lip of linea aspera on middle 1/3 of femur

Innervation – Obturator nerve (L2-L4)

Adductor Brevis

Muscle Type – Hyperactive/Global Stabilizer and Mobilzer

Attachments

Origin – Inferior ramus of the pubis

Insertion – Medial lip of linea aspera on upper third of femur, immediately posterior to adductor longus and pectineus

Functions (pectineus, longus, and brevis)

Unilaterally

• Adduct and flex the thigh
• Equivocal contribution to thigh rotation, depending on position of leg (longus and brevis only)

Bilaterally

• Assist the hip abductors in stabilizing the pelvis about the hip joints against gravity or the ground reaction force when both extremities bear weight

Adductor Magnus

Muscle Type – Hyperactive/Global Stabilizer and Mobilzer

Attachments

Upper Anterior Horizontal Fibers

Origin – Inferior pubic ramus

Insertion – Almost horizontal fibers attaching to just below the lesser trochanter and extending down briefly along the upper portion of the linea aspera

Middle Diagonal Fibers

Origin – Along the ischial ramus between the ischial tuberosity and inferior pubic ramus, sometimes overlapping the upper fibers of adductor magnus

Insertion – Along the linea aspera and down to the adductor hiatus, which is an opening for the femoral vessels to pass through

Posterior Ischiocondylar Vertical Fibers

Origin – Ischial tuberosity area and slightly anterior along the ischial ramus

Insertion – Thick tendon on the adductor tubercle of the medial femoral condyle

Innervation – Obturator nerve (L2-L4) and tibial portion of sciatic nerve (L4-S1)

Functions

Unilaterally

- Adducts the thigh
- Flexes the thigh (upper and middle fibers)
- Extends the thigh (posterior fibers)
- Medially rotates femur
- Laterally rotates thigh, depending on position
- Assists gluteus maximus and hamstring muscles in controlling the tendency of body weight induced hip flexion during the early stance of gait
- Assists adductor longus in controlling abduction and stabilizing the pelvis for weight shift later in gait

Bilaterally

- Assist the hip abductors in stabilizing the pelvis about the hip joints against gravity or the ground reaction force when both extremities bear weight

Functional Groups

Hip Adduction – all adductors and gracilis

Hip Abduction – gluteus minimus and medius, TFL, upper fibers of gluteus maximus,

Hip Flexion and Extension – see iliopsoas

Lateral Hip Rotation – deep six rotators (especially piriformis), long head biceps femoris, posterior fibers of gluteus medius and minimus, sartorius, and to a lesser degree, the psoas major and iliacus

Medial Hip Rotation – TFL, gluteus medius and minimus anterior fibers, medial hamstrings, adductors, gracilis

Myofascial Lines – (adductors) deep front and lateral lines - (adductor longus) front functional line

Dysfunctional Groups

Same as functional group plus Q.L., lateral abdominals, IT band, lateral flexors of the neck, and any other muscle that attaches to the pelvis or sacrum

Description

Although most of the hip adductors are mobilizers during hip adduction, their main duty involves stabilizing the lumbo-pelvic-hip system during weightbearing activities such as running and squatting.

They are also a key component to lateral stabilization of the spine and entire body; unfortunately they are often reciprocally facilitated by weak gluteus medius and minimus muscles, making them a tricky exception to the hypoactive tendencies of global mobilizers.

This reciprocal facilitation causes the adductors to tighten and shorten, both of which overload the ipsilateral Q.L. with hip hiking and the contralateral Q.L. with increased pelvic stabilization during hip abduction, not to mention altered joint mechanics and decreased ROM of the hip and pelvis.

The adductor magnus and hamstrings work closely together. So close in fact that the middle adductor magnus and the short head of the biceps femoris are contiguously attached at the linea aspera of the femur and form an adductor-hamstring muscle that can produce an interdependent force of hip extension and knee flexion.[8,63]

This additional hamstring combo lies beneath the biceps femoris and is an often overlooked division of hamstring strains due to its difficult palpation location. Proper hip adductor functioning is essential to LBD as well as balance throughout the kinetic chain.

- Weak ipsilateral gluteus medius and minimus
- History of hamstring or groin strains
- Sexual tension
- Rigorous soccer playing or horse riding
- Explosive leg movements without proper warm-up, especially abduction
- Slips and falls
- Prolonged sitting with crossed legs
- Referred pain from psoas, vastus intermedius and medialis, sartorius, and gracilis
- Bent over walking posture (mostly magnus)
- Excessive foot pronation
- Tightness in the front functional myofascia line

- Overloads the ipsilateral Q.L. as a mobilizer and the contralateral Q.L. as a stabilizer during standing hip abduction - unilateral
- Inhibits ipsilateral gluteus medius and minimus
- Decreased lateral stabilization (essential for sports)
- Can imitate a mid-lumbar spine lesion from its bilateral pain referral[8,202]
- Pain and tingling in the groin from nerve entrapment by adductor magnus[8]

- Intrapelvic or anterior knee pain from TP's[8]
- Pubic stress symphysitis or fracture[8]
- IT band overload
- Hip and S.I. joint dysfunctions
- Elevates ipsilateral ilium – unilateral
- Improper gait patterns

Individual Assessments

ROM (thigh abduction), posture (iliac crest level and femur rotation), PMAP (hip abduction), and testing for hip abductor weakness (side lying and standing) assessments are described in chapters 12 and 13.

Corrective Actions

1. Improve any pain, faulty postures (utilize a pillow between the knees when sleeping on side) and bad habits, i.e. prolonged sitting with crossed legs, playing sports without stretching hips, etc.
2. Apply manual therapy if adhesions or TP's exist in the adductors, hamstrings, Q.L., and other influential areas such as along the related myofascia lines.
3. Use PMAP to strengthen the gluteus medius and minimus, in weightbearing and side lying positions.
4. Stretch adductors, especially with active techniques that utilize gluteus minimus and medius contractions.

Quadratus Lumborum (Q.L.)

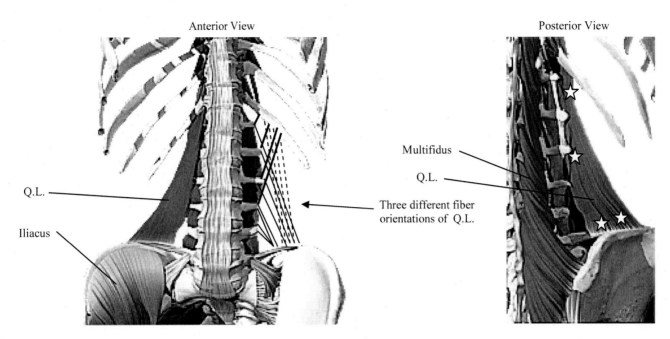

Anterior View

Posterior View

Q.L.

Iliacus

Three different fiber orientations of Q.L.

Multifidus

Q.L.

☆ = **Trigger Point Tendency**

Muscle Type – Hyperactive/Global Stabilizer and Mobilizer

Attachments

A) Iliocostal fibers (nearly vertical)
Origin - Iliac crest and often iliolumbar ligament
Insertion – Medial half of 12th rib

B) Iliolumbar fibers (diagonal)
Origin - Iliac crest and often iliolumbar ligament
Insertion - Anterior transverse processes of L1-L3, (L4)

C) Lumbocostal fibers (diagonal)
Origin - Transverse processes of L2-L4, (L1/L5).
Insertion – Medial half of 12th rib

Innervation - Lumbar plexus, T12-L3, (L4)

Functions

Unilaterally

- Laterally flexes lumbar spine to same side
- Elevates (hikes) ipsilateral hip (I/O)
- Stabilizes lumbar spine (decelerates lateral bending away from muscle)
- Draws down the 12th rib

Bilaterally

- Extend lumbar spine
- Flex the trunk (in certain positions)
- Stabilize lumbar spine
- Assist in forced exhalation (coughing)
- Acts with inhalation

Functional Groups

See abdominal muscles functional group for details.

Myofascial Lines – deep front line

Dysfunctional Group

This group is in addition to the functional groups above; the contralateral Q.L., diaphragm, gluteus medius and minimus, TFL, and the hip adductors.

Description

Quadratus lumborum is recognized as the *most common muscular cause of LBP* by practitioners who can identify its trigger points.[8] The Q.L. is an integral piece of the muscular foundation for the torso due to its strong connections to the pelvis, lumbar vertebrae, and twelfth ribs and is a major stabilizer of the spine throughout most of its ROM or simply standing.

It can be thought of as three muscles in one because of its different fiber arrangements, which are all enclosed between the anterior and middle layers of the LDF.[137] The three segments of the muscle can then be broken down into two categories 1) global stabilizer or mobilizer - depending on the motion 2) local stabilizer.

The global portion of the muscle is the lateral fibers (ilium to 12th rib), and the local stabilizing portion is the medial fibers (vertebrae to ilium and vertebrae to 12th rib). Richardson et all[138] describe the Q.L. as a global stabilizer and note that it is possible, yet difficult to prove with the present testing methods, for the medial Q.L. fibers to act as a segmental stabilizer. McGill et all[141] also note that the Q.L. is capable of creating segmental stabilization forces through its segmental attachments.

Depending on which fibers are shortened, a resultant lumbar scoliosis can be convex away or towards the shortness. This should be taken into account when applying stretches. For example, if it is obvious that the Q.L. is short but the individual does not feel an adequate stretch during stretching, try variations, different stretches, or applying traction to the iliac crest in order to separate it from the 12th rib and search for the specific angles that are restricted.

Sometimes tight lateral abdominal muscles and fascia can limit the Q.L.'s stretch potential and therefore need to be released prior to stretching the Q.L.

Although it functions as a lumbar flexor and extender, *most of its troubles come from lateral dysfunctions.* Whether it is from a side impact car accident, functional scoliosis, compensating for carrying objects on one side, or an imbalance in hip abduction and adduction, the Q.L. seems to inherit the bulk of the lateral lumbar overload.

A lumbar scoliosis will affect the length and function of the right and left Q.L. more than any other muscle, on the other hand, a tight and short Q.L. can create a functional scoliosis that will improve once the Q.L. is normalized. The cause of scoliosis is sometimes very complex and often requires X-rays to determine the root of the deformity.

Distorted pelvis size, crooked L5-S1 vertebrae, long/short leg, or a combination of these are just some of the causes of scoliosis

Once the Q.L. muscle has active TP's, lumbar stabilization and mobility are greatly reduced. The TP's can refer debilitating pain into the low back and hip that makes walking or rolling over in bed an excruciating event.

Eisler[116,] as translated in Travell and Simmons[8,] described the main body of the Q.L. as sometimes

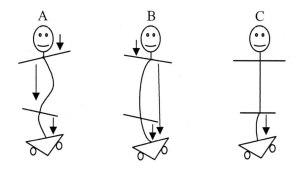

Fig. 11-9 Above are just three possible variations of spinal curvature, there are many more. A short leg could also be the cause of or created by any of the above. Each arrow signifies a tight/short area. The following compensations (tight/short) correspond to the drawings above.

A. Lateral neck muscles and fascia, Q.L., lateral abdominals (right side). Thoracic paraspinals and fascia (left side).
B. Lateral neck muscles and fascia (left side). Q.L., lateral abdominals, paraspinals, latissimus dorsi, and superficial back line of fascia (right side).
C. Q.L. and lateral abdominals (right side).

being anchored extensively to the LDF, and Chaitow and DeLany[4] noted that the Q.L. is wrapped in fascia; this fascial connection reinforces its influence on stabilization. The fascia of the Q.L. is in relation to the colon, psoas, diaphragm, and kidney.[54] Due to their fascia connection, the *Q.L. and psoas are often problematic together.*

Causes of Q.L. Tightness

- Short upper arms (have to lean on arm rests)
- Small hemipelvis
- Weakness in gluteus medius and minimus, which facilitates the ipsilateral hip adductors, and therefore limits abduction of that leg. The Q.L. then compensates with *ipsilateral* hip hiking during abduction, leading to eventual lumbar overload and altered joint mechanics and muscle recruitment patterns (common in sports)
- The above example will also cause the *contralateral* Q.L. to increase its stabilization force in order to maintain trunk stability in the frontal plane if lateral movement is a factor
- ➢ This shows that *both* the right and left Q.L. have to compensate for a weak gluteus medius and minimus, one with hip hiking and the other with stabilization forces
- Dehydration or stressed kidneys
- Lumbar vertebrae or nerve disorder
- Referred pain from longissimus and iliocostalis

lumbothoracis, iliocostalis thoracis, multifidi, psoas, gluteus medius, and R.A

- Lower leg length inequality, which leads to lumbar scoliosis and uneven iliac crest levels
- Bronchitis or prolonged coughing
- Abnormal breathing patterns
- Short and tight rib cage elevators (upper trapezius, levator scapula, and scalenes) that impair breathing patterns and force the Q.L. to overwork in order to depress the rib cage
- Prolonged stooping
- Habitually carrying objects on one side, i.e. purse, child, gym bag, computer bag, etc.
- Walking on uneven surfaces for a prolonged time (beach or a track)
- Any factor that creates abnormal gait patterns or hyperlordosis, i.e. short hip flexors
- Weak abdominals
- Sagging bed

Effects of Q.L. Chronic Tightness

- False leg length discrepancies (hikes the hip and creates illusion of one leg being longer in supine assessment).
- An "S" or "C" curve functional scoliosis compensation pattern (Fig. 11-9)
- Decreased lateral stabilization (very important in sports), also w/bilateral tightness or TP involvement
- Ipsilateral iliacus and psoas tension via the deep fascia connection
- Contralateral Q.L. inhibition and or elongation

- Immobile and dysfunctional lumbar vertebrae (also w/bilateral tightness)
- Inhibition of the ipsilateral gluteus medius or minimus if there is referred pain from Q.L. trigger points
- Along with psoas postural shortening can effect breathing patterns[4]
- Altered gleno-humeral mechanics from a depressed shoulder
- Increased lordosis (bilateral)

*All tightness is unilateral unless specified otherwise.

Individual Assessments

ROM (standing side flexion), posture (iliac crest and rib cage levels, and scoliosis,), PMAP for hip abduction, and muscle testing (supine lateral flexion against ankle resistance) assessments and corrective actions are described in Chapters 12 and 13.

Corrective Actions

1. Improve any pain, faulty postures or breathing patterns, PMAP for hip abduction, and bad habits (i.e. carrying objects on one side only).
2. Stretch and or apply manual therapy to the Q.L., iliacus, psoas major, anterior and lateral abdominals, hip abductors and adductors, erector spinae muscles, and any other relevant area.
3. Balance tension between the left and right Q.L., latissimus dorsi, lateral abdominals, and gluteal muscles with strengthening and stretching exercises.

The Thoracolumbar Paraspinal Muscles

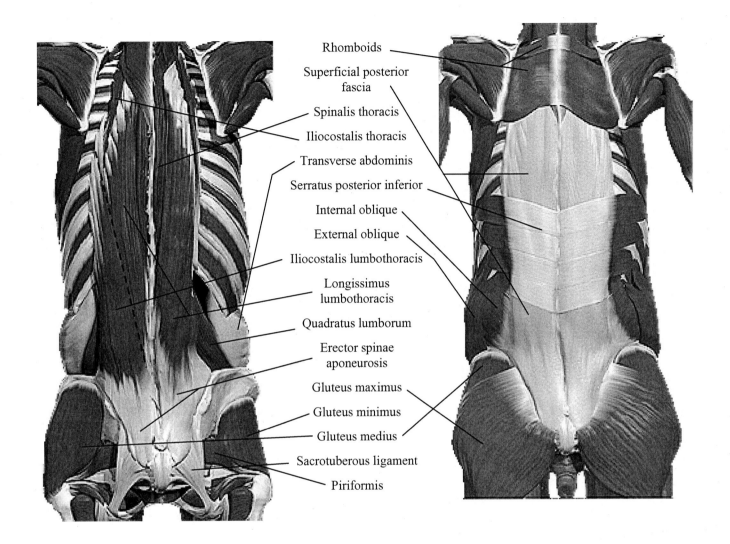

Rhomboids
Superficial posterior fascia
Spinalis thoracis
Iliocostalis thoracis
Transverse abdominis
Serratus posterior inferior
Internal oblique
External oblique
Iliocostalis lumbothoracis
Longissimus lumbothoracis
Quadratus lumborum
Erector spinae aponeurosis
Gluteus maximus
Gluteus minimus
Gluteus medius
Sacrotuberous ligament
Piriformis

Fig. 11-10 The complexity of the paraspinal muscles is obvious here, especially considering that some of layers are not even shown! It may seem ridiculous to break everything up into such specific divisions, but with a deeper look it is apparent that each division has separate functions that are essential in program design for low back disorders.

1st Layer* (most superficial)	**2nd Layer**	**3rd Layer**	**4th Layer**	**5th Layer*** (deepest)
• Latissimus dorsi • Trapezius	• Rhomboids	• Serratus posterior inferior & superior*	• Erector spinae • Spinalis thoracis • Iliocostalis thoracis	• Semispinalis thoracis • Multifidus • Rotatores • Interspinalis • Intertransversales • Lumbar fascicles • Quadratus lumborum

*Not shown

115

Iliocostalis Lumbar Fascicles

Longissimus Lumbar Fascicles

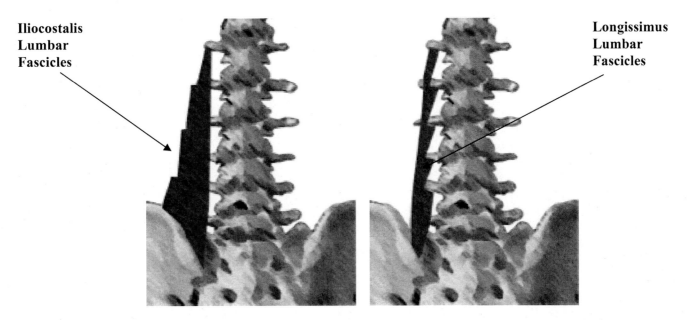

Fig. 11-11 These fascicles are the underbelly of the erector spinae.
Fig. 11-12 The functional unit and all of its components.

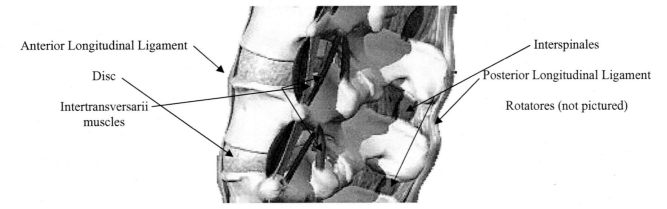

Anterior Longitudinal Ligament

Disc

Intertransversarii muscles

Interspinales

Posterior Longitudinal Ligament

Rotatores (not pictured)

Fig. 11-13 Deep layer; multifidus and Q.L.

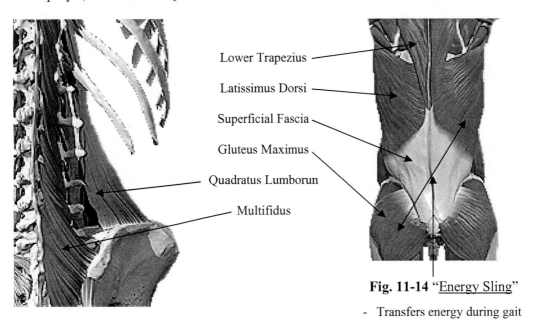

Lower Trapezius

Latissimus Dorsi

Superficial Fascia

Gluteus Maximus

Quadratus Lumborun

Multifidus

Fig. 11-14 "Energy Sling"

- Transfers energy during gait

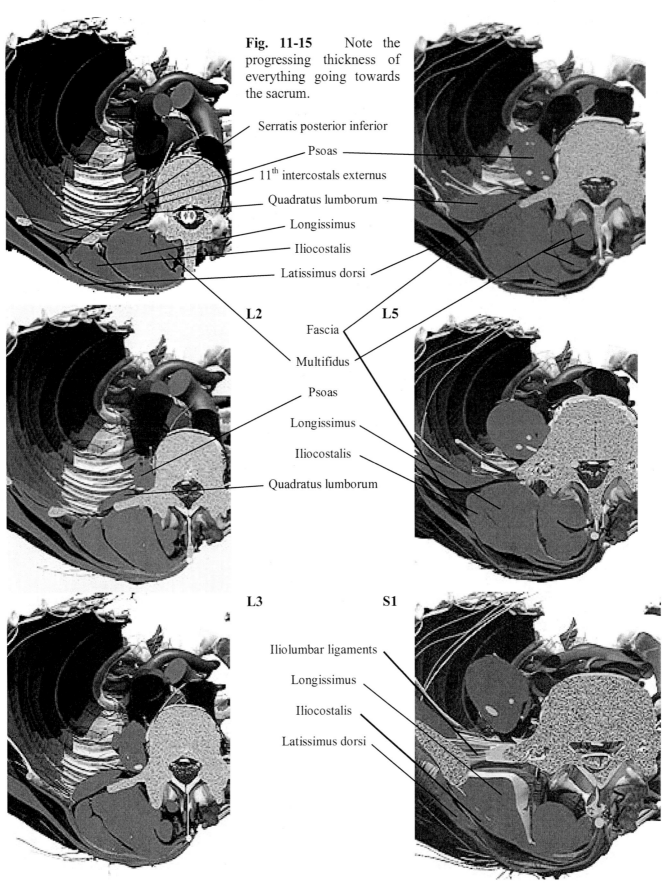

L1

L4

Fig. 11-15 Note the progressing thickness of everything going towards the sacrum.

Serratis posterior inferior

Psoas

11th intercostals externus

Quadratus lumborum

Longissimus

Iliocostalis

Latissimus dorsi

L2

L5

Fascia

Multifidus

Psoas

Longissimus

Iliocostalis

Quadratus lumborum

L3

S1

Iliolumbar ligaments

Longissimus

Iliocostalis

Latissimus dorsi

Divisions of the Thoracolumbar Paraspinal Muscles and Fascia

Box 11 – 2

Superficial Gross Movers
• Latissimus Dorsi*
• Iliocostalis lumbothoracis *(erector spinae)*
• Longissimus lumbothoracis *(erector spinae)*
• Spinalis thoracis
• Iliocostalis thoracis
• Semispinales thoracis**
Deep Intervertebral Stabilizers
• Iliocostalis lumbar fascicles
• Longissimus lumbar fascicles
• Multifidi
• Rotatores
• Interspinales
• Intertransversarii
Lumbar Dorsal Fascia (LDF)
• Superficial layer
• Middle layer
• Deep layer

* The latissimus dorsi is included in this section because of its extensive insertion into the lumbardorsal fascia and the resulting stabilizing extension force it produces on the thoracolumbar spine when it bilaterally contracts.
** Semispinalis thoracis is a gross mover but it is situated deeper with the stabilizers in the fifth layer

Erector spinae, paraspinal muscles, spinal erectors, spinal extensors, and paravertebral group are all names used to describe the muscles along the spine. This of course has lead to confusion whenever one of them is mentioned, and unfortunately this text is going to add to the confusion by changing the names of four of the muscles within these groups.

But, the new names created here should bring clarity to the location and function of some of the individual muscles that make up these complex groups. The names and functions of these muscles are still evolving, as has been shown with recent findings from Nikolai Bogduk[137] and Richardson et all.[138]

The previous names of 1) iliocostalis lumborum (also called iliocostalis lumborum pars thoracis) 2) longissimus thoracis (also called longissimus thoracis pars thoracis) 3) iliocostalis lumborum pars lumborum 4) longissimus thoracis pars lumborum, will be changed in this manual respectively to; 1) iliocostalis lumbothoracis 2) longissimus lumbothoracis 3) iliocostalis lumbar fascicles 4) longissimus lumbar fascicles.

Numbers 1 and 2 have been changed because the originals each describe muscles that arise from lumbosacral area and insert into the thoracic spine, yet one of them is named lumborum and the other thoracic, this is rather confusing. It seems simpler to add lumbothoracic to each (they both attach to the lumbar and thoracic area) and keep their well deserved roots of longissimus (it is longer and along the spine) and iliocostalis (it attaches to the ilium and ribs).

Numbers 3 and 4 have been changed because the ending pars lumborum is long and non-descriptive compared to fascicles, which already has the location described in the beginning of the name (lumbar). *Fascicles*, as described by Bogduk et all[80] are "a bundle of fibers that share the same origin and insertion, such that they exert forces on the same bones".

The complexity of the muscles along the spine can be better understood by separating them into two different groups 1) the superficial gross movers, which consist of long vertical fibers 2) the deep intervertebral stabilizers, which consist of short fibers that run more diagonal than vertical.

These two groups are intimately connected to each other as well as the different layers of fascia. Each muscle's functions will be described below in their appropriate section.

The Superficial Gross Movers

Latissimus Dorsi

Muscle Type – Hyperactive/Mobilizer and Global Stabilizer

Attachments

Origin – Through its medial unity with the LDF it attaches to the spinous processes of T7-L5, posterior 1/3 of iliac crest, and the sacrum

Insertion – Ribs 9-12, inferior angle of scapula (only sometimes), intertubercular groove of humerus, blends with teres major tendon and deep arm fascia

Innervation – Thoracodorsal nerve, C6-C8

Functions

Unilaterally

• Extends (especially past the back), medially rotates

(mostly when arm is abducted), and adducts the humerus
- Depresses and pulls backward on the ipsilateral shoulder and effects spinal posture throughout its entirety
- Side bends the torso to same side
- Assists in hip hiking (I/O)
- Can adduct scapula if attached to it
- Plays an important role in the mechanics and energy flow of walking, along with the LDF and opposite gluteus maximus, fig. 11-14
- Very active with overhead activities; swimming, chopping wood, chin-ups, etc.
- Stabilizes thoracolumbar spine, especially when arm is at side
- Contributes to force closure of S.I. joint during gait

Bilaterally

- Hyperextend the thoracic spine (arms at side)
- Generate lumbar extension moments and posterior shear forces in order to stabilize that area
- Very active during strong expiration (coughing and sneezing) and deep inhalation

Iliocostalis Lumbothoracis

Muscle Type – Hyperactive/Mobilizer

Attachments

Origin – Posterior and medial portion of iliac crest, sacrum, lumbar dorsal fascia (LDF), the spinous process of L5-T11, and sometimes gluteus maximus, also known as the lateral half of the erector spinae aponeurosis

Insertion – Inferior borders of the angles of ribs 6-12 and sometimes 3-12

Innervation – Collectively the erector spinae are innervated by the dorsal rami of spinal nerves, T1-T12, L1-L5, S1-S3

Functions

Unilaterally

- Side bending to same side
- Extension and rotation to same side
- Eccentrically controls deceleration or resists gravity during about the first 45 degrees of flexion and lateral bending to the opposite side, then contributes passive tension for the rest of the ROM

Bilaterally

- Extend the spine
- Anteriorly tilt the pelvis and thus increase lumbar lordosis (I/O)
- Decelerate flexion or maintain stooping of the spine (actively about the 1st 45° of spinal flexion, then passively contribute tension)
- Due to long tendons, they have a high extensor moment to compression penalty ratio (they exert a great extension force without creating great compression loads on the spine)
- Depress lower ribs and assist in coughing and straining to have a bowel movement
- Active during the end of inhalation and extreme exhalation (i.e. coughing)

Longissimus Lumbothoracis

Muscle Type – Hyperactive/Mobilizer

Attachments

Origin – Spinous processes of L1- S5 and across the sacrum to the PSIS, forming the medial half of the erector spinae aponeurosis

Insertion – Tips of transverse processes T1 or T2 – T12 and posterior surface of adjacent ribs T4-12

Functions

It has the same functions as iliocostalis lumbothoracis but with less influence on lateral bending. Collectively, the erector spinae on one side contribute to stabilizing the S.I. joint by creating force closure along with the lats, b.f., and Gmax muscles.

Spinalis Thoracis

Muscle Type – Undetermined/Global Stabilizer

Attachments

Origin – 4 musculotendon strips arising from the spinous processes of T11-L2 and medial portion of the corresponding longissimus muscle

Insertion – 4-8 musculotendon strips into the spinous processes of T1-T4, or sometimes T1-T8, and the corresponding medial border of longissimus

Innervation – Posterior primary divisions of the spinal nerves, as are the rest of the paraspinals

Functions

Unilaterally

- Assists side bending to same side
- Contributes resistance to lateral forward flexion of the spine away from the muscle via the erector spinae aponeurosis

Bilaterally

- Extend the thoracic spine
- Contribute resistance to forward flexion of the spine via the erector spinae aponeurosis

Iliocostalis Thoracis

Muscle Type – Undetermined

Attachments

Origin – Superior borders of ribs 7-12, just lateral to longissimus lumbothoracis

Insertion – Superior borders of ribs 1-6 and transverse process of C7

Functions
Bilaterally

- Extend the thoracic spine

Semispinalis Thoracis

Muscle Type – Undetermined/Global Stabilizer

Attachments

Origin – 5-6 musculotendonous strips arising from the transverse processes of T5 or T6-T10 or T11

Insertion – Spinous processes of C6-T4

Functions
Unilaterally

- Rotates the thoracic and cervical spines to the opposite side

Bilaterally

- Assist extending the thoracic spine

Functional Groups

See the abdominals for details on more groups.

Thoracic extension – erector spinae, latissimus dorsi, iliocostalis thoracis, spinalis thoracis, semispinalis thoracis, and to a small degree the deep paraspinals

Myofascial Lines – (erector spinae) superficial back and spiral lines – (latissimus) arm and back functional lines

Dysfunctional Group

Includes all muscles in the functional groups as well as the; entire posterior vertical (or nearly vertical) lines of fascia, cervical extensors, gastrocnemius (fascial connection), soleus (referred pain into S.I. joint), gluteus medius and minimus, iliacus, transverse abdominis, internal oblique, piriformis, ligaments of the spine and sacrum, pectoral muscles (when short it causes thoracic kyphosis), and the deep paraspinal muscles.

Descriptions

Latissimus Dorsi

The latissimus dorsi is briefly mentioned here for reasons other than its influence on shoulder mechanics and dysfunction. It affects the low back through three main factors 1) it creates an extension and stabilization force on the thoracolumbar spine via its extensive insertion into the LDF, 2) it connects the low back to the arms, and 3) it is part of an 'energy sling' that helps produce movement and transfer tension while creating force closure on the S.I. joint during gait, see fig. 11-14.

The latissimus dorsi is one of only three muscles that contributed to an L4-L5 posterior shearing force during a squat lift of 59.5 lbs (the weight was held in the hands), the other two muscles were the internal obliques and longissimus lumbar fascicles; even during full flexion the latissimus dorsi can produce a posterior shearing force on the lumbar spine.[37] This study points to the fact that the latissimus dorsi is more than just a mobilizer of the arm.

The condition of the latissimus dorsi is essential to the health of the underlying and connecting tissues. For example, if an athlete or worker overuses one muscle more than the other (tennis, volleyball, baseball, painter, brick layer, etc), that side will often become tight and restricted and cause the tissues underneath and nearby to become restricted and dysfunctional as well. This will then lead to an uneven and deficient stabilization system in the thoracolumbar spine, especially in regards to resisting anterior shear forces. Anterior shear forces are one of, if not the most important mechanism in preventing low back injuries.

Causes of Latissimus Dorsi Tightness
• Improper breathing patterns - bilateral
• Scoliosis concave towards the short side - unilateral
• Dominant side used in daily activity – unilateral
• Improper gait patterns – bi or unilateral

Effects of Latissimus Dorsi Tightness

- Altered lumbar joint mechanics – bi or unilateral
- Functional scoliosis concave towards the short side
- Ipsilateral shoulder depression and subsequent neck and shoulder imbalances - unilateral
- Hyperextension of the lumbar spine during overhead activities, i.e. swimming, painting, tennis or volleyball serving, basketball rebounding, etc. – bi or unilateral
- Altered gleno-humeral mechanics
- If one side is tight and the other weak, then it will reduce stability and force closure of the S.I. joint during gait[4]
- Reduced breathing capacity

Individual Assessments

ROM (supine arm flexion) and posture (shoulder level) assessments are described in chapters 12 and 13.

Corrective Actions

1. Improve any pain, faulty habits and shoulder level posture.
2. Apply manual therapy along the back, side, and shoulder; myofascial release is very effective on a tight latissimus dorsi, as well as across to the opposite hip to encourage torso rotation during gait and sports.
3. Stretch the short side.
4. Strengthen the weak side, emphasize integration into daily movements, i.e. walking, squatting, etc.
5. Integrate both sides together as a stabilizing system; standing straight arm pull backs with tubing and squats with arms at side resisting tubing from above are helpful.

The Q.L. is often weak and short on the same side as the weakness and shortness of the latissimus dorsi and it should therefore be corrected in conjunction with the corrective actions mentioned here.

Before the latisimuss dorsi can be trained as a stabilizing unit (right and left side together), the weaker side must be activated so that it is not inhibited by the stronger and more dominant side during routine movements and postures. This can be done by engaging the weak side against resistance and performing functional movements that involve the latissimus dorsi, i.e. 1) squats with arms at side and the weak arm resisting an anterior pull from tubing, while the strong arm is dangling without resistance, 2) strong side straight arm deltoid raises in all directions while the weak arm is at the side resisting an anterior pull from

tubing; this focuses on stabilizing against various forces.

Simply strengthening the weak side with isolated exercises does not engage the neuromuscular system in a manner that will create recruitment patterns which can overcome those of the dominant side and stabilize the thoracolumbar spine during daily movements.

This type of training can take months to achieve noticeable results due to the fact that many athletes have been so dominant on one side for most of their life and continue to do so on a daily basis. Correcting the imbalance between the two sides is not the goal as much as simply activating the weak side in order to enhance spinal stability is.

It is a good idea to continue special training the weak side as long as daily activities favor one side. It is also very beneficial to *stretch the short side immediately before performing exercises* that require great spinal stability, i.e. squats, plyometrics, etc.

Erector Spinae

The erector spinae consists of two muscles (iliocostalis and longissimus lumbothoracis) which are anchored into the sacrum, lumbar spine, and ilium by a broad, strong tendon called the erector spinae aponeurosis.

The longissimus and iliocostalis lumbothoracis muscles insert directly into this tendon, which also is continuous with some gluteus maximus fibers[54] and two separate myofascial lines (spiral and superficial back line) that connect the erector spinae to the sacrotuberous ligament, hamstrings, gastrocnemius, peroneus longus, and the plantar fascia, as well as the cervical and thoracic spine and head.[63]

Because of their extensive contiguity, an injury to the erector spinae can lead to dysfunctions in the LDF and along the related myofascial lines, or vice versa.

The erector spinae are prone to tightness and facilitation[43] with subsequent inhibition of the deeper stabilizers, yet they are often the main target for low back strengthening exercises. This can be injurious unless imbalances are corrected and a detailed understanding of the relationship between the superficial and deep paraspinal muscles is had before assigning specific erector spinae exercises to a problematic low back. See chapter 10 for details on strengthening the low back.

Due to their long lever arms and anatomy, longissimus and iliocostalis lumbothoracic produce the greatest amount of extensor force on the lumbar spine[37,144] with the uppermost segments having little to negative compressive impact on the lumbar spine[144] and the muscles as a whole contributing a minimum compressive penalty on the spine.[37] According to Bogduk et all,[144] the following muscles contribute certain percentages of overall extensor moment at L4-L5;

Total Extensor Moment at L4-L5

- Lumbothoracic Erector Spinae (50%)
- Lumbar Fascicles (30%)
- Multifidus (20%)

Because the erector spinae are 1) often overactive and tight 2) exert the most force on the lumbar spine 3) are unable to control intervertebral segments, stretching them (or massaging if stretching is contraindicated) and activating the deep stabilizers are key factors in avoiding injurious lumbar loads from improper vertebral alignment during daily and athletic activities.

When acting from a reverse origin and insertion (from a fixed thoracic spine), the lumbothoracic extensors can anteriorly tilt the pelvis, which if done too often or against resistance can cause faulty recruitment patterns during spinal extension in the form of a facilitated psoas and inhibited lower abdominals, as well as promoting a hyperlordotic posture. This is a common movement in yoga and physical therapy known as "cat and dog" or "pelvic tilts".

These positions are helpful as gentle movement exercises, but can put an enormous load on the facet joints if done vigorously or too many times. Another way this faulty recruitment pattern can occur is from an already *facilitated psoas muscle that inhibits the lower abdominals and gluteus maximus and creates a lumbar flexion-extension imbalance that anteriorly tilts the pelvis during activation of the erector spinae.*

An important biomechanical factor to note is that during standing spinal flexion the erector spinae have increasing contractile force that is directly proportional to the amount of spinal flexion until about 45°.[7] Then, on the way towards full flexion the ligaments[7] and connective tissue begin to take over carrying the load and the muscles begin to relax.[39,40]

The erector spinae contractions are eccentrically decelerating the torso down to around 45°, where they then start to reduce contractile force until they become "electrical silent."[37]

This electrical silence should not be misinterpreted as being uninvolved with carrying a load. The silent muscles still resist the movement with a substantial passive force during full spine flexion, which needs to be taken into account when constructing an exercise program with a goal of decreased posterior spinal muscle tension.[37] Tight erector muscles and fascia will

create an even greater passive tension on the area and thus increase the chance of injury. The combination of soft tissue and ligamentous interactions during flexion is reversed upon reextension. On a dysfunctional note, *the relaxation of the E.S. during forward flexion can be turned into excitation when pain is present.*[138]

The erector spinae can be completely relaxed when standing erect[142,143] while the multifidi have demonstrated almost uninterrupted patterns of activation during upright postures.[138] This is useful to know when palpating the low back of an upright person.

Causes of Erector Spinae Tightness

- Prolonged or repetitive bending on a daily basis
- Hyperlordotic posture and short psoas
- Joint dysfunctions or pain in the thoracic or lumbar spine
- Soft and sagging mattress
- Referred pain from psoas, multifidi, gluteus medius, R.A., serratus posterior inferior, intercostals, and latissimus dorsi
- Lower leg or pelvis inequality
- Scoliosis
- Latissimus dorsi tightness
- Sudden trauma of bending and lifting too much or in an awkward position, especially while fully flexed
- Total body leaning forward posture
- A closed mind or rigid demeanor; not willing to 'bend' with other's ideas
- Prolonged immobility (sitting, standing, or lying)
- Tight hamstrings, gastrocnemius, or plantar fascia
- Weak gluteus maximus or abdominal muscles
- Prolonged coughing
- No lumbar support or arm rests in chair
- Forward head posture
- Not stretching enough or properly
- Tightness in the contralateral erector spinae
- Improper gait or breathing patterns
- Compensation for inhibited multifidus
- Improper lifting techniques

Effects of Erector Spinae Tightness

- Inappropriate activation and subsequent lumbar spine overload during hip extension
- Excessive facet joint compression
- Trigger points along the erector spinae and referred pain into them, the low back, spine, and buttocks[7]
- Difficulty climbing stairs and rising from seated

- Restricted spinal mobility (inability to touch toes)
- Prone to low back strains
- Tight hamstrings, gastrocnemius, and plantar fascia
- Pain during sit-ups
- Lumbar hyperlordosis and short psoas - bilateral
- Tightness in the opposite side erector spinae
- Unstable force closure on S.I. joint – unilateral
- Improper gait patterns (usually hyperlordis)

Individual Assessments

ROM (sitting and standing flexion), posture (lordosis and kpyphosis), and PMAP (prone hip extension) assessments are described in chapters 12 and 13.

Corrective Actions

1. Improve any pain, bad habits (slouching, improper lifting, ergonomics, soft bed, not utilizing the Gmax while stooping over the sink, etc.), improper breathing patterns, and structural abnormalities. Also, sometimes the association of a more open mind and thus flexible spine is enough to change a restrictive attitude and improve tightness along the back.
2. Apply manual therapy along the erector spinae, spine, posterior hip, Q.L., abdominals, psoas, and wherever else tension is influencing the spine.
3. Stretch (massage if stretching is contraindicated) erector spinae, hamstrings, and gastrocnemius.
4. Strengthen the abdominals if appropriate.
5. Correct influential posture imbalances, i.e. hyperlordosis, forward head, etc.

Most often the erector spinae do not need specific strengthening exercises, instead they need a balanced supporting myofascial system, strong abdominals, regular walking or jogging, exercises that include them but do not place high loads on the lumbar spine (unless daily activities require it, i.e. athletes), and proper lifting and sitting postures in order to be healthy. See chapter 13 &14 for details on strengthening exercises

In cases of LBP or injury, the deep paraspinal muscles, in particular the multifidus, atrophy (due to inhibition) and require special strengthening exercises with the exclusion of erector spinae exercises.[138] See multifidus description below for details.

The Thoracic Erectors

Iliocostalis thoracis, spinalis thoracis, and semispinalis thoracis will be described here together for the function they all have in common, thoracic extension. Some anatomy books consider the iliocoastalis thoracis and spinalis thoracis muscles part of the erector spinae, but they will be considered separately here as a thoracic extensor group to emphasize their main function. It should be kept in mind however that they both can relay stress to and from the erector spinae aponeurosis via their contiguous insertions into the longissimus and iliocostalis lumbothoracis muscles.

Because all three are situated on a kyphotic curve, they are under different stresses then the lumbar extensors and are most often elongated and weak compared to the overactive erector spinae. If these muscles are not strong enough or they are inhibited, then the lower portions of the erector spinae will be left with the duties of extending the spine and resisting flexion forces without the assistance of a tensed posterior passive system coming from the thoracic spine.

The thoracic segments should "lead the way" (along with the legs and abdominal muscles) during spinal extension when coming out of flexion so that 1) the spine can become vertical and shear forces are reduced as soon as possible 2) there is simultaneous tensing of the posterior myofascial system from above (thoracic extensors), in between (abdominals and multifidus), and below (hamstrings and gluteus maximus), meanwhile the smaller lumbar muscles stabilize the lumbar spine in a neutral position and the erector spinae assist the leg muscles in pulling the properly tensed torso upright.

This is very difficult when there is pain in the low back because it causes the superficial lumbar muscles (gross movers) to become overactive and rob the thoracic muscles of their impulses while the deep lumbar stabilizers (mostly the multifidi and T.A.) become inhibited from local pain stimuli.

Increased thoracic kyphosis (usually due to slouching posture) stretches the posterior elements of the thoracolumbar spine and leads to the elongation (eventually becoming permanent) of the posterior passive system all the way down to the sacrum. Slowly overtime or with one traumatic event, this elongation creates laxity in the passive support system, most importantly in the posterior longitudinal ligament (PLL), which leaves it more vulnerable to injury and less able to stabilize the vertebrae against flexion forces.

This is important to the low back because the PLL is 1) capable of producing pain and proprioceptive feedback[145] 2) is thinnest in the lumbar sections (the lower the thinner)[54,145] 3) stabilizes against flexion stress[54,145] 4) is the final barricade to herniated disc material before it reaches the nerve roots and spinal cord. In other words, prolonged or excessive stretching of the PLL due to faulty flexion postures can cause a weakened or damaged PLL that is more likely to cause LBP, disrupt spinal proprioception, and allow herniated disc material to penetrate into the spinal cord and nerve roots.

Therefore, reducing excessive thoracic kyphosis is of the utmost importance in preventative maintenance for the low back and is done by strengthening and activating the thoracic extensor muscles along with practicing good posture during sitting, standing, and lifting.

With practice, an isolated thoracic extension can be done without much involvement from the cervical or lumbar regions and little stress placed on the lumbar spine, see Stage I corrective exercise for details on thoracic strengthening. This is helpful when trying to "wake up" the thoracic extensors from inhibition due to lumbar portion dominance.

It is also important to note that this muscle group is commonly involved with emotional or attitudinal stress that involves a lack of inner strength or pride, i.e. head down and shoulders forward posture. Often times a change in attitude (standing tall with shoulders back) will activate these muscles when exercises fail to do so.

Causes of Thoracic Erector Weakness

- Tight pectorals and excessive thoracic kyphosis
- Overactive erector spinae
- Short upper abdominals
- Referred pain from erector spinae, R.A., latissimus dorsi, multifidi, and intercostal muscles
- Inability to stand up tall and meet challenges, feeling closed off towards others, or feeling the weight of the world on shoulders
- Daily activities that involve prolonged hunching over, i.e. roofer, desk jockey, gardener, crop picker, dentist, being tall and constantly looking down, etc.

Effects of Thoracic Erector Weakness

- Excessive thoracic kyphosis, forward head posture, and compression of the brachial plexus
- Elongation of thoracolumbar posterior passive system
- Mid and low back pain from trigger points in the paraspinal muscles
- Injurious compensations are made in the superficial cervical and lumbar erectors during quick extension movements
- Aches in the thoracic spine from strained posterior ligaments
- Improper breathing patterns

- Poor overall upright balance due to altered center of gravity

Individual Assessments

ROM (sitting and standing flexion) and posture (thoracic kpyphosis) assessments are described in chapters 12 and 13.

Corrective Actions

1. Improve any pain, faulty postures, and bad habits (slouching, improper lifting, ergonomics, poor attitude, etc.).
2. Release any trigger points along the erector spinae, pectoralis major, upper abdominals, or neck flexors.
3. Strengthen with isolated thoracic extensions, then incorporate into functional movements, especially lifting.
4. Stretch pectorals, upper abdominals, and lumbar spine if appropriate.
5. Correct influential posture imbalances, i.e. hyperlordosis, forward head, etc.

These muscles should first be trained in an isolated environment in order to keep the overactive erector spinae from taking over. This can be done by first learning how to activate the transverse abdominis and lumbar multifidi muscles while keeping a neutral spine position, then the thoracic extensors can operate on a stable foundation without any lumbar movement. This exercise takes a lot of practice for some people at first so patience is essential.

The Deep Intervertebral Stabilizers

Iliocostalis Lumbar Fascicles

Muscle Type – Undetermined/Local Stabilizer

Attachments

Origin – Crest of ilium just above PSIS

Insertion – Tips of transverse processes L1-L4 and corresponding posterior surface of middle layer of the LDF, and the iliolumbar ligament

Functions

Unilaterally

- Assist side bending and extension to same side
- Assist in resisting lateral bending, rotation, and flexion away from the muscle

Bilaterally

- Extend the lumbar vertebrae
- Exert a posterior shear force on the lumbar vertebrae, i.e. assist in resisting flexion forces on lumbar vertebrae, but mostly when the spine is extended (lordotic lifting posture)

Longissimus Lumbar Fascicles

Muscle Type – Undetermined/Local Stabilizer

Attachments

Origin – Tips of accessory processes of L1-L4 and posterior surface of the L5 transverse process

Insertion – Just above and medial to PSIS

Functions

They have the same functions as the iliocostalis lumbar fascicles but with less influence on lateral bending.

Lumbar Multifidus

Muscle Type – Hypoactive/Local Stabilizer

Attachments

Origin – Sacrum (as low as S4), erector spinae aponeurosis, medial surface of PSIS, sacroiliac ligaments, and mamillary processes of lumbar vertebrae

Insertion –Spinous processes of superior vertebrae, can span 2-4 vertebrae

Functions

Unilaterally

- Fine tune movements of lumbar flexion, rotation, and side bending

Bilaterally

- Assist extending the lumbar spine
- Control flexion and anterior translation of the vertebrae
- Primarily concerned with stabilization and fine tuning movements between vertebrae

Rotatorers (longus and brevis)

Muscle Type – Hypoactive/Local Stabilizer

Attachments

Origin – Transverse processes of each vertebrae, the rotatores are not always present in the lumbar spine

Insertion – Spinous processes of 1st (brevis) and 2nd (longus) vertebrae above

Functions

Unilaterally

- Gives proprioceptive feedback on intersegmental positions, with an emphasis on rotation
- Assist in contralateral rotation (debatable)

Bilaterally

- Assist extending the spine

Interspinalis

Muscle Type - Hypoactive/Local Stabilizer

Attachments

Origin – One on each side of the lumbar spinous processes connecting it to the adjacent spinous process

Insertion – Spinous processes of adjacent vertebrae

Functions

Same as the rotatores muscles but with more emphasis on extension than rotation

Intertransversarii

Muscle Type – Hypoactive/Local Stabilizer

Attachments

Origin – Pairs of muscles situated medially and laterally that connect adjacent transverse processes

Insertion – Transverse process of adjacent vertabrae

Functions

- Gives proprioceptive feedback on intersegmental positions, most likely focused on lateral bending away from the muscle

Functional Groups

Intersegmental proprioceptive feedback – surrounding fascia, spinal ligaments, joint receptors, and the rotatores, interspinales, and intertransversarii muscles
See abdominals for details on more groups.

Dysfunctional Group

Same as functional group plus the gluteuls, deep posterior myofascial system, and the soleus (referred pain into S.I. joint).

Descriptions

Iliocostalis and Longissimus Lumbar Fascicles

These muscles, or fascicles of the larger lumbothoracic erector spinae, have been anatomically and functionally separated by Bogduk[137]; this separation has improved the understanding of how paraspinal muscles share the responsibilities of different loading situations.

Compared to the lumbar multifidus, these fascicles are better suited for producing extension torque and controlling spinal orientation but probably do not have as much ability for individual segment control.[138]

The lumbar fascicles can create a posterior shearing force on the lumbar vertebrae if the spine is extended[37], but besides the latissimus dorsi, this force is not noticeably assisted by any other paraspinal muscle. However, all three deep lumbar muscles (the fascicles and multifidus) resist anterior translation of the vertebrae during flexion.[138]

Posterior shearing force is necessary to counteract the dangerous anterior shearing forces of forward flexion movements, but the lumbar spine must be extended in order for the lumbar fascicles to have the leverage to exert this force.[37] The internal obliques and transverse abdominus muscles on the other hand can create posterior shearing forces in any posture (via the LDF).[40]

Whether these fascicles become facilitated or inhibited with dysfunction remains undetermined and thus corrective actions are difficult to ascertain. But the relevance of describing these muscles is the fact that with their assistance, the lumbar spine is best prepared to resist anterior shearing forces when in a position of natural lordosis as opposed to flexion. Specific exercises are probably not needed as long as lifting techniques utilize this position.

Lumbar Multifidus

Of all the paraspinal muscles, the lumbar multifidi are the one group that has been scientifically shown to consistently correlate with LBP. While it is common to find structural abnormalities in people *without* LBP, only 1-5% of normal subjects were found to have abnormalities in the multifidus muscle.[154,155]

The lumbar multifidus atrophies quickly (in one person studied atrophy was seen within 24 hours of the onset of pain[146]) and drastically (25% smaller on side of pain at the L5 level[147]) in response to LBP, many times unilaterally. The atrophy is thought to occur so fast because of inhibition, not disuse.[138]

It is the largest muscle crossing the lumbosacral junction[148] and thus is most responsible for stabilizing this area, which coincidently is the most common site (L4-S1) of pathology in low back pain.[138] The multifidi account for about two-thirds of the total stiffness in the spine created by muscular contractions.[149]

Additional to its segmental (vertebrae to vertebrae) attachments, the lumbar multifidi are also segmentally innervated[137,138,148,149], this strengthens the idea that they are capable of fine tuning intersegmental movements. However, even the relatively small multifidus can be broken down into different functions depending on the fibers or fascicles activated.

Richardson et all[138] believe that the superficial fibers produce extension torque and the deep fibers stabilize the vertebrae; this may be one reason why the multifidus muscle has been reported to be overactive in response to disc herniations[258] but in other studies is atrophied in response to disc herniations[197,198] and low back pain.[146,147]

Another reason for the confusion of how to classify the multifidus muscle (as hypo or hyperactive) is that some conclusions were based on EMG results which used surface electrodes; surface electrodes have been found to measure the activity of the erector spinae more than the deep multifidus and are thus not an accurate measure of multifidus activity.[196]

With all that said, there are too many conflicting study's to base a classification on, therefore, clinical wisdom must prevail until further evidence shows agreement on the responses to dysfunction for the multifidus muscle.

This author will base his conclusions on the facts that the multifidus is an obvious essential local one joint stabilizer that becomes deconditioned when sedentary or when training predominantly focuses on the mobilizers, i.e. most athletes or fitness people. Therefore it will be classified as hypoactive.

However, a thought to ponder is that due to its segmental innervation, segmental attachments, and different set of functions depending on fiber location, it is possible that the superficial fascicles or layers of the multifidus could be facilitated while the deeper portion inhibited. In other words, they could have opposite responses to dysfunction, yet still be a part of the same larger muscle. Unfortunately this is impossible to quantify with current technology.

As a unit, the multifidi control lumbar lordosis, increase segmental stiffness, and have the greatest influence on stability in the lumbar spine.[138] Multifidi's impact on stability is reinforced by these findings; 1) multifidus and transverse abdominis activity is independent of the direction of reactive forces[150,151], meaning they stabilize against any force, as opposed to the superficial global trunk muscles which are linked to the direction of forces acting on the spine[150,152,153], meaning they only stabilize against specific forces 2) deep multifidus activity is tonic during repetitive arm movement and in upright postures[151] 3) multifidus has tonic activity during walking.[187]

The multifidus is part of an inner unit that is activated to stabilize against any stress placed on the spine, while the larger and more superficial gross movers mostly react to stresses that oppose their normal function.

Another finding that solidifies the stabilizing role of multifidus is that when stimulated, the mechanoreceptors in the supraspinous ligament, facet joints, and lumbar intervertebral discs have been shown to cause reflex recruitment of the multifidus in order to stabilize the spine.[29]

Fortunately, attaining this segmental stabilization requires only a small percentage of the maximum voluntary contraction of the multifidus, although unstable joints, i.e. sponylolisthesis, lax ligaments, etc, will need additional support. [138]

A study by Hides et all[146] measured the cross sectional area (CSA) of the lumbar multifidus in 26 people with first episode acute unilateral LBP with an average duration of 2 weeks and in 51 normal subjects.

They found that *atrophy of the multifidus occurs on the same side and level of the spine as the pain.* A follow up study by Hides et all[147] measured 39 subjects with acute first episode unilateral LBP and unilateral segmental inhibition of the multifidus. They were randomly placed in a control (non-active treatment) or treatment group (multifidus activation exercises like those in this manual). The following highlights were discovered:

1. LBP subsided in 4 weeks in nearly everybody, regardless of which group they were in.
2. Atrophy of the multifidus occurs on the same side and level of the spine as the pain.
3. Multifidus atrophy normalized in 4 weeks in the treatment group, but atrophy remained in the control group at 10 weeks.
4. The difference in multifidus CSA(%) between left and right side was 5x higher at L5 compared to L2-L4 and S1 (the side with pain was much smaller).
5. 1 year post-treatment, recurrence in treatment group was 30% compared to 84% in control group.

6. 2-3 years post-treatment, recurrence was 35% in treatment group and 75% in control group.
7. After 1 year, subjects in control group were 12.4x more likely to suffer recurrences of LBP than those in the treatment group.
8. After 2-3 years, subjects in control group were 9x more likely to suffer recurrences of LBP than those in the treatment group.
9. *After LBP is no longer present, the multifidus does not automatically return to normal functioning,* specific exercises are necessary to achieve improvement. See pg. 185 for details on specific activation techniques.

Causes of Multifidus Dysfunction

- Low back pain[138]
- Lumbar instability
- Facet syndrome[84]
- Weak abdominals[138]
- Overactive erector spinae
- Poor posture
- Sedentary lifestyle

Effects of Multifidus Dysfunction

- Decreased intervertebral stability
- Prone to low back injury and pain
- Inability to maintain upright lordotic postures and subsequent compensation of superficial paraspinal muscles
- Multifidus myofascial syndrome can imitate sacroiliac syndrome[84]
- Facet syndrome[84]
- Referred pain into the low back and buttocks from TP's[7]

Individual Assessments

The PMAP assessment for multifidus is described in chapter 12. Palpation close to the spine that is tender and refers pain downward is a sign of multifidus dysfunction and trigger point location.

Corrective Actions

1. Improve any pain, faulty postures, bad habits (slouching, improper lifting, ergonomics, soft bed, etc.).
2. Apply manual therapy to any areas that are creating faulty lumbar posture, restricted LDF, or referring pain to the multifidus.
3. Activate the multifidus and transverse abdominis muscles with specific exercises as mentioned on pg.'s

184-185 and follow the guidelines for Stage I of Exercise Progression, then progress accordingly.

4. Once the goal for strengthening the multifidus is attained, performing the exercises 1x per week at the same intensity is all that is needed to maintain the benefits.[149]

5. Manual therapy may need to be applied directly to the deeper paraspinal muscles, including any trigger points in the multifidus, in order to restore proper proprioceptive feedback in the lumbar spine.

Stage I for acute LBP sufferer's should last at least 4 weeks; this is the time it takes for the CSA of multifidus to increase back to normal (see study above). For chronic LBP sufferer's, activation exercises are not enough, the addition of load is necessary to strengthen and increase the CSA of the multifidus[158], such as in Stages III and IV.

Once LBP is present, it doesn't matter what kind of fitness level the person has, the multifidus will be dysfunctional. Roy et all[171] found that *highly trained athletes (male rowers) with LBP had higher fatigue rates in the multifidus than their asymptomatic teammates.*

Therefore, no matter how well trained someone with LBP is, these simple activation exercises are necessary to prevent and improve LBP.

Rotatores, Interspinales, and Intertransversarii

These three muscles are the main source of muscular proprioception for intervertebral movements. They have little leverage to create great motion but are well suited (high muscle spindle density) to relay vertebrae position to the rest of the stabilizing "team".

The rotatores have a misleading name, because they don't seem to rotate anything at all. Donisch and Basmajian[159] believed that the deep paraspinal muscles act by fine tuning small movements between vertebrae, and Mcgill[37] concluded that the intertransversarii and rotatores act as "position transducers in the spine proprioception system".

Basmajian and De Luca[142] experimentally showed through EMG testing that the deep paraspinal muscles were activated with rotation to the opposite side, which is what McGill[37] found with EMG testing of a suspected rotator muscle.

So it seems that instead of creating torque, these muscles react to motion in the vertebrae, as if they were *active ligaments.* This behavior coincides with findings from Nitz and Peck[160] that the rotatores and intertransversarii muscles have 4.5-7.3 times more muscle spindles than the multifidus. Bogduk[137] also

mentions the probable function of the intertransversarii and interspinales muscles is to provide proprioceptive feedback to the nearby muscles via their muscle spindles. McGill[37] showed as well that the rotatores do not activate with isometric twisting force (the abdominal obliques do) but are active in rotation to the opposite side.

This information is significant because it emphasizes the importance of muscular balance throughout the spine as well as having strong abdominals to support the deeper muscles (if the abdominals cannot maintain stability, then excess vertebral motion results and the deep paraspinal muscles become overloaded).

Manual therapy directly on or near the vertebrae is also beneficial in order to release trigger points and restore proper proprioception and coordination throughout the spine and therefore the entire body.

Causes of Intervertebral Muscle Dysfunction

- Low back or spinal pain
- Lumbar instability
- Weak abdominals
- Poor posture
- Sedentary lifestyle

Effects of Intervertebral Muscle Dysfunction

- Decreased intervertebral stability
- Prone to low back injury and pain
- Poor balance, coordination, and proprioception skills

Individual Assessments

Palpation along the vertebrae that produces a local pain is a sign of deep paraspinal muscle involvement (it also points to ligament and facet joint patholgy).

Corrective Actions

1. Improve any pain, faulty postures, and bad habits.
2. Manual therapy if local tender points are palpated.
3. Strengthen the abdominals.
4. Proprioception and stabilization training.

Lumbar Dorsal Fascia (LDF)

Superficial Layer

Attachments

Origin – Serratus posterior, transverse abdominis, internal oblique, the outer lip of the iliac crest, and the aponeurosis of latissimus dorsi

Insertion – Tips of spinous processes at midline of lumbar and sacral vertebrae and their supraspinous ligaments, the ipsilateral erector spinae and gluteus maximus aponeurosis, where it then crosses over to the contralateral latissimus dorsi, gluteus maximus, and erector spinae aponeurosis

Functions

- Relays a stabilizing extension force on the thoracolumbar spine that resists anterior shear forces on the vertebrae, although the spine should be extended for best results
- Relays forces from the arms to the posterior passive system via the lats, i.e. when lifting
- Diffuses tension during gait via movement of the torso on the hips, the faster the gait the better the diffusion (see fig. 11-14)

Middle Layer

Attachments

Origin – Aponeurosis of transverse abdominis and internal oblique, and posterior aspect of Q.L.

Insertion – Tips of lumbar transverse processes and their intertransverse ligaments, 12th rib, and iliac crest

Functions

- Relays a stabilizing extension force on the lumbar spine via activation of the transverse abdominis and internal oblique muscles, regardless of the spine's position
- Works with superficial layer to inhibit expansion of the erector spinae, lumbar fascicles, and multifidus, thus increasing their ability to produce axial tension and stabilization forces

Deep Layer

Attachments

Origin –Lateral lumbocostal arch, anterior aspect of Q.L., and the aponeurosis of transverse abdominis, and internal oblique

Insertion – Anterior aspects of the lumbar transverse processes, iliolumbar ligament, and the iliac crest

Functions

- Works with the middle layer to inhibit expansion of the Q.L., thus increasing its (the Q.L.) ability to

produce axial tension and stabilization forces

Functional Groups

Myofascial Lines – superficial back line, functional back line, and spiral line

Description

Before describing one part of the fascia system (the LDF) it is best to begin by briefly defining some qualities of fascia. Starting at the microscopic level, fascia is one form of connective tissue (mostly collagen fibers) that consists of connective tissue cells specializing in the secretion of a wide variety of substances into the intercellular space.[63]

These secretions supply the bones, ligaments, tendons, and cartilage, thus forming the strong, pliable environment which holds us together and is the medium for all cells to communicate in.[63]

According to Gray[28], "The term extracellular matrix (ECM) is applied to the sum total of extracellular substance within the connective tissue" and "it also provides the physico-chemical environment of the cells imbedded in it, forming a framework to which they can move, maintaining an appropriate porous, hydrated, ionic milieu, through which metabolites and nutrients can diffuse freely."

The connective tissue cells and their secretions have been said to act as our 'organ of form'.[163] This organ of form or connective tissue web separates our fluids into different areas which are all connected to the next, each one organized in a manner that has evolved from genetics and the stresses placed on it, ideally in a manner that allows fluids to flow smoothly and structures to efficiently resist gravity.

The mechanical barriers and immune cells of fascia and connective tissue act as a defense mechanism in cases of infection or toxicity.[4]

Certain stresses, such as sedentary lifestyle, dehydration, or repetitive trauma can cause clogging or adhesions that reduce the stream of nutrients to and from the cells, as well as reduce the extensibility of the fascia[4,63], fortunately, the appropriate manual therapy technique (can reverse these physiologic changes by opening up hydro-attractive channels of flow[118] that will alter the ECM from a gel-like substance to a more liquid state.[4,63,119]

This process is essential to health because the ground substance of connective tissue consists of immune cells among the many other types of cells that are necessary for rebuilding, inflammatory response, sensory input, and more. Fascia also contains proprioceptors (Ruffini and Pacinian corpuscles)[168] and is *likely to play an essential proprioceptive role* in the body, especially in regards to posture.[30,31,32]

Moving on to the macroscopic level, fascia cannot be separated from muscle and is thus often referred to as the myofascial system. The body is physically supported by three main systems, 1) musculoskeletal 2) ligamentous 3) myofascial. Fascia is unique in that it has different layers and is interconnected with the muscles, bones, ligaments, tendons, nerves, blood vessels, organs, skin, and other fascia throughout the entire body.

It can be thought of as an encompassing fibrous network that resembles a giant spider web inside the body, with the holes of the web being filled with organs, muscles, bones, nerves, blood vessels, etc. As Thomas Myers[63] describes it, "There is only one muscle; it just hangs around in 600 or more fascial pockets."

An important difference between muscle and fascia is that *muscle acts like elastic and fascia like plastic.*[63,161,162] This means that a muscle will attempt to recoil back to its original length when stretched, but fascia will lengthen and retain this deformation if stretched slow enough, or tear if stretched too fast.

However, the body will eventually build new fibers and reconnect the newly lengthened area if it is not routinely stretched or mobilized.[63] Because the fascia is continuous from head to toe, dysfunctions or adhesions in one area will eventually travel along the stress lines and layer levels of the connective tissues and create problems at the weakest links, even if they are at the opposite end of the body.

Now back to one small section of myofascia system. The LDF is made up of three layers which start out as a thin deep layer and end up as a thick and strong superficial layer.[169] The LDF, also called the thoracolumbar fascia, is an integral part of lumbar stabilization because of its potential to produce an extensor moment that resists anterior shearing forces on the vertebrae during flexion.[37,40,82,91,106,167]

This stabilizing extension force is best activated while the spine is in a neutral position, but it is possible to activate it throughout all spinal postures via the internal obliques and transverse abdominis muscles.[40]

It is unknown exactly how much extensor moment it can handle, and is even thought to contribute only small or negligible amounts of extension force[164,165,166], but with its amplifying affect on axial stress through contractions of the Q.L., multifidus, erector spinae, and lumbar fascicles, in conjunction with the stabilizing roles of the multifidi and lumbar fascicles, the LDF plays a vital role in stabilizing the lumbar spine, especially against anterior shear forces.

Restricted or tight LDF can be the result of many dysfunctions that can then lead to new dysfunctions, i.e. a short and tight latissimus dorsi can cause the LDF to strain and lead to altered force closure of the S.I. joint and eventually plantar fasciitis on either or both sides.

This chain of events must be broken down in order to find the cause; releasing restricted LDF gives only temporary relief (and is possibly harmful if it is serving to protect underlying tissues) if a muscle or tight fascia elsewhere is the culprit.

In a study of individual muscle and passive tissue forces and moments during *full flexion*, McGill[37] found that the LDF created more compression and force than any muscle while assisting the Q.L., internal obliques, latissimus dorsi, lumbar fascicles, and articular ligaments in resisting anterior shearing forces.

The interspinous, supraspinous, and posterior longitudinal ligaments contributed the most individual forces and compression during full flexion, although the LDF created a little more force than the posterior longitudinal ligament.

Causes of Restricted LDF

- Short latissmus dorsi
- Short biceps femoris
- Dehydration
- Nearby instability
- Poor posture
- Poor nutrition
- Sedentary lifestyle

Effects of Restricted LDF

- Decreased intervertebral stability – mostly with a unilateral restriction
- Altered joint mechanics in the thoracolumbar and lumbosacral spines during gait or any other motion that involves the arms and the torso
- Prone to low back injury and pain
- Decreased ability to re-hydrate the low back during and after rigorous activity, therefore leading to premature fatigue and soreness

Individual Assessments

Palpate the LDF by utilizing myofascial release (MFR) hand positioning (see pg.'s 175-176) and noticing any restrictions. There should be a natural 'give' in the underlying tissues when myofascial release techniques are applied.

Corrective Actions

1. Improve any pain, faulty postures, gait patterns, or bad habits (sedentary lifestyle, not enough water, dominant latissimus dorsi, etc.).

2. Learn how to properly activate the CORE.

3. Stretch any short influential muscles, such as the hamstrings and latissimus dorsi.

4. Strengthen latissimus dorsi and abdominal obliques if needed

5. Apply MFR and other appropriate manual therapy techniques to the LDF and any other influential restricted areas.

Gluteus Maximus

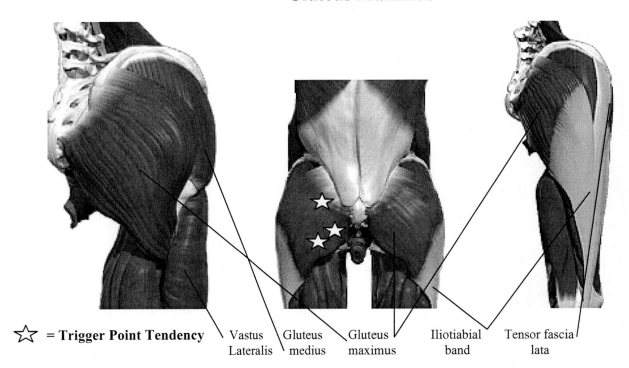

☆ = **Trigger Point Tendency**   Vastus Lateralis   Gluteus medius   Gluteus maximus   Iliotiabial band   Tensor fascia lata

Gluteus Maximus

Muscle Type – Hypoactive/Global Stabilizer and situational Mobilizer (hip extension with knee flexed)

Attachments

Origin – Posterolateral sacrum, sacral and gluteus medius fascia, lumbar fascia (LDF), sacrotuberous and sacroiliac ligaments, side of the coccyx, erector spinae aponeurosis, and the posterior border of the ilium and iliac crest

Insertion – The bulk of the muscle attaches into a thick tendinous band that fuses with the iliotibial band of the TFL, while the deep lower fibers attach into the gluteal tuberosity between the insertions of vastus lateralis and adductor magnus

Innervation – Inferior gluteul nerve (L5-S2)

Functions

Unilaterally

• Powerful extender of the thigh during strenuous activity; jumping, running, standing from seated position, climbing hills or stairs, etc.
• Assists lateral rotation of the thigh
• Assists hip abduction (mostly upper fibers)

Bilaterally

• Same as unilaterally plus the following;
• Assist in maintaining erect posture while standing and walking (I/O)
• Stabilize the pelvis through an elastic sling that connects one shoulder to the opposite femur via the gluteus maximus, LDF, and contralateral latissimus dorsi; this relationship is essential during gait
• Assist in trunk extension by pulling down on the pelvis, especially in the last few degrees of extending out of a flexed position (I/O)
• Posteriorly tilt the pelvis (I/O)

Functional and Dysfunctional Groups

See the abdominals, iliopsoas, and hip adductors for details on functional groups for hip flexion, extension, and abduction, and spine extension and flexion, hip rotation, and tilting of the pelvis

Myofascial Lines – back functional line and lateral line

Description

The gluteus maximus is an important assistant to the spinal extensors and a main mobilizer of hip extension, especially with intense activities. It plays an essential role in maintaining upright posture while standing and walking; unfortunately it is often weak, which

132

overloads the erector spinae and hamstring muscles and creates excessive forces in the lumbar spine.

Once this muscle is weak, it forces the erector spinae muscles to constantly pick up the slack during forward bending (leaning over the sink, walking uphill, lifting techniques, etc.), which causes them (erector spinae) to become chronically sore, tight, and tired.

It also forces the hamstrings to overwork during hip extension, not to mention the extra work that the erector spinae muscles have to do to stabilize the pelvis during this movement; this faulty recruitment pattern results in lumbar extension during hip extension and unnecessary stress in the lumbar spine.

In order to achieve low back health, it is necessary to have a strong gluteus maximus that activates during lifting techniques and hip extension, as well as walking and standing postures.

Causes of Weak Gluteus Maximus

- Prolonged sitting or laying, sedentary lifestyle
- Overactive hip flexors and hyperlordosis
- Overactive erector spinae and hamstring muscles
- Pelvic asymmetries or local joint dysfunctions or pain

Effects of Weak Gluteus Maximus

- Low back pain
- Decrease hip extension and therefore decreased ability to stabilize against flexion forces
- Altered muscle recruitment during hip extension that results in high loads in the lumbar spine
- Decreased hip flexion if muscle is also tight from adhesions
- Difficulty rising out of chairs, walking uphill, climbing stairs, etc., all of which are likely to cause pain when active TP's are present in the muscle[8]

- Altered gait patterns, leading to compensations in the contralateral latissimus dorsi and ipsilateral hamstring muscles that eventually effect their resting length
- Allows anterior tilting of the pelvis and a resulting hyperlordosis and overactive psoas
- Inferior migration of the ipsilateral pelvis, resulting in a lowering of the gluteal fold and ilium[55]
- Increased lumbar lordosis with scoliosis resulting towards weak side[55]
- Slight flexion of all major joints in the lower limb[55]
- Lowered hip during standing/walking on weak side

Individual Assessments

ROM (hip flexion), posture (knee flexion, ilium height, femur rotation, lordosis, gluteal fold, and lumbar scoliosis), and PMAP (prone hip extension) assessments are described in chapters 12 and 13.

Corrective Actions

1. Improve any pain, faulty postures (hyperlordosis, forward head, thoracic kyphosis, etc.) or bad habits (sleeping on back or side without pillows under or between legs, sitting on a wallet in the pocket, etc.).
2. Apply manual therapy where appropriate to improve pain and compensations, especially in the hip flexors, hamstrings, and erector spinae.
3. Strengthen/activate the gluteus maximus with simple, isolated exercises, as well as practice activating it during gait.
4. Stretch the hip flexors into hip extension, but only as far as the gluteus maximus can control, i.e. use active stretching techniques and make sure that the erector spinae are not activating and causing lumbar extension.
5. Progress strengthening exercises to include lifting techniques and explosive movements.

The Deep Six Hip Stabilizers

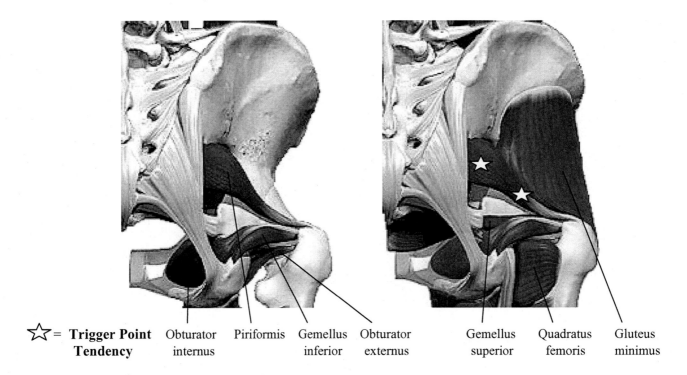

☆ = **Trigger Point
Tendency**

Obturator
internus

Piriformis

Gemellus
inferior

Obturator
externus

Gemellus
superior

Quadratus
femoris

Gluteus
minimus

The Deep Six Hip Stabilizers

- Piriformis
- Gemellus Superior
- Obturatur Internus
- Gemellus Inferior
- Obturatur Externus
- Quadratus Femoris

The piriformis will be the focus here, but it cannot be talked about without mentioning the other five muscles that work closely together with the piriformis in extending, rotating, and stabilizing the hip. The six muscles listed above are commonly referred to as rotators, which they are, but as Thomas Myers[204] points out; "…their primary role is that of stabilization, and particularly, stabilizing the hip in an extended position on the femur." and "….they are so important to good posture and dynamic core support….".

Anatomically, the other five muscles are located just below the piriformis, some of them merging together at their attachment sites and others commonly absent in some people. These muscles seem to act more like local stabilizers while the piriformis acts like both a global stabilizer and mobilizer.

The piriformis is the most troublesome muscle out of the group because of three main differences 1) it is the only one to attach to the sacrum 2) it consistently houses trigger points 3) it is capable of causing neural entrapments.

As a whole, these six muscles seem to act as the rotator cuff of the hip joint, mainly preparing and stabilizing the joint for action. They can create movement, such as lateral rotation, in certain positions but they are best equipped as stabilizers.

Piriformis

Muscle Type – Hyperactive/Global Stabilizer and situational Mobilizer

Attachments

Origin – Anterior surface of the sacrum around the second and third anterior sacral foramina; some fibers may attach to the margin of the greater sciatic foramen at the capsule of the S.I. joint and to the sacrotuberous ligamament

Insertion – Medial superior surface of the greater trochanter, often times blending together with the common tendon of obturator internus and the gemelli muscles

Innervation – Sacral plexus (L5-S2)

Functions

- Laterally rotates the femur, mostly when it is already extended*
- Medially rotates the thigh once it's flexed past 60º
- Abducts the thigh when the hip is flexed 90º
- Brings the posterior inferior pelvis and sacrum towards the ipsilateral trochanter, rotating the trunk away, i.e. when standing on 1 leg (I/O)
- Assists in locking the S.I. (piriformis only) joint and stabilizing the pelvis*, ensuring a stable foundation as the other leg is mobilized (soccer kick)
- Stabilizes the bottom of the spine, via the sacrum, by making small adjustments to side leaning – left muscle resists leaning to the left
- Alternates contractions during gait in order to lock the S.I. joint in the support phase or heel strike

Bilaterally

- Keep the sacrum (piriformis only), pelvis, and hip joints locked (similar to force closure) into a stable, yet mobile position while the mobilizers extend the body from a flexed or bent over position*
- Posteriorly tilt the pelvis (I/O)
- Maintain spinal extension by bringing the ischial tuberosities towards the back of the greater trochanters, i.e. standing posture*
- Can create counter nutation of the sacrum (tucking the tail under)

* All of the deep six hip stabilizers share this function.

Functional Groups

See the abdominals, iliopsoas, and hip adductors for details on functional groups for hip extension, rotation, and abduction, and spine extension and flexion, and tilting of the pelvis

Myofascial Lines – The piriformis and other deep hip stabilizers do not belong to any true myofascial lines due to their virtually perpendicular angle to the length of the body, but their influence on overall hip and low back tension is undeniable

Dysfunctional Group

Same as functional groups.

Description

The piriformis will be briefly described here separately because of its troublesome reputation. It is an important muscle in certain unspecific LBP cases because it can cause "Piriformis Syndrome", which has so many symptoms they almost seem unrelated, see "Effects of Piriformis Tightness" for symptoms.

Travell and Simmons[8] have listed three conditions that possibly contribute to piriformis syndrome; 1) referred pain from TP's in the piriformis 2) nerve and vascular entrapment at the greater sciatic foramen by the piriformis 3) S.I. joint dysfunction.

Chaitow and DeLaney[4] also note that the piriformis syndrome is commonly caused by entrapment of the many neurovascular bundles, including the sciatic nerve and more.

It seems that some people are more prone to developing this syndrome because of their anatomical makeup, which can consist of the sciatic nerve, or parts of it, running inferior, superior, or through the piriformis muscle; the most common is running anterior (inferior) to it, with the other variations occurring much less often.[8]

Although this syndrome is not common, it is crucial to identify it, or any other kind of neural entrapment, because they do not often respond well to exercise, only stretching and manual therapy seem to help.

The tendency to develop TP's in this muscle is most likely due to its wide variety of responsibilities it has, especially stabilizing the S.I. joint, not to mention the fact that it is situated in a spot in the pelvis where referred pain is commonly located, thus allowing it to become influenced by referred pain.

Causes of Tight Piriformis

- Compensation for weak gluteals or bicep femoris
- Side leaning posture (towards the tightness)
- Underlying bursitis
- Prolonged driving with the foot and leg externally rotated
- Extremely pronated foot
- Referred pain from erector spinae, multifidi, Q.L., gluteus medius, minimus, and maximus, soleus, and pelvic floor muscles
- Running with severe pronation or medially rotated legs
- Poor sleeping postures
- High heeled shoes
- Prolonged hip flexion with abduction, such as having the legs in stirrups for examination
- Slips and falls onto the buttocks
- Resisting a slip or fall, especially when on one leg
- An "uptight" or submissive attitude, i.e. "tight ass" or someone with their tail tucked between their legs

Effects of Tight Piriformis

- Piriformis syndrome, which includes[8]; pain in the low back, groin, buttocks, back of thigh and leg, foot, and in the rectum during defecation, swelling of the limb, sexual dysfunctions, tender piriformis to palpation, and pain and weakness against resisted thigh abduction at 90° hip flexion
- Restricted and or painful hip ROM
- A backwards tilted sacrum (counter nutation) - bilateral
- Person compensates by standing more on the other leg[55]
- Compressed and dysfunctional S.I. joint
- Lumbar and sacral curves are reduced[55] – bilateral
- Decreased sacral stabilization and therefore spinal stabilization, and an increased workload for the synergistic muscles, such as the erector spinae and gluteus maximus during re-extension from a flexed position

Individual Assessments

ROM (there are four different tests) and posture (ASIS height, pelvic tilt, femur and foot rotation, and lordosis) assessments are described in chapters 12 and 13.

Corrective Actions

1. Improve any pain, bad habits (sitting on wallet in back pocket, prolonged leg crossing), postures (place a pillow in between the knees while sleeping on side), and neurological symptoms.
2. Apply manual therapy where appropriate to improve pain and compensations, especially in the mid to lower buttock region and muscles that refer pain to that area.
3. Stretch the piriformis and balance muscle tension surrounding the lumbo-pelvic-hip area.
4. Learn to activate the CORE muscles in order to stabilize the lumbo-pelvic-hip area before movement and assist in force closure of the S.I. joint. See pg.s 206 and 233 for specific piriformis exercises.

Tensor Fascia Lata (TFL)
And
The Iliotibial Band (ITB)

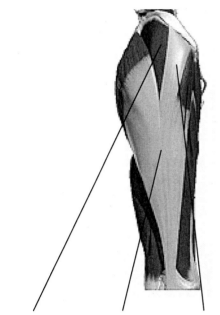

Gluteus medius   Iliotibial band   Tensor fascia lata

TFL

Muscle Type – Hyperactive/Mobilizer

Attachments

Origin – Outer, anterior lip of the iliac crest and into the lateral ASIS region and deep surface of fascia lata

Insertion – Into the ITB about 1/3 the way down the femur, although length can vary dramatically

Innervation – Superior gluteul nerve (L4-S1)

Functions

Unilaterally

• Flexes, abducts, and medially rotates the thigh at the hip
• Assists the gluteus minimus and medius muscles in stabilizing the pelvis against the tendency to fall away from the stance leg
• Stabilizes the knee through the ITB
• Anteriorly tilts the ilium
• Controls leg movement during gait

Bilaterally

• Same as unilateral plus the following
• Cause hyper-lordosis by anteriorly tilting the pelvis

ITB

Muscle Type – Tendonous sheath

Attachments

Origin – Spans across the iliac crest from the PSIS to the ASIS, via the TFL the gluteus maximus muscles

Insertion – Lateral tibial condyle and lateral patellar retinaculum (superficial fibers), lateral femoral condyle and linea aspera (deep fibers),

Functions

• Relays tension from the TFL and gluteus maximus muscles to 1) mobilize the thigh on the hip 2) stabilize the pelvis and knee once it is tensed

Functional Groups

See the iliopsoas and hip adductors for details on functional groups for hip flexion, extension, ab/adduction, rotation, and tilting of the pelvis.

Myofascial Lines – spiral and lateral lines

Dysfunctional Group

Same as functional groups plus the Q.L. and lumbar paraspinal muscles.

Description

The TFL and ITB are well known trouble makers for those who repetitively flex their thigh, i.e. runners and cyclists, wreaking havoc on the lateral thigh, hip, and knee. Once the TFL becomes overactive and the ITB irritated, prolonged activity is almost impossible without severe pain, usually in the form of tendonitis at the lateral knee or a solid mess of adhesions along the lateral thigh and ITB.

The tendonitis can be caused by the taut band rubbing on the insertion point at the knee joint, which if repeatedly done will create friction and eventually local inflammation. This sets up the low back for a stressful compensation pattern in which the many muscles surrounding the pelvis have to protect the knee from pain.

LBP caused by TFL tightness usually involves many deep rooted and chronic compensation patterns around the pelvis that take quite some time to correct, especially if the individual continues to perform the aggravating activity. This is not uncommon with people training for marathons who will continue to train in pain and reinforce the faulty movement patterns, which can persist long after the training and pain.

Good history taking with each client is essential for finding the right evidence. For example, if the professional knows that an individual who has LBP for no apparent reason has trained in pain in the past, even if the pain was not in the low back, then there is a good chance that chronic faulty recruitment patterns and their subsequent altering of joint mechanics have slowly created a tight and painful low back. This sort of knowledge can make the person who is in pain feel much better about their situation now that they have some idea of the cause. It also helps to create the corrective actions program by giving incite on how much time could be involved with such chronic faulty recruitment patterns.

A normal TFL is essential for lateral stability in sports such as tennis, soccer, water polo, football, martial arts, and more. All athletes should be assessed for TFL involvement with LBP or knee pain.

Causes of Tight TFL

- Weak gluteus minimus and medius
- Weak gluteus maximus
- Tends to compensate with overactive hip flexors and or Q.L.
- Underlying bursitis
- Referred pain from the Q.L.
- S.I. joint dysfunction
- Prolonged sitting, especially with crossed legs

Effects of Tight TFL

- Low back pain
- Referred pain deep into the hip and down the thigh from TP's[8]
- Difficulty sleeping on that hip[8]
- Underlying bursitis
- ITB friction syndrome at the origin or insertion

- Inhibited gluteus medius and minimus muscles during hip abduction, causing subsequent medial rotation and flexion of the thigh during that motion; the Q.L. is also likely to become overactive and assist hip abduction with hip hiking
- S.I. joint dysfunction
- Piriformis syndrome
- Adductor and hamstring strains

Individual Assessments

ROM (side lying leg drop), posture (ilium height, knock-knees, femur rotation, and lordosis), and PMAP (hip abduction) assessments are described in chapters 12 and 13.

Corrective Actions

1. Improve any pain, bad habits, or influential postures (hyperlordosis, femur rotation, etc.).
2. Stretch the TFL, non weightbearing stretching positions are ideal so as to not activate the TFL which would try to stabilize the pelvis.
3. Stretch and or apply manual therapy to the TFL, Q.L., hip adductors, abductors, extensors, flexors, and rotators, and the low back.
4. Practice PMAP for hip abduction.

Gluteus Medius and Minimus

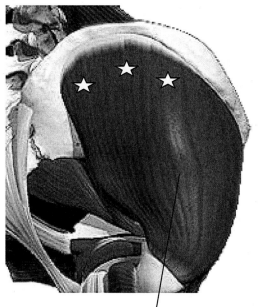

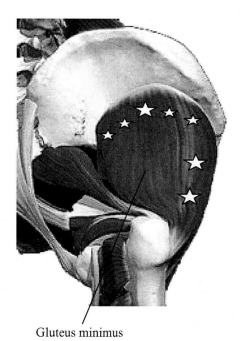

☆ = **Trigger Point Tendency**   Gluteus medius   Gluteus minimus

Gluteus Medius

Muscle Type – Hypoactive/global stabilizer and mobilizer

Attachments

Origin – Outer surface of the ilium along the anterior three-fourths of the iliac crest, between the anterior and posterior gluteal lines, and the gluteal aponeurosis

Insertion – Posterosuperior angle and the lateral surface of the greater trochanter

Innervation – Superior gluteul nerve (L5-S1)

Functions

Unilaterally

- Most powerful abductor of the thigh
- Flexes and medially rotates the femur (anterior fibers)
- Extends and assists lateral rotation of the femur (posterior fibers)
- Essential stabilizer of the pelvis during single limb weight bearing, preventing the pelvis from dropping excessively toward the unsupported side (I/O)
- Major lateral stabilizer of the pelvis

Gluteus Minimus

Muscle Type – Hypoactive/global stabilizer

Attachments

Origin – Outer surface of ilium between the anterior and inferior gluteal lines

Insertion – uppermost anterior surface of the greater trochanter, deep and anterior to the piriformis

Functions

- Same as gluteus medius but more as an assistant

Functional Groups

See the iliopsoas and hip adductors for details on functional groups for hip flexion, extension, ab/adduction, and rotation.

Myofascial Lines – no true lines identified

Dysfunctional Group

Same as functional groups plus the Q.L. and lumbar paraspinal muscles

Description

The gluteus medius and minimus are essential weigthbearing muscles which easily become victims of a sedentary lifestyle. They are very important stabilizers in standing and walking postures and once they become weak or inhibited, they also become very susceptible to TP's and tightness.

The tendency to sit for most of the day and then participate in strenuous activity such as hiking, running, or sports, is a common way to overload the gluteus medius and minimus muscles. This overload usually leads to 1) the development of TP's 2) compensations throughout the lumbo-pelvic-hip region 3) a main source of LBP.

The best way to avoid overloading these muscles is to stay within the limits of the body while exercising (duration, effort, difficulty, and frequency) and perform specific stretches and exercises that maintain balance throughout the kinetic chain.

The gluteus medius and minimus function similarly but have very different referred pain patterns from TP's. Gluteus medius refers pain mostly in the local area of the hip, sacrum, low back, and buttocks, while gluteus minimus refers pain into similar spots as well as down the posterior and lateral aspects of the leg.[8]

Sometimes the referred pain can be mistaken for *sciatica, lumbar facet joint, and S.I. joint pain patterns*.[8] Because the gluteus medius is generally the most powerful abductor of the leg[8,28,61,142], any dysfunction in it is usually coupled with Q.L., TFL, and gluteus minimus compensations.

When both legs are grounded the abductors and *contralateral* adductors work synergistically to stabilize the pelvis[4,206], however, when a leg is in the motion of ab or adduction the *ipsilateral* abductors and adductors are antagonists to one another. Therefore, when one side (abductor) is dysfunctional it can affect both right and left adductors.

The gluteus minimus and medius are often inhibited and cause facilitation of the adductors, making for an unstable ankle, knee, hip, and low back during running, jumping, or prolonged walking.

Athletes who need explosive lateral movements must have a strong gluteus minimus and medius on both sides, otherwise Q.L. and TFL compensations will create hip hiking and unwanted femur rotations which lead to poor balance and increased lumbar spinal loading.

Causes of Weak Gluteals

- Sedentary lifestyle or prolonged non-weightbearing positions
- Faulty alignment of the femur in the hip joint
- Overactive TFL
- Tight adductors
- Overactive pirifomris[41]
- Referred pain from piriformis, R.A., Gmax, iliocostalis lumbothoracis, and especially Q.L.
- Underlying bursitis
- Sprained ankle (cannot bear weight on that leg)
- Excessive pronation overloads the gluteals and often causes TP's and tightness-weakness in them

Effects of Weak Gluteals

- Low back, hip, buttocks, lateral thigh and leg pain referred from TP's that can mimic sciatica[8]
- Sprained ankle
- Overactive/tight adductors (both sides)
- Overactive ipsilateral Q.L. and lateral obliques, and possibly on the contralateral side with chronic situations
- Decreased lateral and or stance stability (pelvis sidebends away from weakness) and increased lumbar stress during lateral motion
- S.I. joint dysfunctions
- Difficulty sleeping on involved side if TP's are present[8]

Individual Assessments

ROM (hip adduction), posture (ilium height and femur rotation), strength (Trendelenburg test), and PMAP (hip abduction) assessments are described in chapters 12 and 13.

Corrective Actions

1. Improve any pain, faulty postures[8] (increase base of support during standing, place a pillow between the knees when sleeping on one side, sit down to put on pants if unstable, orthotics for pronation when necessary, etc).
2. Apply manual therapy to any muscles that are causing pain and problems in the area; stretching of the gluteus minimus and medius are recommended at first to reduce tension, but the long term goal is usually strengthening, not lengthening these muscles.
3. Follow the guidelines in chapter 13 for strengthening the gluteus medius. Utilize both standing and side lying positions.
4. Stretch adductors (w/active gluteal stretches), TFL, lumbar paraspinals, and any other influential muscles.

Hamstrings

"The Strained Three"

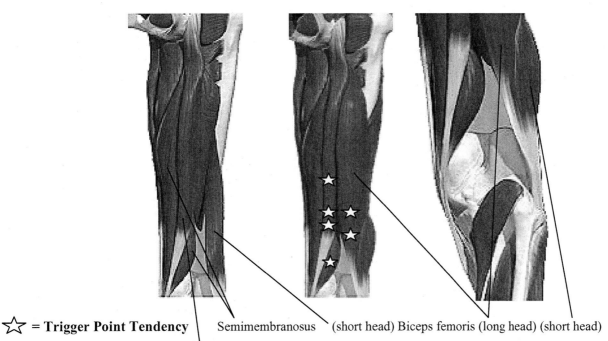

☆ = **Trigger Point Tendency**   Semimembranosus   (short head) Biceps femoris (long head) (short head)

Semitendinosus

Biceps Femoris

Muscle Type – Hyperactive/Mobilizer

Attachments

Long Head

Origin – Posterior aspect of ischial tuberosity, common tendon with semitendinosis, and the sacrotuberous ligament

Insertion – Lateral aspect of the fibula and tibia heads

Short Head

Origin – Lateral ridge of the linea aspera and the lateral inter-muscular septum, very close to the middle adductor magnus

Insertion – Fuses with the long head tendon into the same insertion point

Innervation – Sciatic nerve (L5-S2)

Functions

Unilaterally

- Extends and laterally rotates the thigh at the hip

- Flexes and laterally rotates the lower leg at the knee*
- Restrains the tendency toward hip flexion (caused by the weight of the trunk) during the stance phase of gait, standing, and forward bending
- Assists adduction of the thigh
- Assist posterior tilting of the ilium
- Assists stabilizing the S.I. joint via the sacrotuberous ligament

Bilaterally

- Same as unilaterally plus the following;
- Assist posterior tilting of the pelvis
- Raise the trunk from a stooping position, especially with straight legs
- Restrain the tendency toward hip flexion (caused by the weight of the trunk) during standing and forward bending

* Includes short and long head, all other functions are long head only

Semitendinosis

Muscle Type – Hyperactive/Mobilizer

Attachments

Origin – Posterior aspect of ischial tuberosity via the common tendon with long head of biceps femoris

Insertion – Curves around the posteromedial tibial condyle and attaches to the proximal medial tibia

Semimembranosus

Muscle Type – Hyperactive/Mobilizer

Attachments

Origin – Posterior aspect of the ischial tuberosity, lateral and deep to the common tendon of the biceps femoris and semitendinosis

Insertion – Posteromedial aspect of the medial condyle of the tibia

Functions

• Both of these muscles function just like the long head of the biceps femoris with the exception of influencing medial rotation instead of lateral
• The biceps femoris also has more influence on the low back and rotational function of the entire body through its association with the myofascial spiral line

Functional Groups

See the abdominals, iliopsoas, and hip adductors for details on functional groups for hip flexion, extension, abduction, and rotation, and tilting of the pelvis

Myofascial Lines – superficial back (hamstrings) and spiral lines (biceps femoris)

Dysfunctional Group

Same as functional groups plus the gastrocsoleus complex

Description

The hamstrings are constantly being treated for those with LBP because they always seem to be tight and painful when stretched. It can be difficult to assess whether tight hamstrings are creating the problems for LBP or are a protective mechanism used by the body to actually protect the injured lumbar spine from excessive stress, such as when forward bending.

In the latter case it is best to find the source of pathology before simply stretching or releasing what might be the body's last line of defense in resisting injurious motions in the lumbar spine. It is usually a good idea to save the hamstrings towards the end of treatment so that they can normalize with the corrections of other muscles that influence the position of the pelvis and thus not be so tight when treated.

The hamstrings are similar to the posterior muscles of the neck because they both are commonly overloaded by gravity and dominating flexor muscles, and they are part of the posterior myofascia continuum.

The fascia of the hamstrings, which is often strained or too tight, transfers tension through the sacrum and erector spinae via the superficial fascia surrounding the sacrotuberous ligament and the sacrum.[63] Therefore, *hamstring tension can cause low back pain and stiffness as well as protect lumbar and pelvic pathologies.*

Stretching the hamstrings is most beneficial when the entire superior and posterior fascia system is included in the stretch, as in downward dog or forward flexion. Those with nerve damage should be careful to not overstretch the sciatic nerve and spinal cord during total body flexion stretches.

See 'The Tight Hamstring' on pg. 41 for more on the confusion about tight hamstrings.

Causes of Tight Hamstrings

• Weak gluteus maximus
• Weak lower abdominals
• Weak gastrocnemius
• Sciatica
• Lumbar or pelvic pathology that requires protective tightness
• Prolonged sitting, especially with the bottom of the thighs compressed against a hard chair
• Forward leaning posture (torso and or head)
• S.I. joint dysfunctions
• Postural overload (hyper-lordosis) by dominant hip flexors
• Running, especially sprinting, with too tight of hip flexors or insufficient warm-up
• History of hamstring strains or tears
• Erector spinae tightness
• Referred pain from the piriformis, gluteus minimus and medius, and gastrocnemius
• Repetitive or heavy lifting with straight legs

Effects of Tight Hamstrings

• Low back pain and stiffness

- Pain and possibly a limp with walking[8]*
- Pain in the buttock or back of knee during sitting and difficulty rising from a seated position[8]*
- Mimics "growing pains" in kids[8]*
- Difficulty touching toes during forward bending with knees extended
- Hamstring strains or tears
- Alters hip and lumbar extension patterns and leads to increased lumbar spinal loads
- Myofascial rigidity along the posterior aspect of the body, from head to toe
- Plantar fasciatis
- Dysfunction of lumbo-pelvic rhythm
- Trigger points can lead to referred pain in the buttock, upper calf, and posterior knee regions[8]
- Adductor magnus tightness
- Inhibition of gluteus maximus

* If TP's are present

Individual Assessments

ROM (hip flexion with knee extension), posture (knee flexion, ilium height, femur rotation, and lordosis), and PMAP (prone hip extension) assessments are described in chapters 12 and 13.

Corrective Actions

1. Improve any pain, bad habits (chairs with hard edges or that are too high), postures (leaning forward and hyper-lordosis), and fualty PMAP for hip extension.
2. Improve any influential factors (S.I. joint dysfunction, short hip flexors, weak gluteus maximus, gastrocnemius or abdominals, referred pain from other muscles, improper warm-up before sprinting, etc.).
3. Stretch and apply manual therapy to the hamstrings and posterior myofascia system if indicated; note that the lateral hamstrings are commonly tighter and require stretching of the leg across the body combined with flexion at the hip.

The Gastrocsoleus Complex

"The Rigid Foundation"

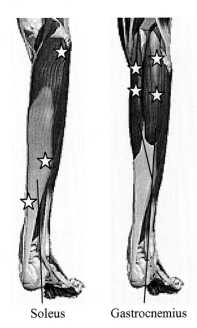

Soleus   Gastrocnemius

⭐ = **Trigger Point Tendency**

Gastrocnemius

Muscle Type – Hyperactive/Mobilizer

Attachments

Origin – Each head (lateral and medial) attaches to its corresponding femoral condyle via a strong, flat tendon, and to the capsule of the knee joint

Insertion – Merges with and on top of the soleus to form the Achilles tendon, which attaches to the posterior aspect of the calcaneus

Innervation – Tibial nerve (S1-S2)

Functions

- Plantar flexes the foot (standing on balls of feet)
- Inverts the foot (similar to supination)
- Stabilizes leg and body against forward leaning postures and stresses
- Stabilizes the knee and ankle during ambulation
- Assists knee flexion weakly
- Most active during explosive or sudden movements

Soleus

Muscle Type – Hyperactive/Global Stabilizer and Mobilizer

Attachments

Origin – Posterior surface of fibula head, along the proximal third of the medial tibia border, and the fibrous arch between the proximal tibia and fibula

Insertion – Blends together with the underside of the gastrocnemius tendon to form the Achilles tendon

Functions

- Plantar flexes the foot (standing on balls of feet)
- Inverts the foot (similar to supination)
- Stabilizes leg and body against forward leaning postures and stresses
- Stabilizes (along with tibialis anterior) against forward and backward sway during quiet standing
- Stabilizes the knee and ankle during ambulation
- Most active for stabilization purposes
- Musculovenous pump for lower leg

Functional Groups

Plantar Flexion – plantaris, peroneus longus and brevis, flexor hallucis brevis and longus, tibialis posterior, flexor digitorum lingus

Dorsi Flexion – extensor digitorum longus, peroneus tertius, extensor hallucis longus, tibialis anterior

Supination – tibialis posterior and anterior, extensor hallucis longus, flexor hallucis longus, flexor digitorum longus, plantaris

Pronation - proneus longus, brevis, and tertius, extensor digitorum longus

Myofascial Lines – superficial back line (gastrocnemius)

Dysfunctional Group

Same as functional groups, plus the muscles involved with ambulation.

Description

There is some confusing literature about certain functions of the gastrocsoleus complex, also called the "triceps surae". EMG study's appear to show that it is not very active, if at all, during the "push-off" phase of walking or running[207,208], but it is active throughout the stance phase as a knee and ankle stabilizer.[208,209] It was even concluded that there seemed to be no such thing as a push-off phase because of the inactivity in the lower leg muscles.[207]

On the other hand, *Gray's Anatomy*[28] notes: "Gastrocnemius provides force for propulsion in walking, running, and leaping. Soleus is said to be more concerned with steadying the leg on the foot in standing" Later saying "....soleus probably [also] participates in locomotion and gastrocnemius in posture."

Gray's anatomy often has the most intelligent theories on muscles and their functioning because they are primarily based on the anatomy and biomechanics of the body as opposed to EMG results or other study's that involve the functioning of dysfunctional people (neuromuscularly speaking of course).

For instance, an EMG study that measures the activity of the gasctrocsoleus complex may be misinterpreted because of people who have inhibited gluteus maximus muscles (very common) and decreased hip extension during gait (very common). These two factors would encourage the use of the hip flexors to overpower gait mechanics and become the main movers in a forward propelling system. This of course is dysfunctional because it inhibits the other part of the pattern which should be the gluteus maximus extending the hip and initiating (along with the contralateral latissimus dorsi) the push-off phase, which would utilize the gastrocsoleus complex. This is a very simple description of an extremely complex action (gait).

This push-off sequence is essential for the low back because it encourages the 'energy sling' during gait and without it the hip flexors are overworking during ambulation and creating excessive spinal loads. It is difficult to say what the proper form of walking should be, but by practicing the different methods of walking one can get a feel for what is best.

Try for yourself and see which feels more efficient, it may take some practice to learn how to properly utilize the gluteus maximus, contralateral latissimus dorsi, and gastrocsoleus complex, but once learned, it usually feels a lot easier and more comfortable on the low back, not to mention it naturally speeds up the pace by increasing hip extension and thus lengthening the stride. See pg. 26 for more on gait patterns.

The gastrocnemius is also a contributor to total body stability by way of controlling forward sway against sudden movements. For instance, it was shown that gasctrocnemius EMG activity occurred prior to that of the local upper extremity muscles during sudden forceful movements of the hands and arms.[210] Keep in mind that the gastrocnemius functions best at the ankle when the knee is extended, and the soleus is relatively unaffected by knee position.[8]

Another confusing dilemma with the gastrocsoleus complex is that it is usually tight and short, but also weak, especially in the medial fibers, which allows the lower leg to externally rotate and come up onto the lateral side of the foot while rising onto the balls of the feet. Unfortunately treatment protocols often neglect the strengthening component and focus on stretching.

It is invaluable to be able to raise one's own body weight onto the balls of the feet, yet this frequently cannot be done properly. It is a simple exercise that should be included in almost any program, as opposed to the strengthening exercises that utilize machines to strengthen the gastrocsoleus complex. The latter methods do not involve the entire kinetic chain with balancing and controlling body weight as the former does.

In summary, the gastrocsoleus complex is important to the low back because 1) it affects gait patterns, in particular hip extension 2) they are directly connected through the superficial posterior myofascia system 3) it assists in restraining the tendency to lean forward 4) it stabilizes the leg, and therefore the spine, during ambulation 5) it can cause improper lifting techniques when short (see below).

Causes of Tight Gastrocsoleus Complex

- Prolonged running or walking, especially on uphill or slanted surfaces and without proper stretching
- Prolonged forward leaning postures, i.e. standing over the sink[8]
- Referred pain form the gluteus minimus[8]
- Wearing high heal shoes[8]
- Prolonged shortened positions, i.e. during sleeping or sitting with the legs up
- Tight sock bands around the mid-calf area[8]
- Improper gait or running patterns, i.e. dominant hip flexors and inhibited gluteus maximus
- Emotional stress, asthma, fatigue and allergies are all related to a dysfunctional gastrocsoleus complex due to its relationship with the adrenal glands[211]

Effects of Tight Gastrocsoleus Complex

- Low back pain and stiffness from improper lifting techniques due to restricted ankle dorsi flexion[8]
- Edema and pain in the foot and ankle from upper soleus trigger points[8]
- Referred pain into the heel, mid-calf, and S.I. joint from soleus trigger points[8]
- Pain in the posterior knee and bottom of the foot from gastrocnemius trigger points[8]
- Calf cramps, especially at night (gastrocnemius)[8]
- LBP getting out of a chair without arm rests (gastrocnemius)[8]
- Shin splints[8]
- Plantar fasciitis
- Increased hip flexion during uphill walking from the lack of dorsi flexion available.

Individual Assessments

ROM (dorsi flexion), posture (knee flexion and forward lean), and strength (toe raises) assessments are described in chapters 12 and 13.

Corrective Actions

1. Improve any pain, poor habits (high heels shoes, prolonged plantar flexion positions, leaning over sink, etc.) and postures (forward leaning).

2. Stretch and or apply manual therapy to the gastrocsoleus complex, superficial posterior myofascia system, and any muscles that are referring pain to the posterior lower leg.

3. Practice proper gait patterns, focusing on the hip extension and push-off phases.

4. Strengthen the gastrocsoleus complex progressing from 1) two legged standing toe raises 2) one legged standing toe raises; also make sure that the dorsi flexor muscles are strong enough to balance the pull of the plantar flexors.

5. Travell and Simmons[8] offer the following helpful strategy in keeping the soleus vascular pump working during prolonged periods of inactivity: during sitting or lying, alternate plantar and dorsi flexion of one foot followed by the other, repeat about six cycles every half hour to ensure efficient blood flow out of the lower leg.

Chapter 12 Low Back Assessment

The assessments in this chapter can be used for thorough evaluation of the general population and those with LBP. An assessment of nearly the entire body is necessary to get an idea of all the possible causes for a LBD, as well as many other seemingly isolated disorders. Fortunately, this plethora of tests is not needed for everyone. Many individuals will present an uncomplicated case and require fewer tests to be performed, while others will challenge the evaluator with the "simple backache" that has not improved with any prior treatments.

A detailed history of the person and knowledge of injury mechanisms are the most important facts in determining the appropriate tests for each individual, and thus efficiently utilizing time.

The reason for so many tests is that the low back can be a mystery to even the most sophisticated technological assessment. It is common for asymptomatic individuals to have the same structural abnormalities as those with symptoms. In fact, disc herniations have been found on MRI scans in many asymptomatic individuals.[80]

A comprehensive evaluation of soft tissue, structure, and function is needed to rule out and narrow down the possible causes of dysfunction. The history of an individual and knowledge of injury mechanisms will help decide which tests are most appropriate and provide direction for the assessment by giving clues about which tissues are most likely involved with an injury or pain syndrome and which are not.

For instance, if a truck driver with 20 years on the job suddenly has LBP for no apparent reason, then there is a good chance that muscle atrophy in the spine and disc problems from the years of seated vibration are a main factor and should thus be taken into account. But, if someone has acute LBP after improperly lifting a heavy object with their spine flexed and twisted, then annular tears and possibly intersegmental soft tissue tears are likely the main contributors to the pain.

The former example could probably benefit from exercise while the latter would first need to rest until the acute phase of healing is finished; both should first be referred to a licensed practitioner to learn the extent of the disorder.

It is not within the scope of personal trainers to diagnosis with these assessments, but it is within their scope to evaluate and screen each person for red flags, such as disc herniations and the like.

Classifications of Low Back Disorders (LBD's)

Classifying a LBD is a controversial task that has resulted in very general terms that are hard to argue due to the lack of evidence supporting most LBD's. For the benefit of all involved, this manual has created specific classifications based on neuromuscular and musculoskeletal dysfunctions.

There are only a few accepted classifications for a LBD. Here are two well respected examples.

British and American Classifications[41]

1. Simple backache
2. Nerve root pain (<5%)
3. Serious spinal pathology (<1%)

Quebec Task Force Classification of Spinal Disorders[51]

1. Pain without radiation
2. Pain + radiation to extremity, proximally
3. Pain + radiation to extremity, distally
4. Confirmed nerve root compression
5. Spinal stenosis
6. Postsurgical < 6 months
7. Postsurgical > 6 months
8. Chronic pain syndrome
9. Other diagnosis (tumor, infection, fracture, rheumatologic, disease, etc.)

With close inspection one can detect that there is something missing from these classifications; most of them don't tell about the nature of the cause, instead they focus on the symptoms or situation of the person. It is well known that treating symptoms often ignores what is responsible for the symptoms in the first place. As stated brilliantly by Adams and Bogduk et all[80];

"It is important to appreciate that pain is a symptom which may reveal little or nothing about the nature of any underlying disorder or disease."

In the British and American classifications, 94% of LBD's are confined to one classification, a "simple backache." These categories are so general because they are based on the medical profession's need for proof. And because there is no accepted way to validate the involvement of certain dysfunctions as the main cause of LBP, most cases are labeled as "simple" or non-specific.

Unfortunately this philosophy does not produce a

treatment plan other than general exercise, ice, heat, rest, and medication. Exercise Progression simply *works on correcting neuromuscular and musculoskeletal dysfunctions while taking into consideration the source and type of pain, along with the phase of healing, nutrition, and psychological factors.*

It is understandably difficult to diagnose something that cannot be concretely verified, but because rehabilitative exercise and manual therapy are already known to improve LBD's, it seems sensible to further sub-classify the "simple backache" into categories that facilitate exercise programming by describing what type of intervention they require, i.e. musculoskeletal and or functional.

Because a single cause is rarely found for LBD's, it is essential to find as many influential dysfunctions as possible in order to decipher the hierarchy of general and local adaptation syndromes. Important dysfunctions or adaptations can then be sub-classified under the "simple backache." This provides a more detailed description of the person's condition and training needs.

Box 12-1 is meant to compliment the "nerve root pain" and "serious spinal pathologies" classifications that are already commonly used. It should be noted that the peripheral nerve entrapment sub-classification of soft tissue differs from "nerve root pain."

The sub-classifications can be added together to give an even more specific description, such as; Simple backache: repetitive strain/chronic, neuromuscular (weak CORE), and structural (vertebral instability).

These sub-classifications are a product of Exercise Progression and are not used in the medical profession, yet. They should not be used for anything other than creating a specific exercise and manual therapy program. Guidance and exercise clearance from a qualified professional are required when pain or pathology is present. The specific contraindications and corrective actions for many of the sub-classifications can be found in chapter 13.

Sub-classifications of the "simple backache"

Box 12 -1

Kinetic Chain	Physiological	Psychological
Soft tissue* Structure* Neuromuscular	Nutrition Cardiovascular system Internal systems etc.	Somatization Depression Fear/Anxiety Inability to cope etc.

* These are also sub-classified by cause (repetitive strain or traumatic injury) and phase (acute, subacute, or chronic)

These sub-classifications are the same as the classifications for "non-serious pain syndromes" described on pg. 22. See pg.'s 22-23 for more details on these sub-classifications, except the structural aspects, which are unique to the low back and are as follows.

Structural

- Facet joint pathology
- Scoliosis
- Stenosis
- Spondylolisthesis
- SI joint syndrome
- Disc or joint degeneration
- Hypermobility
- Hypomobility

Key Links to LBD's

Box 12-2

Lifestyle	Physical Findings
Prolonged sitting or standing	Upper and lower crossed syndrome
Insufficient or improper stretching	Excessive pronation
Sedentary	Altered hip extension, abduction, and trunk flexion firing patterns
Daily repetitive bending or twisting	TP's in Q.L., E.S., psoas, gluteuls, abdominals, or deep paraspinals
Too frequent or too intense of activity	
Obesity	Short adductors, psoas, gastrocsoleus, E.S., pirifomis, and hamstrings
Poor body awareness	
Lack of nutrition, especially water	Weak one leg balance test
Improper breathing	
Poor sleeping patterns	Weak abdominals
Improper lifting, bending, sitting, or standing.	Poor leg strength and stamina
Stressful daily life along with poor coping mechanisms	Short leg
	Any serious spine pathology

Key Links

Knowing where to look and then what to focus on once dysfunctions are found is a key to unlocking the door that leads to LBP relief. Experience shows that only about 20% of painful spinal syndromes can be diagnosed as having any pathoanatomic origin[52], this means that 80% experience pain without any signs of structural pathology.

These numbers are useful to keep in mind when searching for the causes of LBP, especially when the assessment concludes nothing out of the ordinary. In these cases, lifestyle key links can be the missing piece to improvement. The following are some key links for the low back and are a priority in corrective actions.

The following assessments do not include the history, which is detailed in chapter 2 and always taken first.

Assessment Categories

1. Red flags
2. Neurological tests
3. Structural tests
4. Posture/Gait
5. ROM
6. Palpation
7. Breathing
8. Muscle testing
9. Functional strength tests

Red Flags

- Illness or other symptoms of disease are present along with the back pain.
- Pain is severe even during rest.
- Swelling and redness accompany the pain.
- Unable to walk on tip toes or heels due to weakness (indicates nerve root problem).
- Single leg raise (SLR) elicits a sharp pain or pain before 20°.
- Sharp pain cannot be relieved in any position.
- Acute problem without diagnosis or referral from a specialist.

Neurological Dysfunction Tests

The neurological tests on pg. 150 should be performed if symptoms go below the level of the buttock crease.[1] Otherwise, the therapist's intuition is the best guide on when to use them. The supplementary tests are intended to follow up positive neurological tests in order to rule out other influences. Dermatome and reflex testing are also recommended but are left out of these assessments because they are best suited for a licensed specialist.

The first six nerve root tests are muscle strength tests and are positive if the test action is weak, but if only *pain* is elicited on these first six tests, it often indicates pathology in the surrounding joints or muscles, not at the nerve root. If LBP is present in the low back during any of the last three tests (which are all passive ROM), it can be from neurological, muscular, or structural origin.

Sciatica symptoms must be distinguished from simple nerve entrapment (peripheral) by mainly the piriformis, referred pain from the gluteus minimus muscle, or more serious involvement at the spinal cord, vertebrae and discs (nerve root). True sciatica is not common, only about 2-5%, and is usually associated with herniated lumbar discs between 40 and 45 years old.[80]

Nerve root pain is commonly associated with numbness in the same areas as the pain and is usually down the leg and into the foot along the sciatic nerve where it is more intense then the corresponding LBP.[4] If there is obvious and palpable irritation and inflammation surrounding the sciatic nerve at the piriformis and or down the leg along its path, then it rules out the gluteus minimis as the primary factor and points to a peripheral and or nerve root cause. If this irritation is accompanied by desensitization to feeling i.e. can barely feel a pin prick or light touch, then it points to a spinal nerve root dysfunction, not peripheral.[1]

Structural Pathology Tests

The structural tests on pg.'s 152 and 153 are useful to see what is going on inside the spine and its joints. The first five tests are positive if pain is induced. Again, the tests do not assure anything, but they do help create limits and goals for exercise, along with clues to the structural integrity of the spine and its interaction with surrounding muscles. The supplementary tests and findings are intended to follow up positive joint tests in order to rule out other influences.

Posture

Posture should be assessed in two different positions. First, by letting the person assume the most comfortable posture, which accentuates habitual and compensatory imbalances. Second, have them assume a posture with the feet about shoulder width apart and pointing forward (up to 10° of external rotation is acceptable), this position allows for the identification of true postural abnormalities, i.e. an elevated hemipelvis. Observing the first posture requires only a glance in order to get an idea of the compensations, while the second posture requires a detailed analysis of structural landmarks.

Posture is observed from four different views; anterior, posterior, left side, and right side. It is a good idea to view the posture from a distance and then up close.

Anterior

- Feet (pronated/supinated) & (toeing in/toeing out)
- Knees (bowlegged/knock-kneed)
- Femur rotation
- ASIS height
- Iliac crest levels
- Pelvic rotation
- Torso rotation
- Shoulder elevation
- Arm rotation
- Head tilt & rotation (L/R)

⇒ Posture is continued on page 153.

Neurological Assessment

Box 12-3

Nerve Roots	Test Action[3]	Supplementary Tests
L2	Hip Flexion	Palpate L1-L3 for abnormalities. Check lumbar and hip ROM to rule out arthrokinetic or neuromuscular inhibition.
L3	Knee Extension	Palpate L2-L4 and patella. Check lumbar, hip, and knee ROM.
L4	Foot Dorsi Flexion	Palpate L3-L5 and ankle. Check hip, knee and ankle ROM.
L5	Extension of Big Toe	Palpate L4-S1. Check knee and ankle ROM.
S1	Hip Extension	Palpate L5-S2. Check lumbar and hip ROM and PMAP for hip extension.
S2	Knee Flexion	Palpate S1-S3. Check lumbar, hip, and knee ROM.
L5, S1, and S2 (sciatic nerve)	Supine Straight Leg Raise (SLR)	This pain is easily distinguished from hamstring or muscle tightness by its intensity, but can commonly be confused with a sacroiliac dysfunction. See page 151 for more details.
L2-L4 (femoral nerve)	Prone Knee Bending	Palpate entire lumbar region for abnormalities. Check lumbar, hip, pelvis, and knee ROM.
Cervical and Lumbar (spinal cord and sciatic nerve)	Sitting slump (slouch) with SLR.	Palpate the paraspinal muscles along entire spine as well as the posterior fascia system for trigger points and tightness. Check flexion and extension ROM of the cervical, thoracic, and lumbar spine, as well as at the hip, pelvis, knee, and ankle.

Hip Flexion
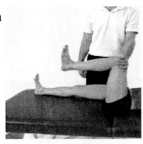

Big Toe Extension
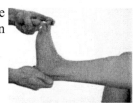

Straight Leg Raise (SLR)
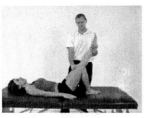

Knee Extension
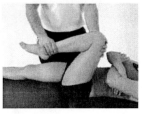

Hip Extension
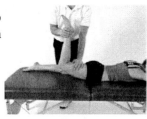

Prone Knee Bending
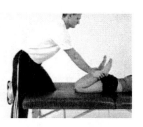

Dorsi Flexion
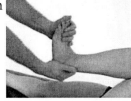

Knee Flexion
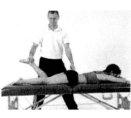

Sitting slump (slouch)
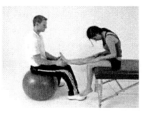

The Straight Leg Raise (SLR) Test

The SLR is one of the most commonly used orthopedic tests for determining the origin of low back and/or radiating leg pain. It is a relatively simple test to administer, yet has very complex results.

The lumbar nerve roots have a narrow range of movement for stretching and are not brought into tension and stretched by the SLR until 35° to 70° of the leg raise have been reached.[279] If there is compromise of the normal space (i.e., disc bulge, inflammation) this space is used up and the pain will manifest more quickly, thus giving a positive test for pain.

It is essential to perform follow-up tests for clients with a positive SLR, as nerve root compression can mimic sacroiliac inflammation. Different authors have various opinions on the results of an SLR test. Below is a compilation of findings;[279,280,281]

0 to 35° = nerve root compression/extradural involvement
35 to 60-70° = indicates sacroiliac or disc disease
beyond 60-70° = lumbosacral conditions

The following tests are used to clarify the results from the SLR and determine any other sources of pain.

Goldthwaite's Test: Place your hand under the person's lumbar spine and locate the lumbosacral spinous processes. As you lift the leg to a point of pain, feel for motion between these segments. If pain is experienced before the spinous processes separate, this suggests the dysfunction is in the sacroiliac joint. If the pain occurs simultaneously with the motion of the lumbar segment, the pathology is more likely in the lumbar spine.

Neck flexion: Once the leg is raised to the point of pain, instruct the person to lift their head, bringing the chin to the chest. If this movement is limited or increases the pain in the lower back or leg, inflammation of the nerve root is likely.

Bragard's Sign: If the SLR is positive, lower the leg on the tested side to just below the point of pain and quickly dorsiflex the foot. If the pain is replicated or increased, this suggests sciatic neuritis (irritation of the nerve).

SLR w/external rotation: If the SLR is positive, lower the leg on the tested side to just below the point of pain and externally rotate the leg. An increase in sciatic pain signifies piriformis syndrome.

Sicard's Sign: If the SLR is positive, lower the leg to just below the point of pain and quickly dorsiflex the great toe. If the pain is duplicated or increased, this suggests sciatic radiculopathy (irritation at the nerve root).

Cox Sign: If the person raises the affected hip off the table instead of flexing the hip, this indicates prolapse of the nucleus into the intervertebral foramen (IVF).

Seated SLR (Lesegue Sitting Test): With the person seated, the affected leg is raised to the point of pain and considered positive if pain is reproduced or increased in the lower back or leg. The patient may lean back to avoid pain; this would also be considered a positive finding. Pain with a SLR should be reproduced with the seated SLR.

Deyerle's Sign: With the person seated, the affected leg is raised to the point of pain. The knee is then slightly flexed and pressure is applied into the popliteal fossa. If the radicular symptoms are increased, the test is positive for sciatic nerve irritation above the knee due to stretching of the nerve over an abnormal mechanical obstruction.

Well Leg Raise: The SLR is performed on the unaffected leg. If pain is referred back to the symptomatic side, this indicates nerve root compromise by an extruded disc.

Fajerstajn's: This test is the same as Bragard's, but performed on the unaffected side. Pain produced with this maneuver suggests intervertabral disc syndrome or dural adhesions.

Vleeming's Active SLR: This test is discussed in detail by Dr. Craig Liebenson in the Feb. 24, 2003 issue of *DC*. It is the same as the SLR, except the client moves their own leg. Pain or poor motion control with the maneuver suggests SI joint dysfunction or compromised hip flexors.[282]

While all of these tests may seem ridiculously extensive, they are the key to narrowing down the cause of that elusive "simple backache." It is also important to note where the pain goes during these assessments. Is it in the back, the buttock or the leg? Does it go down to the knee or foot? Does it cause tension or pulling up into the neck? These notes are invaluable for documenting the severity of a person's complaints and show the progressive response to care.

What is the use of all these tests (neurological and structural) if an MRI, X-ray, or doctor's diagnosis often fall short of helping the situation? That is precisely the point! We should not focus on what is going on in the spine as much as we focus on how the body reacts to different movements.

The goal is not to diagnose, rather to create an exercise program that utilizes the best positions for each individual to allow for proper healing to occur. For instance, there are common exercise guidelines for disc herniations and the like, unfortunately everyone is different and diagnoses are often incorrect or invalid. Therefore, finding each person's limitations for movement will enable the professional to design programs that will not aggravate the situation and thus allow the pathology to heal. Simple? Yes. Are these tests performed often? No. Why not? I wish I knew. Let's change that.

Structural Assessment

Box 12-4

Structural Pathology	Test Action	Supplementary Tests or Findings
Spondylolisthesis (A)	One leg standing lumbar extension.[3]	Check gluteuls, hip flexors, adductors, all lumbar and thoracic paraspinal muscles, Q.L., and abdominals for trigger points, hypersensitivity, and tightness. Also check S.I. joint function, related vertebral motion by palpation, and PMAP for hip extension and abduction, and trunk flexion.
Facet Joint (B)	One leg standing lumbar extension w/rotation.[3]	See above
Spinal Segment-Stability (C)	Prone bilateral knee flexion with applied lumbar pressure.[3]	See above
Spinal Segment-Stability (D)	Prone on table with legs on ground and applied lumbar pressure, then lift legs.[3]	See above
Stenosis of Intervertebral- Foramen and Facet Joint (E)	Standing lumbar side flexion with rotation and overpressure.[3]	See above
Iliosacral Movement (F)	Standing flexion. If one of the PSIS moves more anterosuperiorly, then the test is positive on that side.[4]	A positive test can be from a "fixed" iliosacral junction, a tight contralateral hamstring, or a tight ipsilateral Q.L. If one or both hamstrings are tight, they can cause a false-negative test.[4]
Iliosacral Movement (G)	Stork test. Standing while flexing knee and hip to 90°. The PSIS on the side being moved should move inferiorly and medially.[4]	If the ipsilateral PSIS moves superioly it indicates an iliosacral dysfunction[4], which is something that can later be compared for improvement after certain muscles have been balanced. This and the previous test should be compared with the static posture of ASIS symmetry. See corrective actions on pg?
Sacroiliac Movement (H)	Seated flexion. If one PSIS moves more superior, it suggests ipsilateral sacrioiliac restriction.[4]	A tight Q.L. can cause a false-positive test.[4] The main difference between this test (sacroiliac) and the previous two (iliosacral), is that this test is more concerned with sacral movement and the other two with movement of the hemipelvis.
Altered Spinal Mechanics	Compare spinal rotoscoliosis during sitting and standing flexion	If the rotoscoliosis (seen with exaggerated paraspinal muscles on one side which resemble a hump) is greater during standing flexion, then muscular compensations in the lower body and pelvis are suspected. But if it is greater during sitting flexion, then a spinal dysfunction is likely the primary factor.[57]

Structural Assessment
(Box 12-4)

A

E

B

F

C

G

D

H

Posture (continued)

Posterior

- Feet/Achilles tendon (pronated/supinated)
- Gluteal folds
- PSIS asymmetry

- Iliac crest level
- Rib cage level
- Lumbar scoliosis
- Thoracic scoliosis
- Full spine curvature
- Scapula rotation
- Scapula ab/adduction
- Scapula elevation
- Shoulder elevation
- Head tilt (L/R)
- Head rotation

Side (R/L)

- Knees (flexed/hyperextended)
- Pelvic tilt [anterior (lordosis)/posterior (sway or flat back)]
- Thoracic curvature(normal/kyphosis)
- Shoulder (anterior/posterior)
- Head (anterior/posterior)
- Head tilt (up/down)

Common Postural Faults

Before beginning the postural evaluation it is essential to know what ideal posture looks like and to be aware of the following faulty postures which are commonly seen in individuals who are asymptomatic or symptomatic. This is another reason why it is a good idea to assess everyone; it could save them from future injuries and symptoms. These postures, along with each fault found in the following assessments, will be further described in this chapter and chapter 12.

The layer syndrome (modified from Jull and Janda 1987)

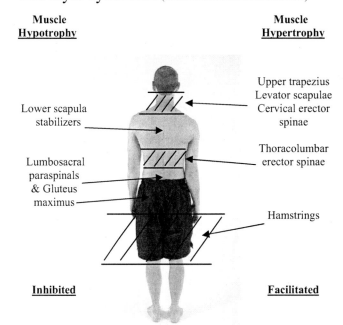

Muscle Hypotrophy		Muscle Hypertrophy
		Upper trapezius Levator scapulae Cervical erector spinae
Lower scapula stabilizers		
		Thoracolumbar erector spinae
Lumbosacral paraspinals & Gluteus maximus		
		Hamstrings
Inhibited		**Facilitated**

153

Ideal posture
Side view

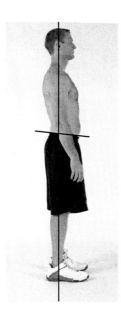

Head: Neutral position
Cervical spine : Normal curve (extension)
Thoracic spine: Normal curve (slight flexion)
Lumbar spine: Normal curve (extension)
Pelvis: Neutral position
Hip joints: Neutral position
Knee joints: Neutral (neither flexed or extended)
Ankle joints: Neutral position (leg perpendicular to sole of foot)

The pelvis should be a little bit more posterior

Upper/Lower Cross Syndrome
Side view

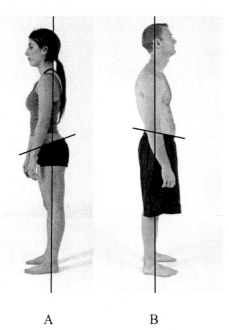

A   B

Head: Forward
Cervical spine : Hyperextended
Thoracic spine: Hyperflexed (excessive kyphosis)
Lumbar spine: Hyperextended (hyperlordotic)
Pelvis: Anteriorly tilted
Hip joints: Flexed
Knee joints: Slightly hyperextended
Ankle joints: Slight planter flexion

Flat Back
Side view

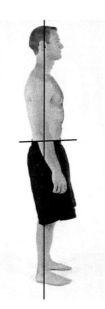

Head: Varies
Cervical spine : Varies
Thoracic spine: Upper portion is hyperflexed, lower portion is straight
Lumbar spine: Flexed (straight)
Pelvis: Posteriorly tilted
Hip joints: Extended
Knee joints: Varies
Ankle joints: Varies

Tight hamstrings and a posteriorly tilted pelvis play key important roles in a flat back posture. So does a "tight ass" mentality.

Sway Back
Side view

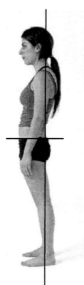

Head: Forward
Cervical spine : Slightly extended
Thoracic spine: Hyperflexed
Lumbar spine: Increased flexion with flattening lower portion
Pelvis: Posteriorly tilted and anteriorly displaced
Hip joints: Hyperextended
Knee joints: Hyperextended
Ankle joints: Neutral.
A sway that begins lower than the knee joint is a forward lean posture.

Forward Lean
Side view

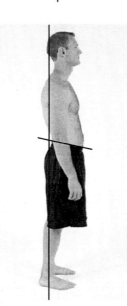

Head: Forward
Cervical spine : Slightly extended
Thoracic spine: Hyperflexed
Lumbar spine: Hyperextended (hyperlordotic)
Pelvis: Anteriorly tilted
Hip joints: Flexed
Knee joints: Varies
Ankle joints: Varies
Feet are usually pronated (flattened) from the displaced forward weight of the body.

154

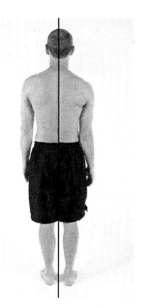

Right Handed Posture
Posterior view

Head: Varies
Shoulders : Right side lower
Thoracic spine: Curved concave right
Lumbar spine: Curved concave right
Pelvis: Right side higher
Short/Tight Muscles: (R) lats. Q.L., lateral abs, hip adductors, tibialis posterior (L) hip abductors, peroneus longus/brevis,
Long/Weak Muscles: same as short/tight, but opposite side

Lazy Posture
Side view

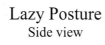

Head: Forward
Cervical spine: Hyperextended
Thoracic spine: Hyperflexed
Lumbar spine: Flattening (flexing towards straightened)
Pelvis: Slight posterior tilt
Hip joints: Extended
Knee joints: Varies
Ankle joints: Varies

Think of the muscles as clothes and the bones as the coat rack. That is what "lazy" posture is like. The muscles are just hanging (relaxing/giving in) there. Awareness and effort usually improve this situation.

Lordosis
Side view

Head: Varies
Cervical spine : Varies
Thoracic spine: Usually more flexed
Lumbar spine: Excessive extension
Pelvis: Anteriorly tilted
Hip joints: Flexed
Knee joints: Varies
Ankle joints: Varies

Layer Syndrome

This is very similar to upper and lower cross syndromes, but less specific. It is a great visual for how the body does get tight and weak in seemingly alternating areas on the body. This "syndrome" affects virtually everyone in varying degrees. Another name for it could be "sitting syndrome."

Upper/Lower Cross Syndromes

Although these syndromes are not always expressed together, it seems best to talk about them in combination because they facilitate each other, depending on which one started first. This is another "sitting syndrome" issue. Depending on the person's history and present habits, they will be prone to upper or lower cross syndrome, usually one more than the other.

These postures will take over the entire body's structure if left uncorrected for long enough. The stresses caused by either of them will spread all the way up, or all the way down the body's musculoskeletal system. Over time they can even permanently alter the joint mechanics throughout the body, especially in the spine.

As with most postures, the secret to fixing them isn't simply corrective exercises. As you can see in the images for upper/lower cross syndrome on pg. 154, those two people also have the ability to assume other postures, such as flat and sway back, and even ideal posture.

So what does that mean? This is the most important concept of posture to understand. It is an ATTITUDE and awareness. Those people in the images have tendencies, just like everyone else, to succumb to gravity and have poor posture. It is not unique for someone to have more than one posture. Unfortunately it is not very common for people to know that they have more than one posture and that each of them is associated with a different feeling or attitude or situation they experience.

The realization of those key tendencies can be the difference in actually changing someone's posture much more than the exercise themselves.

Flat Back Posture

This posture is less common than the others, but still an issue with many people. The causes are widespread and can be from having an uptight (tight-ass) attitude, issues with holding things in (squeezing the buttocks and not wanting to let go, even going back to potty training issues), or from physical habits that encourage that posture. Weak hip flexors are also a common contributor.

Sway Back Posture

Sway back, lazy posture, flat back, and forward lean posture are all very alike but have important differences.

Box 12-5 *Key Distinctions*

POSTURES	Posterior pelvic tilt	Anterior pelvic tilt	Forward body sway	Hyper-extended hips	Flat lumbar spine
Flat Back	X			X*	X
Forward Lean		X	X		
Sway Back	X		X	X	X**
Lazy	X***			X*	X**

* Hips are only extended, not hyperextended
** Spine is flattening, not yet flattened
*** Only slightly tilted

Sway back posture can be from repetitively leaning the knees or hips against things when standing, i.e. the sink. This posture places significant stress on the anterior hip and sacroiliac joints and the external oblique muscles. The posterior deviation of the thoracic spine often causes the illusion of lordosis.

Forward Lean Posture

This posture can be called "the ski jumper" for the resemblance of the forward lean of jumpers to gain wind resistance. It creates very poor balance and extreme stress on ankle, hip, sacroiliac, and lumbar joints. This posture is unique from the other three because of its lumbar extension stress.

Lazy Posture

Another way to say lazy in this case is lack of awareness. It is almost as if the pelvis is a tripod that the body is *resting* on. Muscle weakness is a likely cause here, especially in the endurance of the stabilizers.

POSTURAL ASSESSMENT

Anterior View

Because the use of a plumb line is not always possible, this posture assessment will focus on observations without it, but may make occasional references to it. It is imperative to have a picture of a plumb line in the observers mind when viewing posture. From the side view, placing one finger just anterior to the malleolus and placing another finger from the other hand at the mid-hip area will allow for an imaginary line to be drawn up to the shoulder and head.

Feet (pronated/supinated)

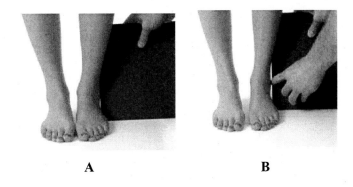

A   **B**

Fig. 12-1   A is ideal alignment. B shows how to slide the finger in to check for a space between the lateral malleolus and straight edge (clipboard in this case).

While standing upright with the feet about 3-5 inches apart, place a straight edge (a ruler works well) on the ground touching the lateral side of the sole of the foot beneath the malleolus. It should align vertically while touching the ground, the lateral aspect of the foot, and the lateral malleolus. If there is a gap between the lateral maleolus and the straight edge, then the foot is pronated. If there is a gap between the lateral foot and the straight edge, then the foot is supinated.

Notice if the person's natural tendency is to stand with the feet wide apart. Although this creates a wider foundation, it forces the muscles to work harder to maintain it. Try it yourself and feel how much easier it is to stand with the legs closer together than farther apart. This is especially important for those with LBP.

Also notice any forward leaning posture, this is usually a contributor to pronation.

Feet (toeing in/toeing out)

Each foot should be pointed straight or slightly rotated laterally. On average, it is acceptable to have up to 10° of toeing out (foot is pointed laterally), but any "toeing in" is dysfunctional. Because there is no rotation of the knee when it is extended in a standing position, as well as no rotation of the ankle[49], it can be concluded that any abnormal toeing in or out is usually a result of femur rotation at the hip joint.[4]

Knees (bowlegged/knock-kneed)

While these two faults are commonly hereditary and structural, it is possible for certain postures to create these imbalances. As mentioned by Kendall and McCreary[49], hyperextended knees along with lateral rotation at the hip can cause the appearance of knock-knees, while hyperextension and medial rotation can cause a bowlegged appearance. If the knees are flexed, the appearance will be in reverse in relation to the hip rotation mentioned above.

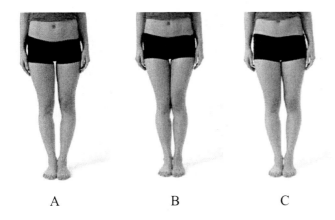

A   B   C

Fig 12-2   A is semi-bowlegged or someone standing with hyperextended knees. B shows knock-knees or flexed knees. C shows normal knees. This is a person with normal knees, and therefore A and B would appear more exaggerated in real cases.

These examples are postural defects and can be improved by stretching and strengthening the appropriate muscles, but genetic and structural abnormalities usually require more drastic measures such as wedges on the heels of shoes.

To determine a bowlegged or knock-kneed posture, have the person stand with both feet and knees together. If the knees cannot touch, then a bowlegged posture is present. If the knees are together but the feet cannot touch, then a knock-kneed posture is present. The feet and knees should touch (although this can be difficult if the upper legs are large) if the knees are normal.

Femur rotation

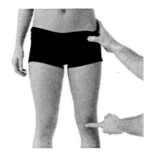

Fig. 12-3

An imbalance here is commonly in conjunction with, but not always, toeing in or out and pronation or supination. To check for femur rotation, observe the knee caps. If they are pointing outward, then the femur is laterally rotated, if inward, then the femur is medially rotated.

Once the center of the knee cap is found, observe which direction it points. The pelvis is stabilized by the examiner to keep the person balanced in case of a jerk reflex and to relate it to the position of the knee.

This person was assessed in her most comfortable position (to view any habitual postural stresses; this allowed the evaluator to learn that she often stands with hyperextended knees), which was feet together. Her femurs should also be assessed with the feet a few inches apart to note any changes.

Pelvic Assessment

The following three part pelvic assessment can be confusing and difficult to grasp until all components are fully understood and the ability to remember and integrate each finding is had. Assessing the pelvic region thoroughly involves three waves of tests, performed in the following order, yet interrupted by other assessments throughout;

1.   Structural dysfunction

A.   Stork test
B.   Standing flexion
C.   Seated flexion

2.   Standing asymmetry

A.   ASIS height – anterior view
B.   Iliac crest levels – anterior view
C.   ASIS vs. PSIS heights. (pelvic tilt) – side view

3.   Supine asymmetry

A.   ASIS height
B.   Iliac crest levels
C.   Pelvic rotation
D.   Inflare/outflare
E.   Shear dysfunction ("upslip" or "downslip")

The structural dysfunction assessments are near the beginning of the assessment and demonstrate which hemipelvis is dysfunctional, (see the individual tests on pg.'s 151 and 152 for details). These results are later used to determine the side of asymmetry in the supine assessment. The supine assessment gives a much clearer picture of the true structural asymmetry in the pelvic area because little to no lower leg inequalities or habitual compensations can interfere with results.

The next wave of pelvic assessing begins right here in the posture section. The standing position gives hints about dysfunctions and abnormalities, but mostly shows the postural compensations to leg length inequalities (LLI) or patterns of habitual use, or gives clues about which muscles may be weak or tight.

If a noticeable asymmetry exists in the standing assessment, the findings should be recorded and saved for later. At this point, asymmetry only shows that there is an imbalance between the two hemipelvis's; what type of imbalance is to be later determined in the supine assessment.

To sum it up; the structural pelvic assessment points to *which side* is dysfunctional; the standing assessment gives an idea about *which muscles* are imbalanced; the supine assessment tells *what type* of dysfunction it is.

The rest of the low back postural exam continues in order until the pelvic tilt in the side view is reached. Then the third and final standing pelvic assessment begins. Once finished their, the assessment continues until the ROM assessment is reached, and then the last wave of pelvic assessing begins. These are described on pg. 168.

The reason that the pelvic tests are not done in immediate succession of one another is because the entire assessment of the low back flows smoother when it is done with less moving back and forth from sitting to standing to lying. This way of assessing requires that the examiner keep a picture in their head and on paper of all the results that accumulate throughout the assessment and make quick judgments of priority areas to assess.

ASIS height

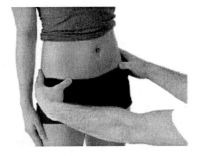

Fig. 12-4

This test compares the left and right ASIS. Simply place the thumbs on both ASIS's (the pointiest bone protruding from the anterior pelvis) and the rest of the fingers on top of the iliac crests. This gives a feel for the position of the entire pelvis. The iliac crest position is noted in the following test. Note which side (ASIS) is higher or lower here.

Iliac crest levels   anterior ◄───► posterior

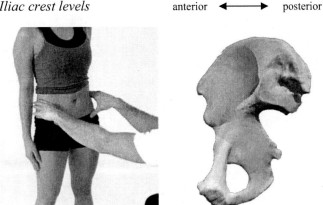

Fig. 12-5   **Fig. 12-6**

Assessing the level of the iliac crests is best done by comparing the anterior and posterior observations. Otherwise, a rotated hemipelvis can give the illusion of a lower or higher iliac crest. For example, if one hemipelvis is rotated anteriorly, it can seem lower from the anterior view and higher from the posterior view; this is due to the curvature of the bone.

To observe each iliac crest's height, place the index fingers into the lateral abdomen (soft place) just above the pelvis. Then tug downward, and depending on the size and shape of the person, it will be easy or difficult to find the top of the iliac crests. It is useful to also use the thumbs to feel the ASIS's at the same time so an idea can be had of the overall orientation of each hemipelvis.

Remember, just because one side is higher, doesn't mean that that hemipelvis is higher. It could mean that it is rotated anteriorly. Because the posterior portion of the ilium is naturally higher, see fig. 12-6, it can make the entire ilium seem higher when it is rotated anteriorly. This could also give the illusion of the opposite asymmetry when observing it from the back because the higher portion is more anterior and a lower part is now being palpated instead of that higher crest.

The asymmetry of iliac crest heights can be a result of numerous causes, including; LLI, small hemipelvis, faulty postural habits, scoliosis, iliosacral dysfunctions, and sacroiliac dysfunctions. Iliac crest asymmetry is a very important postural dysfunction due to the compensation scoliosis "C" or "S" curve it can produce. These curves can have drastic effects on the rest of the body, especially the Q.L. muscle and lateral stability.

The most common cause of iliac crest level asymmetries is compensations due to bad posture, although structural abnormalities are more common than rare. Around 10% of the normal population is believed to have LLI of 10mm[8], while 20-30% of people examined in an orthopedic practice had a small hemipelvis, in conjunction with or separate from a LLI, with the smaller hemipelvis usually on the shorter leg side.[56]

To learn the cause (structural abnormality or postural) of the asymmetry, multiple observations are necessary to identify a structural abnormality. It is best to assume that the cause is postural while trying to prove otherwise with the observations because the only way to be sure it is a postural cause is to rule out all structural abnormalities.
The following are observations, clues, and tests for structural anomalies that influence iliac crest levels and are all based on the findings of Travell and Simons.[7,8]

Observations

1. A small hemipelvis can produce a compensatory scoliosis when sitting and standing, but a LLI produces one only when standing, unless the curve has become osteoarthritic and therefore more permanent than functional.
2. A LLI provokes symptoms primarily when standing, while a small hemipelvis can cause pain during sitting, standing, and lying supine.
3. A LLI does not always cause pain or discomfort. It is common for people to live happily with their imbalance until something happens to aggravate the situation, such as a slip and fall or car accident. Then, the Q.L. is the muscle that is most often overloaded.

Clues to LLI

1. It is not uncommon to have a smaller hemipelvis, upper arm, and face on the same side as the shorter leg.
2. During standing posture, the arm on the short leg side

hangs away from the body while the other arm rests against the body.

3. One iliac crest is lower*, in conjunction with a low opposite shoulder.

4. One PSIS is lower.

5. A compensatory scoliosis curve that is emphasized when bending forward by a prominent rib cage on one side.

6. When standing, body weight rests mostly on the short leg, while the other leg is positioned more anterior or diagonal, and likely flexed.

7. A lift (under the heel) of appropriate height seems comfortable and corrects any compensatory scoliosis and iliac crest and shoulder height discrepancies. This can be reinforced by adding the lift to only the other side and noting the discomfort it creates.

8. When standing, one knee is taller than the other, and possibly an ankle as well.

9. All of the above point to a LLI, but the only way to be sure is to measure an X-ray of the leg.

*An iliac crest height asymmetry does not signify a LLI, only the possibility of one. There are numerous pelvic dysfunctions that can tilt the pelvis in the absence of a LLI.

Tests for Structural Abnormalities

1. *Small hemipelvis.* Discerning a small hemipelvis from a pelvis that is merely twisted around the horizontal axis through the sacroiliac joints is best described by Travell and Simons[7] as follows.

"Such an obliquity is detected by placing the thumbs on the posterior superior iliac spines and resting the hands over the crests of the ilia, pointing each index finger to an anterior superior iliac spine, fingertips at equal distances from the spines bilaterally. When the seated patient rocks the pelvis backward, the relative heights of the anterior and posterior spines are noted on each side of the pelvis. Then the patient rocks the pelvis forward for comparison. When all points on one side are lower than the corresponding points on the other side, regardless of the position of the pelvis, that half of the pelvis is smaller. If, however, one anterior spine dips much lower than the other when the pelvis rocks forward, the pelvis is twisted."

2. *Small vertical hemipelvis* (sitting). Observe the person from behind while they are seated and notice any shoulder tilting, the smaller pelvis being tilted lower, and a compensatory "S" curve scoliosis. Attempt to correct these by sliding a lift under the ischium of the short side. If this improves the imbalances then a small vertical hemipelvis is possible, and probable if it's in conjunction with the previous test being positive. To be sure the proper side is deemed short, place the lift under the other side and notice the difference, which is usually discomfort and pain if it is placed under the larger side.

3. *Small anteroposterior hemipelvis* (supine). This abnormality causes discomfort while sleeping supine and places great stress on the Q.L. In the supine position, the smaller pelvis will be more posterior and respond well to a lift placed under it. Make sure the correction is right by placing the lift under the other side and noticing the difference, which is usually an exaderation of the imbalance and symptoms.

4. *Short upper arm.* One or both arms may be short, which forces the person to lean sideways to reach the armrest of most chairs, which aggravates the Q.L. muscle. A short arm is when the elbow does not reach the iliac crest when the arm is hanging down by the side.

5. Once a structural abnormality is indicated, apply manual therapy to the Q.L. and other influential areas to restore balance, then reassess for pelvic symmetry. If asymmetry still exists, then a structural abnormality is probable, or more manual therapy is needed. It can take up to four weeks before chronic asymmetry is corrected or noticeably improved by manual therapy and corrective exercising.

Pelvic rotation

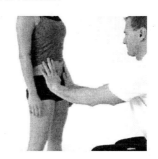

Fig. 12-7

Pelvic rotation in the standing posture assesses the balance of influential musculature more than it does the structural asymmetry of the pelvis, which is best done in a supine position. That is why this test is not included as part of the standing pelvic assessment.

Observe any pelvic rotation by placing the palms of the hands vertically over each side of the anterior hip, overlapping the psoas and iliacus muscles. This placement gives a good feel of the position of the pelvis. Sometimes the imbalance is so obvious that it can be seen without having to palpate. Note whether each side is rotated forward or backward (anterior or posterior).

Torso rotation

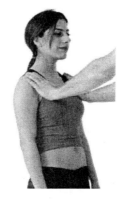

Fig. 12-8

Place the hands on the anterior shoulders and note the relationship between left and right. The torso is rotated anterior on the right if the right shoulder is forward and the left shoulder is posterior, *and* the midline of the torso is also rotated. The illusion of a rotated torso can be created by only one anterior shoulder. This illusion is different because one shoulder is forward, but the other shoulder is not posterior.

Shoulder elevation

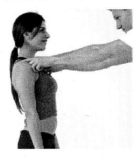

Fig. 12-9

Shoulder height discrepancies are easily observed by placing a finger atop of each acromium process (bony process on top of each shoulder) and comparing heights, although this can be misleading if the individual has injured their AC joint in the past.

Arm rotation

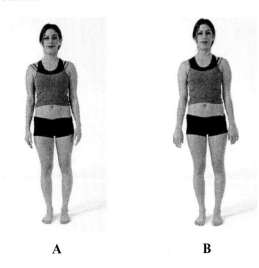

A   B

Fig. 12-10   A shows normal hand and arm position while B shows extreme anterior rotation.

Observe the hand and knuckle positions. If more than the thumb, index finger, and half of the middle finger's knuckle are showing, then the arm is medially rotated. Tight pronator muscles should be checked for tightness because of their influence on forearm rotation. A medially rotated arm is often in conjunction with, or due to, a forward shoulder. A laterally rotated arm is rare.

Head tilt and rotation (L/R)

Observe if the head is leaning or rotated to one side. Do not use the ears as a reference for tilting because they can be uneven themselves.

Posterior View

Feet/Achilles tendon (pronated/supinated)

The achilles tendon should be vertical. A pronated foot will have the appearance of an achilles tendon that bows

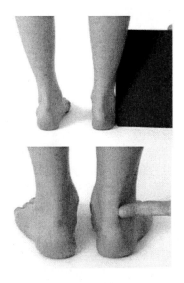

inward (convex medially), while a supinated foot has an achilles tendon that bows outward (convex laterally). This observation should be together with the placement of a straight edge, as in the anterior view.

Fig. 12-11

The top view shows a slightly bowed in (pronated) Achilles tendon, yet a "normal" positioning of the lateral malleolus. The bottom view confirms this with a close-up of the curve.

This confliction of findings is caused by the semi bowing-out (hyper-extended knees in this case) of this person's leg, which forces the lateral malleolus to be more lateral than a normal pronated foot.

Gluteal folds

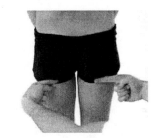

Fig. 12-12

Place fingers along the fold-lines of the buttocks and compare sides.

The folds should have similar qualities, but an anteriorly rotated innominate will give the appearance of a crease with less depth, and a posteriorly rotated innominate will produce a deeper and more apparent fold or crease.[4] Any difference in the level of height can be due to LLI, laterally tilted pelvis, or a weak gluteus maximus.

PSIS symmetry

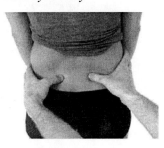

Fig. 12-13

This observation is to confirm the results of the ASIS findings and involves comparing the heights of the two sides. To find each PSIS, palpate the general area by rubbing in small circular motions with the thumbs until the protrusion is found. Take the measurement with the thumbs directly under each prominence. Note whether they are the same height, same distance from the midline, or more anterior or posterior.

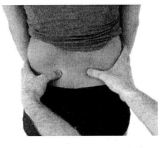

Iliac crest levels
Fig. 12-14

Same process as the anterior view, but from behind. Remember to imagine the image of the hemi-pelvis to give you an idea of whether one is higher or simply rotated. This hand position can be used to get the image, while a hand position more like fig. 12-15 can be used to feel the top of the hemi-pelvis.

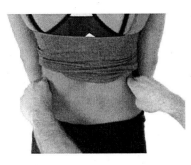

Rib cage level

Fig. 12-15

The 12th rib is the bottom of the rib cage and thus the ideal landmark to measure the rib cage by. Unfortunately it is much more difficult to palpate than the 11th rib. Therefore, under the assumption that there is no asymmetry between the 11th and 12 ribs of each side, this assessment will utilize the 11 rib as a landmark. If the examiner has the skill to palpate the 12th rib, then by all means use that landmark.

To find the 11th rib, place the lateral aspects of the index fingers on the lateral and somewhat posterior part of the rib cage, above the 11th rib. Then slide the fingers down the lateral rib cage until they come to the narrower and softer region of the mid-section. Approximate the fingers together firmly while pressing slightly upward until the 11th rib is felt. This may take a few tries with obese individuals. Be careful not to press any tissues into the tips of the floating ribs, as they can be quite sharp.

Note the height of each side and relate them to the height of each iliac crest to get a picture in the mind of how the trunk is situated on the pelvis. Then create an even larger picture by performing the next assessment, scoliosis.

Scoliosis

Scoliosis is a condition in the spine that produces an abnormal lateral (left to right) curvature of the spine and vertebral rotation that are usually in the thoracic and or lumbar regions.

It can be either functional (the spine is normally straight but a curve has resulted due to compensating for other abnormalities, i.e. bad posture, and can be corrected once the main cause is treated) or structural (the spine is set into this curvature forever, but this does not mean that excess tension cannot be relieved by employing the appropriate strategies).

The lateral spinal curve can be in the shape of a "C" or can be a combination of two curves that result in an "S" shape. These curves can be caused by congenital, developmental, or degenerative influences, with the cause usually unknown and classified as idiopathic scoliosis.

Right thoracic scoliosis is the most common type of scoliosis.[259] The ensuing convex curve to the right forces the involved vertebrae to side bend left and rotate right, as well as push the erector spinae muscles laterally.[260] Thoracic scoliosis is also the most likely to progress into a serious deformity, especially in females.[259] Also, a right concave side is more often than not related to right handedness.

Detecting these curves is fairly easy in mild to moderate cases because the individual is often already aware of it and their clothes wear unevenly. If it is not this obvious or the person is unaware of their abnormality, then a few tests and observations are needed to learn if and where the curve is.

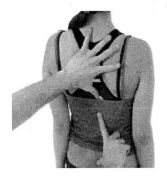
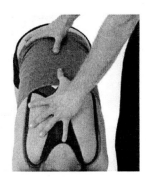

A   B

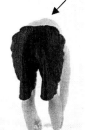

C

Fig. 12-16   A and B show the finger placement to test for any curvature. C shows the posterior "hump" that is on the convex side of a curve and is due to posteriorly rotated ribs on that side.[259]

1. Run two fingers down the spine, starting at C7 and ending at the sacrum, while holding one of the individual's shoulders to stabilize them against the firm pressure. This may take a couple of times to get a feel of the curvature.

2. The first test can be confirmed by placing a finger on C7 and the corresponding thumb on T6. Then place the other pinky finger on T12 and the thumb on L5. This should form a straight line and can be even further confirmed by drawing a dot on each spinous process and noting the symmetry.

3. Have the person bend forward as if to touch their toes, and notice any "humps" or areas that appear larger on one

side of the spine, usually in the thoracic area. The posterior "hump" is on the convex side of the curve and is due to posteriorly rotated ribs on that side.[259] This rotation will also cause the chest or breast to be relatively "indented" on that side.

4. The ribs, and thus the chest or breast, on the side of concavity will be pushed and rotated anteriorly, crowded together, and more pronounced because of the vertebral rotation.[259]

5. A true structural curve will not straighten out during lateral or forward flexion.[260] A non-structural or functional curve will be corrected or improve with lateral or forward flexion.[58,260] The lateral flexion should be to the convex side in order to improve the curve.

6. LLI are commonly involved with functional scolioses.[8,260]

Use these observations to differentiate any curvatures for the thoracic and lumbar regions. Remember, the observations only show signs of a curvature, not what areas need to be corrected. Often times LLI, poor postural habits, foot pronation, and uneven iliac crest levels need to be addressed before focusing directly on the spine. Scoliosis assessment and corrective actions should involve the entire body and all of its parts.

Scapula rotation

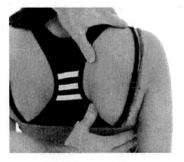

Fig. 12-17

First find the medial border of the scapula, then place one finger or thumb from each hand at approximately mid level of the medial border. Slide one digit upward and the other downward until they each come to a place where the medial border starts to deviate laterally, stop at this point. Both of these points are short of the superior and inferior angles, but are used as reference points here because of the difficulty in palpating the superior angle of the scapula through the upper trapezius and levator scapula.

These two points (inferior and superior digits) should form a vertical line. It can be tricky if the reference points used by the digits are too far superior or inferior because of the curving shape of the scapula. If the bottom digit is more lateral than the top digit, then the scapula is superiorly rotated. If the bottom digit is more medial, then the scapula is inferiorly rotated.

Scapula ab/adduction

The scapulas should lie about 5cm from the medial border of the scapula.[62] This distance is approximately the width of the three middle fingers (the size of the fingers of the

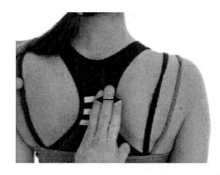

Fig. 12-18

individual being assessed; sometimes the evaluator's fingers are much larger or smaller than the person being evaluated) when they are placed together.

The scapulas should lie flat on the rib cage, but with abducted scapulas, the medial border of the scapula is often more prominent and in conjunction with or a result of a forward shoulder. An abducted scapula has a medial border that is situated more than 5cm away from the spine.

Adducted scapulas are closer to the spine than normal and are less frequent than abducted scapulas. This can be a result of the typical military posture that was once held by voluntary muscle contractions and has now become an involuntary postural adaptation. This posture is commonly involved with an elevated scapula as well.

Scapula elevation

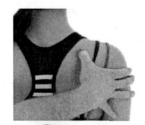

Fig. 12-19

The scapula is situated between the 2nd and 7th to 8th ribs.[54] Observe the level of the scapula by first finding T2 (have the person tuck their chin which shows the protrusion of C7, then slide the finger two vertebra down to T2). With firm pressure, locate the superior angle of the scapula and compare its height to T2.

Be aware of mistaking a rigid knot in the levator scapula for the superior border or being fooled by an illusionary asymmetry in scapula height due to uneven shoulder heights.

An elevated scapula is higher than T2 and associated with forward shoulders and abducted scapulas. A depressed scapula is below T2 and associated with a

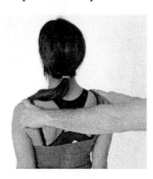

downward sloping of the shoulders. The latter example is rare.

Shoulder elevation

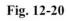

Fig. 12-20

Place fingers on the acromium processes (bony parts of the top of the

162

shoulders) and compare the heights of each side.

Head tilt and rotation (L/R)

See anterior view.

Side (R/L)

Knees (flexed/hyperextended)

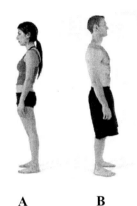

A　　**B**

Fig. 12-21 A shows hyperextended knees while B shows flexed knees.

Good alignment of the knee will show a plumb line that passes from just in front of the lateral malleolus and slightly anterior to the midline of the knee.[49]

Deviation of the knee posterior to the plumb line (or relative to the front of the malleolus) is indicative of hyperextension of the knee. Extreme hyperextension of the knee will place the ankle joint into plantar flexion.[49] Deviation of the knee anterior to the front of the malleolus indicates a flexed knee.

Pelvic tilt

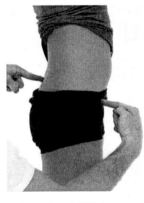

Fig. 12-22

This test is the third and final test in the standing pelvic evaluation and it sheds some light on whether one hemipelvis (innominate) is asymmetrical or the entire pelvis is tilted.

The ASIS and PSIS on one side must be palpated and compared for relative height. The normal relationship is when the ASIS is equal to or no more than a half an inch inferior to its corresponding PSIS.[4]

If both ASIS's are more than a half an inch inferior to their PSIS's, than there is an anterior tilt of the pelvis, which is associated with an increased lumbar lordosis, as well as pronated feet, upper crossed syndrome, and many other asymmetries and dysfunctions.

If the ASIS is superior to the PSIS, then there is posterior tilt, which can be a result of at least two different postures, a sway or flat-back posture. See pg. 154 for pictures of sway and flat back postures.

If only one hemipelvis is tilted, then the pelvis is not considered tilted. Instead, there is an innominate, or hemipelvis asymmetry or dysfunction. Whichever side is

not of normal proportion (ASIS vs. PSIS height) is the side of dysfunction, and therefore is deemed as rotated superiorly or inferiorly.[4] Therefore, both sides need to be measured to assure findings; otherwise it is easy to measure only one side, find it to be tilted, and assume that the entire pelvis is rotated.

A pronounced lordosis is an obvious sign that both sides, and therefore the whole pelvis, is anteriorly tilted; whereas a dysfunctional hemipelvis does not necessarily increase lordosis.

These results should match up with the three structural test findings. For example, if the right hemipelvis is noted as dysfunctional in the structural assessments, it should also be the right side that was found to be dysfunctional in the standing pelvic tilt assessment.

Again, if both sides are dysfunctional in the standing assessment, then the entire pelvis is either anteriorly or posteriorly tilted. If only one side is dysfunctional, then only that hemipelvis is rotated.

Thoracic curvature

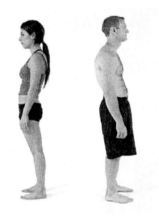

Fig. 12-23

These pictures show excessive thoracic curvature, among other things.

A normal thoracic curvature is one that is slightly kyphotic (convex posteriorly). The upper abdominals are frequently dominant in posture faults such as upper cross syndrome and cause subsequent inhibition of the thoracic extensors.

Take note of any excessive curvature that is seen as a protrusion or hump. This posture is associated with forward shoulders, scapulas, and head, as well as elevated scapulas.

Shoulder (anterior/posterior)

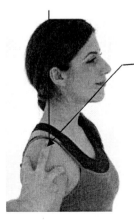

Fig. 12-24

The middle of the shoulder should line up with the middle of the ear, middle of the hips, and just anterior to the lateral malleolus.

Care must be taken to not compare the shoulder position to only that of the head, because a forward head will make the shoulders appear posterior. They must be compared to hips, feet, and head in order to tell where the asymmetry is stemming from.

The greatest signs of a forward shoulder are the presence of thoracic kyphosis and or abducted scapulas. Certain postural faults can displace the entire body forward and make interpreting the alignment of the shoulder, hip and foot landmarks tricky. A rotated torso can also give the appearance of a posterior or anterior shoulder.

Any deviation forward and the shoulder is considered anterior. Any deviation backwards and it is considered posterior. It is rare however that the shoulder is posterior.

Head (anterior/posterior)

The back of the ear should line up with the point just anterior to the medial malleolus,[49] see fig. 12-24 It is common to have the head forward from this point and therefore be considered anterior. It is rare to have a posterior head. An anterior head posture is associated with forward shoulders and thoracic kyphosis.

Head tilt (up/down)

A normal head position is one that is horizontally level, with no upward or downward deviation of the chin. The cervical curve should also be slightly convex anteriorly.

Gait

Gait should be observed from the front, back, and side, including shoes on and off if time permits. The following alignments should occur naturally.

Level head
Level shoulders
Arms swing opposite of the legs
Torso rotates opposite of the hips
Hip extends and toes push off
Knees point forward without rotating
Feet pointing relatively forward (up to 10° of external rotation is acceptable)
Time spent on each foot should be equal
The torso rotation should initiate the arm swing, not vice versa
The lumbar spine should be naturally curved
There should be no leaning to one side

ROM

A smooth flow can be accomplished if the following order is used. Start from standing and finishing with lying prone. Because of this flow and that of the entire low back evaluation, the pelvic assessment is included in the supine section, even though it is a postural assessment.

Standing

- Standing lumbar flexion
- Standing lumbar extension
- Standing lumbar extension with rotation
- Standing lumbar side flexion (L/R)

Sitting

- Sitting lumbar flexion (straight legs)
- Sitting lumbar flexion (legs bent, off table)
- Sitting torso rotation
- Neck ROM
  - flexion
  - extension
  - lateral flexion
  - rotation

Supine

- Leg length
Pelvic assessment
  - ASIS height
  - Pelvic rotation
  - ASIS flare
  - ASIS, PSIS, pubic ramus
- Hip flexion
- Hamstring
- Piriformis
- Hip adduction/abduction
- Psoas
- Rectus femoris
- Gastocnemius
- Soleus
- Pectoralis minor
- Latissimus dorsi
- Pectoralis major
- TFL (on side)
- Torso twist (on side)

Prone

- Femur rotation
- Quadriceps

Descriptions of each ROM Assessment

ROM can be limited by muscle tightness and or joint pathology. The end feel of the ROM is a good indicator of what type of problem is present. An abrupt stop in ROM indicates a structural influence while a springy or pliable resistance at the end range indicates a soft tissue restriction.

164

For some situations (cold day out, person has been sitting all day prior to assessment, etc.) it is beneficial to repeat certain tests a few times or even have the person warm up with some aerobic activity before the entire assessment in order to loosen up the joints and surrounding tissues to their normal working capacity.

Standing

Standing lumbar flexion

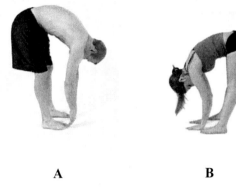

A   **B**

Fig. 12-25   A shows a hypermobile thoracic spine. B shows very flexible hamstrings and lumbar spine. Note the difference between the direction their lumbar spines (A is angled upward and B downward). Check out how pronounced the differences are when these two people perform the sitting lumbar flexion test, fig. 12-28.

The knees should be straight and feet slightly apart. The person is instructed to bend forward towards the floor and let the arms hang downward. This test can be hindered by the inability or excessive ability to bend at the hips, which gives the appearance of an inflexible or flexible spine respectfully. The proper way to bend at the hips sometimes has to be taught and can take more than one session to learn. If this is the case, focus on observing the curve of the lumbar spine.

Bent knees can signify soft tissue restriction anywhere along the posterior connective tissue system, although the tightness is usually coming from the hamstrings and or gastrocsoleus complex. *Leaning to one side during the first part of forward flexion but then returning to the midline is indicative of a short psoas muscle on that side.*[8]

The main goal of this, and the other two sitting flexion tests, is to learn where the ROM is limited and where it is excessive or normal. It is quite easy to bend down and touch the floor with a tight lower back as long as the hamstrings and or the thoracic spine are flexible enough to allow it.

The areas of restriction can be clarified by looking at the actual curve in the lumbar spine, which should be slightly flexed at the end ROM of flexion. It is common to see someone who can touch the floor, yet their lumbar spine is straight. A closer look will show that their thoracic spine is hypermobile and or the hips have rotated so much that the spine appears closer to the ground and therefore more flexible.

The palm of the examiner's hand can be placed on the lumbar spine during flexion to feel for any vertebral gapping or movement. Lack of movement suggests low back tightness.

With all that being said, this test is difficult to judge only the low back on and is better suited to paint a picture of how the entire posterior soft tissue system works together and how much body control the person has.

Standing lumbar extension

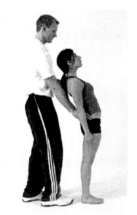

Fig. 12-25

Start in the same position as the flexion test, then ask the person to extend backwards as far as possible, which should be 25° according to the normal values stated by the "Guides to the Evaluation of Permanent Impairment"[66] as referenced in Liebenson (1996).[41] S.I. and facet joint dysfunctions can limit this ROM and also cause pain on one or both sides of spine, as well as radiating downward. Make sure that the person doesn't push their pelvis anteriorly to gain ROM.

The examiner should be ready to support the person in case they lose their balance.

Standing lumbar extension with rotation

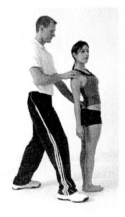

Fig. 12-26

This is the same as the standing extension test with the addition of rotation to each side. ROM is not so much a factor with this test as is the presence of pain. When extending and rotating to the right, this test can;
1. Aggravate TP's in the left psoas, lateral abdominals, or Q.L. and cause LBP on the left.
2. Aggravate a dysfunctional S.I. or facet joint on the right (possibly on left) and cause LBP on the right (possibly on left).
3. Aggravate the Q.L. or deep paraspinal muscles on the right and cause LBP on the right.

4. Aggravate sensitive facet joints and cause local or referred pain down into the hip and buttocks.

Standing lumbar side flexion (L/R)

Fig. 12-27

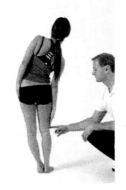

First, correct any iliac crest level difference by placing an appropriate size lift under the short side's foot. With the feet shoulder width apart, ask the person to bend laterally without deviating forwards or backwards or lifting their foot and slide their hands down the side of each leg. Normal ROM is when the finger tips reach just past the knee.[4] Be aware of short or long upper arms affecting the test. The key is the end feel of the ROM. Restriction in this test points to shortness in the Q.L. and or lateral abdominals.

Sitting

Sitting lumbar flexion (straight legs)

A   B

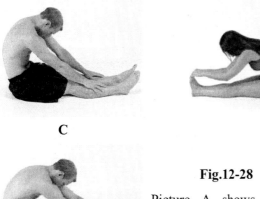

C

Fig.12-28

Picture A shows extremely tight hamstrings (hips can't rotate anteriorly), calves (feet unable to dorsi-flex), and lumbar spine is tight (goes straight without flexing), along with a hypermobile thoracic spine. B shows normal hamstrings and calves, but above average spine flexibility. C is now warmed-up and shows no obvious signs of limited ROM, although hypermobility in the thoracic spine is a sign of compensating for tightness elsewhere along the same stress-lines of tissues or structures, i.e. lumbar spine.

Sit on the floor or a hard surface (a soft surface will induce pelvic rotation) with the legs straight and toes pointed upward. Instruct the person to lean forward as if to touch their toes, ideally T.A. activation (abdominal hollowing) occurs at this point. The knees should not bend and the pelvis should not tilt.

Kendall and McCreary[49] state that "The ability to touch fingertips to toes is a desirable accomplishment for most adults." This ability of course includes a balanced flexibility between the legs, hips, and spine.

This test shows where tension resides in the posterior muscles and structures. Results should be compared to those of the standing and sitting tests.

The following findings are clues to muscle tightness during the sitting flexion test;

• Tight gastrocnemius will not allow the feet to point upward.

• Tight hamstrings cause the pelvis to rotate posteriorly and low back to be positioned posterior to the buttocks.

• Tight low back erector spinae muscles create the appearance of a flat lumbar spine.

• Always be aware of individuals with an imbalance between structural torso and leg length. This will give the illusion of tight or flexible muscles, i.e. someone with a long torso and short legs is more able to touch their toes.

• If pain is present or worsens in the low back during head flexion, then soft tissue (fascia, muscles, or nerves) are suspected to be strained.

Sitting lumbar flexion (legs hanging off table)

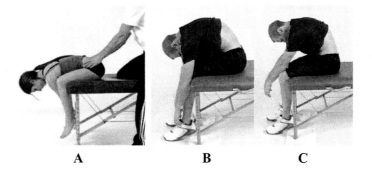

A   B   C

Fig. 12-29

Picture A shows extreme lumbar flexion, while B appears to exhibit normal lumbar ROM, but it is all at the hips. C shows the same bend if the hips did not move. Both B and C had no lumbar vertebral motion.

This test isolates the mobility of the lumbar spine and erector spinae because of the bent knees. Have the person sitting with their knee crease at the edge of the table and knees flexed with the legs dangling. It is often helpful to instruct them to apply light downward pressure on the iliac crests in order to stabilize the pelvis on the table while they attempt to flex the spine and bring the head to the knees. If this flexion attempt does not reverse the lumbar curve then the erector spinae are likely short in this area.[4,12]

Take note of any flat areas of the spine and differences between the thoracic and lumbar mobility. Flat areas are evidence of tight erector spinae and or restricted vertebral segments. Often times there is a compensatory hypermobility (resulting in kyphosis) of the thoracic spine in order to make up for the immobile lumbar spine.

Sitting torso rotation

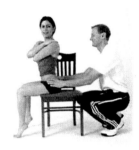

Fig. 12-30

The person is sitting with the hips and knees bent approximately 90° and the hands atop each opposite shoulder. Instruct them to rotate the torso as far as possible without deviating into flexion, extension, or side bending. The normal ROM is 45° in each direction.[41] Note any asymmetry between sides. <u>Feet should be flat.</u>

Neck ROM

The measurements for neck ROM should be taken while the *person is seated* with the shoulder girdle stabilized. Pain during these tests can be from TP's in the muscles or structural dysfunctions such as facet syndrome, immobile vertebrae, displaced vertebrae, etc. Structural dysfunctions that cause pain require referral from a specialist before starting an exercise program that involves the neck.

Neck Flexion

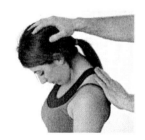

Fig. 12-31

According to Chaitow and DeLaney[11], "The chin (mouth closed) should easily touch the sternum". A ROM of about 50° is normal for flexion.[11,52]

Neck Extension

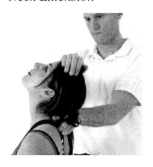

Fig. 12-32

Normal ROM for neck extension is 70°.[11,52] Another way to measure it is to stick your finger right above C7 as they are extending. They should be able to pinch your finger.

Neck Lateral Flexion

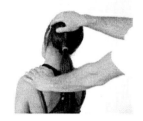

Fig. 12-33

A normal ROM for lateral flexion is about 45°.[11,52] If the side being tested is the same side that is stabilized by the examiner's hand, then the upper trapezius is being evaluated, but if the opposite side is supported then the cervical spine is being assessed.[11]

Neck Rotation

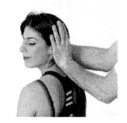

Fig. 12-34

A normal ROM for neck rotation is 85°.[11,52]

Supine

Leg length test

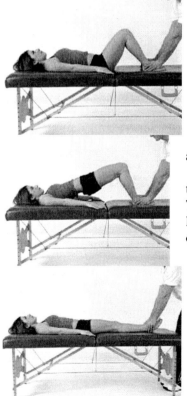

Fig. 12-35

Before evaluating the supine pelvis and leg length, it is best to align the body by doing the preparations described in box 12-5. This alignment will yield more accurate results for assessing a supine pelvis.[4]

Compare the levels of the two medial malleoli. They should be at equal levels. If they are not, this observation only shows that the legs are uneven, from what can only be known after correcting any influential muscle tension (usually in the Q.L., psoas, and or piriformis) or a measurement done on an X-ray of the leg.

If after correcting

myofascial tension the LLI disappears, then it is likely that it was a functional (due to pelvic asymmetry), not structural LLI.

Box 12-5 (Fig. 12-35)

Aligning the pelvis prior to supine assessment

1. Lying supine, flex both knees and place the feet together flat on the table at midline.
2. Raise the hips of the table slightly and then lower them back on the table and flatten the legs out.

The pelvis

This is the third part of the pelvic assessment. The first two were in the structural and posture assessments. Assessing the supine pelvis involves *feeling how it moves and responds to palpation in specific directions*, and seeing if any postural distortions are present, such as;

- innominate tilt - anterior/posterior
- pelvic rotation – right/left
- innominate rotation – inflare/outflare
- innominate shear – "upslip"/"downslip"

The following supine observations will allow the examiner to figure out the orientation of the pelvis as a whole and as a hemipelvis. Their results should be compared to those of the standing assessment, any differences in results requires re-assessing for validation. If the results are still different in the two positions, then the reason should be figured out. Some possibilities are joint laxity in the hip or S.I. joint, a larger gluteus maximus on one side (causing that innominate to appear more anterior in the supine assessment), or someone laying more to one side on a soft table that is indented in the middle from overuse (causing the innominate towards the edge of the table to appear more anterior and rotated medially).

The alignment described in Box 12-5 levels out the pelvis and makes for a more accurate assessment.[114] This should be done prior to any supine pelvic or leg length assessments.

ASIS height

Compare the heights of the ASIS's on both sides. In order to figure out which side is inferior or superior. Refer to the results of the stork and standing forward flexion tests. The side that was dysfunctional is the side that is displaced.

This test should be performed standing (A) and supine (B) for complicated situations in order to

This observation gives information about whether or not and which way (anterior or posterior) the hemipelvis is tilted.

Fig. 12-36   *ASIS Height*

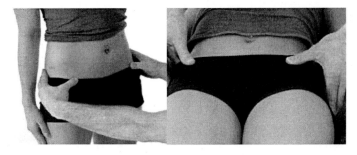

A   B

Pelvic rotation

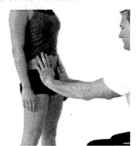

Fig. 12-37

This test can be done standing or supine, with the same hand position. Supine observation shows a truer structural imbalance, and the standing test shows more how the body compensates throughout it entirely.

Place the palms on each ASIS. The observer is looking for one ASIS to be more anterior than the other (higher off the table when supine with the ipsilateral buttock having more clearance between it and the table); this signifies an anteriorly rotated pelvis. This is different from a flared hemipelvis because both ASIS are equidistant from the midline of the body.

These observations give information about whether or not and which way (right or left) the entire pelvis is rotated.

ASIS flare

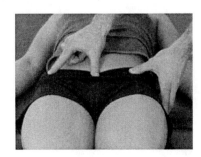

Fig. 12-38

Each ASIS is compared to the midline of the body, usually the umbilicus; they should both be equidistant from the center of the body. Any deviation laterally is an outflare and any deviation medially is an inflare of the innominate.

The side that is inflared will have an ipsilateral buttock with more clearance between it and the table (test by sliding the hand under each side). This should be differentiated from pelvic rotation, which assesses rotation of the entire pelvis, not just one hemipelvis, and has both ASIS equidistant from the body's midline.

The side that is most dysfunctional is the side that moved most superiorly on the stork and or standing flexion tests. Although it is possible to have an inflare on one side

and an outflare on the other.[4]
This observation gives information about whether or not and which way (laterally or medially) each hemipelvis is rotated.

ASIS, PSIS, and pubic ramus ("upslip"/"downslip")

Fig. 12-39

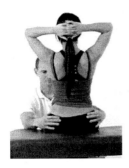

Grab the tops of the iliums with the thumbs and as much of the pelvis as possible with the bottom fingers. If small hands and a large pelvis are a problem, then use both hands to measure one side at a time, palpating the top of the ilium and the ischial tuberosity (sit bone).

If the ASIS, PSIS, and pubic ramus of one hemipelvis are all more cephalad than their contralateral landmarks and no rotation of the innominate is apparent, then that side is considered an "upslip" or superior innominate shear.[4] There should be palpable tension on the side of the "upslip".

This observation gives information about whether or not and which way (upwards or downwards) each hemipelvis is subluxed or sheared.

Hip flexion

Fig. 12-40

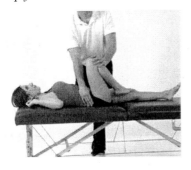

The person is supine on a firm surface with the non-examined knee bent and foot flat on the ground *or* that hip is held in flexion by the person's hands if the previous method did not flatten out the lumbar spine. The examiner places a hand on the examined side's iliac crest and ASIS to feel for any pelvic rotation. The other hand of the examiner brings the examined bent leg into hip flexion (cup the posterior knee crease if knee pain is present). The range is noted once hemipelvis tilting begins. The normal range for hip flexion is 120°.[53]

Hamstrings

Lying supine, bend the non-tested knee so that the foot rests on the table (this eliminates any influence on pelvic rotation by a short psoas). Raise the tested straight leg until the resistance barrier is met or pelvic compensations begin. Normal ROM for this position is 90°[43], although it is often said that a normal range for males is 70°. Any pain in this test signifies nerve

Fig. 12-41

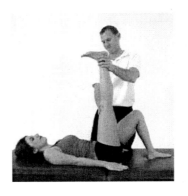

influences or the stretch was past the muscle's limit.

Compare results for clarification to the sitting flexion test on pg. 153.

Piriformis

Piriformis tightness is difficult to separate from tightness in the other five deep hip external rotators, but its irritability is usually distinct. To test for piriformis (and the other lateral rotators) shortness and involvement, any or all of the following four tests can be used.

Test # 1

Fig. 12-42

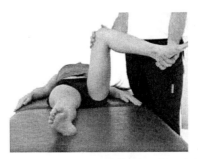

Bring the tested leg of the supine person up to about 60° of hip flexion. Make sure that the tested leg is in no more than 60° of hip flexion.

Beyond 60° of flexion the piriformis turns into a medial hip rotator.[65] Rotate the femur internally (foot moves away from the midline) until the resistance barrier is felt. Normal ROM is 40-45° for internal rotation. The end ROM should be springy; if a sudden stop in range and or pain in the posterior hip and buttock occur, then piriformis, S.I. joint, or hip joint adhesions/dysfunction are likely.

Test # 2

Fig. 12-43

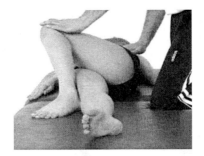

(piriformis # 2)

Place the tested leg of the supine person over the opposite straight leg with the foot lying flat next to the non-tested knee.

Apply force to the knee in the direction of adduction. The movement should be smooth with a gradual increase in springy resistance towards the end range. A sudden

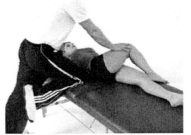

stop in range or pain in the posterior hip and buttock are signs of piriformis, S.I. joint, or hip joint adhesions/ dysfunction involvement. The total ROM (ideal = about 45°) is not as important as the feel of this stretch.

Test # 3

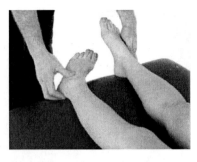

Fig. 12-44

(piriformis # 3)

With the person supine, passively rotate their tested straight leg, which is flat on the table, medially until resistance or discomfort is felt. The leg should rotate enough to allow the foot to touch the opposite ankle (180°), without any compensation in the pelvis. The end range should have the same feel as the first test. Any rigidity or pain is a sign of piriformis or sometimes the posterior fibers of the gluteus medius and mimimus being involved.

Test # 4

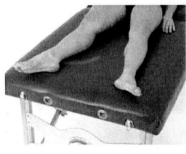

Fig. 12-45

While lying supine, the affected leg will be "naturally" rotated excessively outward during a relaxed posture if the piriformis is tight. The example in this picture is tight. The other tests are needed to confirm or deny the finding here.

Hip abduction

There are four main tests for adductor tightness. Any pain during the tests should be further assessed to find its origin. Check the piriformis and movements of the hip if pain is present. The first test assesses the entire adductor group while the second, third, and fourth tests assess more specific fibers of the group and their interaction with the rest of the body. The second, third, and fourth tests should be done in a smooth succession and are useful for narrowing down areas of tightness when applying manual therapy or if the first test causes pain (likely due to piriformis involvement or hip joint adhesions/dysfunction) and interferes with the true length of the adductors.

Test # 1

With the person supine, the examiner stabilizes the opposite side with one hand and slides the tested leg into flexion and abduction with the other while placing the

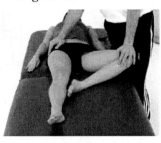

Fig. 12-46

person's foot flat against the opposite knee of their extended leg (this technique assesses the shortness of all three major adductors[8]).

When stabilizing the opposite pelvis, the tested thigh should be approximately 5-10° off the table, or about a flat hand's width of clearance beneath the proximal half of the thigh.

The foot can then be placed further up the thigh to involve more of the ischiocondylar fibers of the adductor magnus. Any pain or limitation in this position can be caused by TP's in the vasti, especially the vastus medialis.[8]

Test #2

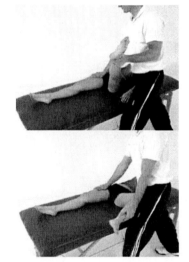

Fig. 12-47

(A = top: B= bottom)

With the person supine, grab the ankle of the tested side and stabilize the non-tested pelvis by applying pressure to the mid thigh of that side.

Flex and abduct the tested leg approximately 45° in each direction, with the non-tested leg lying flat and extended (fig. A). This position mainly tests the ischiocondylar fibers of the adductor magnus, as well as the gracilis and medial hamstrings.

If 45° of abduction cannot be reached, then, besides the adductors, the hamstrings, gracilis, or myofascia (in the superficial back or deep front lines) are possible contributors to tightness.

To differentiate where the limitation is coming from, flex the tested knee at the position of restriction (as in B). If the ROM now increases, hamstring, gracilis, or myofascial shortness was the cause for restricted movement, not adductor tightness.

Test # 3

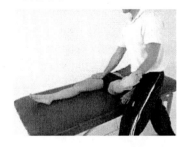

Fig. 12-48

This test utilizes the same positioning as test # 2, with the addition of increasing abduction to 60-70°. This position tests all three adductor muscles. Again, differentiate any restriction by flexing the knee as in the previous test.

Test # 4

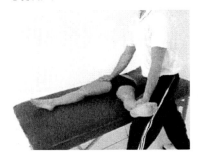

Fig. 12-49

Start at the end position of test # 3, then lower the leg towards the floor to approximately 30° to test for shortness in the adductors longus and brevis, and pectineus.

❖ All four adductor tests and ROM's are adapted from Travell and Simon's[8], with the author's addition of the medial hamstrings and myofascia involvement in test #'s 2 and 3 by flexing the leg; utilizing leg flexion to rule out the hamstrings is modified from Janda[43] and Chaitow and DeLaney,[4] who both used tests without any leg flexion.

Hip adduction

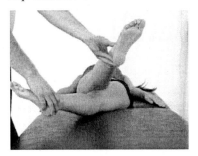

Fig. 12-50

With the person supine and both legs straight, raise the non-tested leg just enough so that the tested leg can be passively moved underneath it.

The tested leg should be able to adduct across the body approximately 30° without causing that hip to compensate.

This test should be compared to the results of the TFL ROM test in order to clarify or rule out TFL involvement.

Psoas

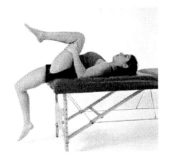

Fig. 12-51

This is a normal psoas and hip flexor test.

Although no test singles out the psoas, the following tests will consistently find psoas shortness.

Lying supine with the buttocks near the edge of the table, ask the person to grab the non-tested knee and pull it up towards their chest enough so that their back is flat, but not so much so that the lumbar spine is flexed (buttocks comes off the table).

The tested leg, which is hanging off the table, should normally be parallel to the table with the knee naturally bent to 80°. The thigh should also be able to move into slight extension, about 10°, with light pressure from the examiner.[4]

If the thigh is parallel to the table but the knee is not naturally flexed to about 80°, then the rectus femoris and TFL are tight.

If the thigh is above the table but the knee is naturally flexed to 80°, then the psoas is probably the main tightness.

If the thigh is above the table and the knee is not naturally flexed to about 80°, then the psoas, rectus femoris, and TFL can all be tight and therefore additional tests are needed to rule out the normal muscles. This can be done by straightening the leg to see if the ROM improves. If so, it was the rectus femoris and TFL that were tight. If the leg is still higher than the table with the straight leg, then the psoas are short.

If in any of the above tests, no matter what the result, the thigh cannot be moved into 10° of extension with light pressure from the examiner, it is a sign of hip flexor tightness or hip joint adhesions or dysfunctions.

Rectus femoris

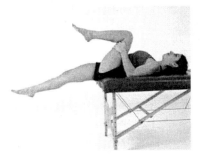

Fig. 12-52

Same as in the psoas test. If the thigh is parallel to the table but the knee is not naturally flexed to about 80°, then the rectus femoris and TFL are tight. The rectus femoris and TFL are considered normal in length if the knee can naturally flex to 80°.[49]
This test shows tight rectus femoris and perhaps TFL.

Gastrocnemius

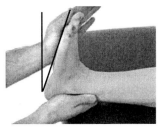

Fig. 12-53

This is about 20° of dorsi flexion, which is ideal.

The feet should be over the edge of the table enough so that the Achilles tendon is not pressed against the table. To make things ergonomically efficient the following method is recommended and is adapted from Chaitow and Delaney.[4]

To test the right side, the right hand of the examiner cups the individual's right heel and lightly grasps the Achilles tendon. While the right hand pulls on the heel, taking the slack out of the gastrocnemius, the left palm pushes on the ball of the right foot, keeping the foot in a neutral position (no inversion or eversion).

The normal ROM is 0° with minimal force applied and up to 20° with moderate force. 0° is when the foot is perpendicular to the lower leg.

Soleus

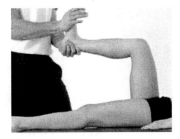

Fig. 12-54

The same test as gastrocnemius but with a passively flexed knee.

Pectoralis minor

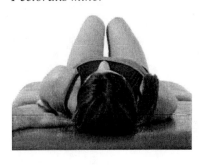

Fig. 12-55

Observe the posture of the supine person and notice the position of the shoulders. A shoulder that is off the table or has excessive space underneath it indicates a short pectoralis minor.[49] The person in this photo has an exaggerated tight left pectoralis minor.

Latissimus dorsi

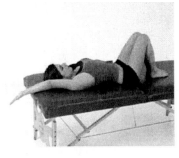

Fig. 12-56

With the person supine, knees bent, and feet flat on the table, ask them to keep their lower back flat while placing both arms straight above their head so that they will lay flat on the table with the palms facing upward.

They should be positioned on the table towards their feet enough so that their arms can lie flat on the table.

If one arm cannot lie flat on the table (180°) and or it slides laterally (into adduction) down the table, the latissimus dorsi and or pectoralis major are tight.

Tightness in the latissimus dorsi (and teres major) is associated with the arm bending at the elbow and sliding down the table into slight adduction[4], as well as not allowing the shoulder to lay flat. The pectoralis major is also associated with not allowing the shoulder to lay flat.[4]

Pectoralis major

Test # 1

Use the same test as latissimus dorsi above.

Test # 2

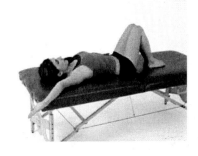

Fig. 12-57

This test is for the lower fibers.

The test can also be modified to test specific fibers of the muscle.

To test the upper fibers of pectoralis major, lie in the same position as the latissimus dorsi test, but place the tested arm into 90° of abduction (perpendicular to the body). The arm should be able to lie flat on the table. Shortness in the upper fibers will cause the arm to rest above the surface of the table.

To test the lower fibers, lie in the same position and place the arm into about 135° of abduction, see abovedf. The arm should be able to lie flat on the table. Shortness in the lower fibers will cause the arm to rest above the surface of the table.

These two tests are adapted from Kendall and McCreary[49], with the addition of the specific degrees of movement, which are similar to those in the pictures used by the noted authors. However, the authors did not mention specific degrees of motion.

TFL (on side)

Test # 1

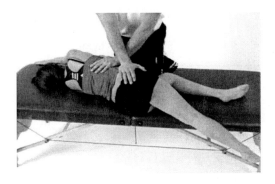

Fig. 12-58

The individual should be side lying with their back near the edge of the table. The tested leg is on top and straight and the non-tested leg is bent on the bottom to stabilize the body. The examiner stands behind the person (not shown here because of view obstruction) while supporting the top pelvis with one hand and applying downward pressure on the lateral knee with the other hand so that the leg moves downward behind the body.

The thigh should be in neutral between lateral and medial rotation and in slight extension.

The normal ROM for this test allows the toes to move beneath the table. If this ROM is not possible with the pelvis fixed, a short TFL and iliotibial tract are likely.[49]

The above test assesses the TFL muscle and entire length of the IT band including its fibers that cross the knee joint). In order to distinguish between the two, the TFL and upper fibers of the IT band can be assessed by using the following test, which is adapted from Chaitow 2001.

Test # 2

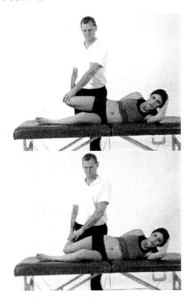

Fig. 12-59

(keep the head relaxed and down on the table)

Have the person assume a side lying position and hold their non-tested bottom leg into about 90° of hip and knee flexion.

Hold their top leg at the ankle and knee so that it is in a neutral position, i.e. no abduction or adduction or flexion or extension of the hip.

Carefully flex the top knee to 90° without altering the position of the hip. Continue holding the ankle as you release the knee and let the leg lower to its resting position.

Ideally, the leg should lower easily with the knee close to resting on the table; the person in the photo above has a relatively flexible TFL and negative test. Jerky movements point to a dysfunctional TFL while the inability of the knee to touch the table points to a short TFL. The IT band and lateral fascia are taken out of this test by bending the knee.

Be aware of people with wide hips which can prevent the knee from touching the table and cause a false-positive test result.

Torso twist (on side)

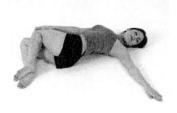

Fig. 12-60

The individual should be side lying on the non-tested side with the knees bent to 90° near the edge of the table and the arms

out at 90° of flexion lying on top of each other on the table (picture not shown). Instruct the person to rotate backwards so that their arm is straight and in a diagonal angle, about 135° of abduction (see fig. 12-60). The shoulder should be able to touch the table with the knees together.

If the shoulder cannot reach the table, then the pectoralis minor and torso portion of the "front functional line" of myofascia are likely to be restricted.

If the top knee comes up off the bottom knee, then the low back and possibly the pectoralis minor and "front functional line" are restricted.

Prone

Femur rotation

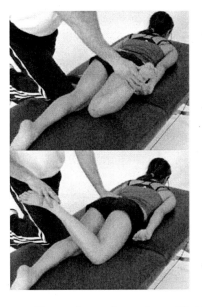

Fig. 12-61

With the person prone, the tested knee is flexed 90° and the leg in 0° of abduction, while the nontested leg is placed in 30° of abduction.[52] The pelvis is firmly stabilized by the examiner's hand while the other hand passively rotates internally and externally the leg until the contralateral pelvis begins to move.[52] The normal ranges[52] are;

- Femur internal rotation - 38-45° (top photo)
- Femur external rotation - 35-45° (bottom photo)

The end feel of ROM is very important in these tests because arthritis, adhesions, or degeneration in the hip can also cause decreased external and internal rotation. These abnormalities cause a much more abrupt stop in motion. Extreme limitations in hip ROM point to more structural influences than muscular, although both can coexist.

Quadriceps

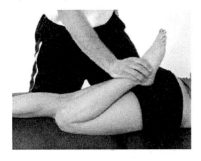

Fig. 12-62

With the person prone, flex the knee of the tested leg until the resistance barrier is met. The foot should be able to come very close to, if not touch the buttocks and have a springy and painless end feel of ROM.

Obstacles for this test are large thighs and knee problems.

Palpation

These are the areas that should almost always be palpated for a LBD. A more specific palpation assessment can take place if there are other priority areas that show up in the assessment.

Anterior

Sternum

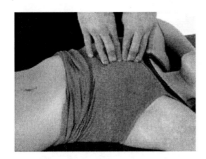

Fig. 12-63

Tenderness often reveals improper breathing patterns and forward shoulders posture.

Abdomen

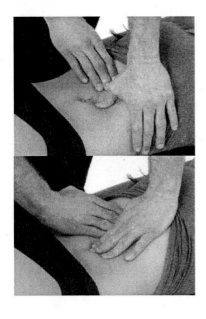

Fig. 12-64

Tenderness can be from organ stress or abdominal muscle TP's. Tug on the skin and underlying tissues to feel for adhesions and tightness in all directions.

The bottom photo shows a tug from up to down, diagonally. This tests for adhesions along the spiral and diagonal lines of fascia.

Pelvis/Hip

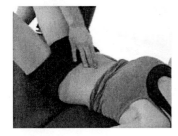

Fig. 12-65

Look for tender hip flexor and oblique TP's along the lower lateral quadrant of the abdomen and on the ASIS and AIIS of the ilium.

Side

Greater Trochanter

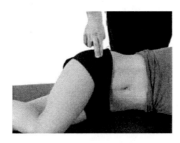

Fig. 12-66

Tenderness can signify hip (bursitis, arthritis, etc.) or soft tissue (trigger points, ligament strains, etc.) problems. Q.L. TP's can refer tenderness here.[8]

Gluteus Medius/Minimus

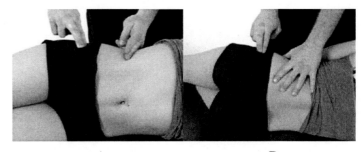

A   **B**

Fig. 12-67 Anterior and posterior views of the palpation.

These muscles harbor TP's that are frequently involved with LBP and sciatica. They are located along the ridge of the ilium bone and the nearby surroundings, fanning down over the hip joint.

TFL

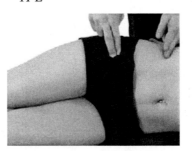

Fig. 12-68

This muscle is often overactive and tender, and requires attention.

The left hand in the photo is showing the crest of the ilium.

TFL

It is also a good idea to palpate down the lateral thigh to get an idea of the tension along the IT band.

Q.L.

A   **B**

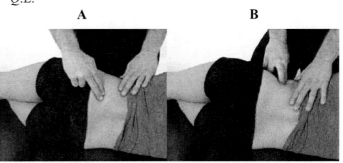

Fig. 12-69

Trigger points and adhesions are common in the Q.L. muscle but difficult to locate because of the erector muscles and fascia overlying it. Local tenderness must be discerned from kidney stress. The thumb of the left hand in the photo is showing the last rib.

Posterior

Lumbar Spinous Process

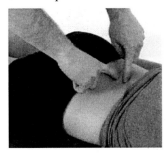

Fig. 12-70

Palpate for depth (spondylolisthesis) and tenderness.

Lumbar Facet Joints

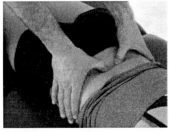

Fig. 12-71

Although difficult to palpate, overlying muscle spasm or tenderness can indicate an underlying pathology. A lumbar facet joint pathology can refer pain to the surrounding areas, as can the overlying muscles.[41] The pain referred from facet is most often downward, and hardly ever upward.[44]
The thumbs in this photo are just lateral to the spinous processes.

Posterior Fascia

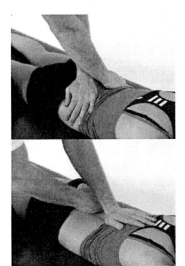

Fig. 12-72

The top photo shows how to assess tension from top to bottom, i.e. vertical tension along the spine.
The bottom photo shows the positioning for assessing lateral tension, i.e. the corset-like structure of the interconnected abdominal and lumbar fascia.
There should be a natural give to the tissues. Experienced hands will detect dehydration and abnormal stiffness.

Erector Spinae

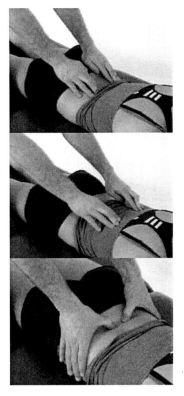

Fig. 12-73

A

Shows palpation of the lumbar longissimus and iliocostalis.

B

Shows palpation of the thoracic portion of the erector spinae muscles.

C

Shows a more specific palpation of the iliocostalis muscle.

* Look for tender nodules, rope-like muscles, and general stiffness in these areas.

Piriformis

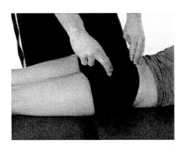

Fig. 12-74

The sciatic nerve runs through this muscle sometimes and is often very sensitive to touch. Take care to not irritate the nerve. It is not uncommon to have the person tense up their glutes and make this a difficult palpation to interpret. In that case the ROM test is the best gauge for tightness.

Ischial Tuberosities

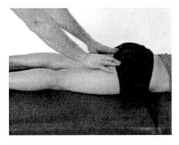

Fig. 12-75

This tests for tightness in an area that is an anchor point for many tissues that traverse the entire posterior body; such as the fascia from the erector spinae and hamstrings, and local ligaments. Tightness here points to many different causes, but it is usually a sign that the hamstrings and erector spinae should be stretched.

Hamstrings

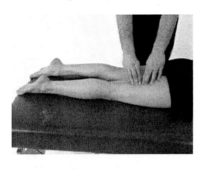

Fig. 12-76

Make sure to palpate both the lateral and medial portions of this muscle. Trigger points are common in the belly (middle) of the muscle even though pain is often in the attachment points. Tightness and tenderness here are common from too tight of hip flexors and poor posture. Therefore simply stretching this area will not resolve the problem; the hip flexors and posture must be addressed first.

Gastrocsoleus Complex

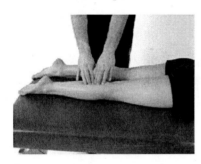

Fig. 12-77

Feel for tender nodules and overall stiffness. This area is a common root of many imbalances.

Plantar Fascia

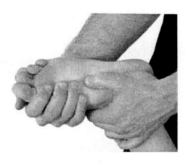

Fig. 12-78

Feel for pliability and tender points. An inflexible foot equals a stiff foundation that creates compensations elsewhere.

Breathing

Upper chest or abdominal breathing is commonly replacing diaphragmatic breathing, which is due most likely from the influences of stress and bad posture. Improper breathing affects the entire spine and its surrounding musculature. A low back dysfunction can influence breathing or vice versa by way of the psoas and Q.L., which are both posture and respiratory muscles that have a tendency to shorten.

Breathing is easily observed and trained while in the supine position (fig. 12-79), but any position will do. Simply place one hand on the stomach and the other on the sternum, feeling and watching for the abdomen to start rising first and the rib cage to expand soon after.

Fig. 12-79

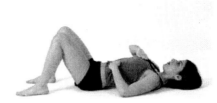

The shoulders should rise slightly upwards towards the end of an inhalation, allowing this movement to be felt just superior to the clavicle.

Many people cannot accomplish this without taking deep and unnatural breaths, which is definitely incorrect and counter productive because of the increased tension it creates.

Practicing breathing can be a very frustrating endeavor. It is common for people to try too hard by tightening their lips, tensing other areas of the body, or breathing through their mouth even though they normally breathe through their nose. These are all compensations and are not desirable.

Another goal is to have the inhalation be very similar to the exhalation in regards to time (3-7 seconds in, pause, 3-7 seconds out) and force (inhaling hard and exhaling softly is a common compensation).

Improper breathing patterns need to be identified because they are associated with upper crossed syndrome, neck pain, headaches, chest pain, and thoracic outlet syndrome.[41]

Muscle Testing

LBP causes a number of compensations throughout the neuromuscular system, creating a range of dysfunctions that seems to vary depending on the person's activity and pain level and lifestyle. Richardson et all[138] note a continuum of dysfunction for those with LBP that they describe as the following.

"At one end of the continuum is the patient with lack of control in muscles of the local system but minimum compensation by the global muscles. In fact, these patients may exhibit lack of strength and endurance of their antigravity and even global muscles.

At the other end is the patient with low back pain with lack of control in muscles of the local muscle system, and maximum compensation and overactivity in the global system. The presentation of most patients with low back pain probably lies somewhere between the two extremes. Clinical practice suggests that patients with maximal compensation in the global muscle system offer the greater challenge to the therapeutic skills of the practitioner, as these patients appear to have greater problems."

It is this author's experience that 1) this continuum is based on activity and pain levels (see fig. 12-80) and 2) the reason for the greater difficulty in those with overactive global muscles is that these people (athletes, very active people, or those in extreme pain) have deeply engrained faulty neuromuscular recruitment patterns.

Motor Control Continuum for LBP

Sedentary →	Average	Extreme (activity/pain)
↓ local control	→	↓ local control
↓ global compensation	(in-between)	↑ global compensation

Fig. 12-80 Unless specifically trained, the ability to control important local stabilizers diminishes the more we sit and the less we do, as does our strength and endurance in the global muscle system. On the other hand, the more activity we engage in, or pain we have, without training the local stabilizing system, the more the global system will compensate with faulty recruitment patterns and rob impulses from the local neuromuscular system.

Ask any experienced coach or teacher and they will tell you that it is much easier to learn new things than unlearn old habits and patterns.

The tests in this section evaluate function and strength of one muscle at a time, while the functional tests that follow evaluate more of the fitness, coordination, and endurance levels of a muscle group in relation to daily activities. This section is mainly manual muscle testing and is used for gaining immediate results that confirm the level of functioning (inhibitions, weakness, pain, etc.) in the neuromuscular system that was found in the prior assessments (posture, ROM, etc.).

These quick tests are ideal for those who apply manual therapy because they can *pin-point* dysfunction and be used to show signs of improvement immediately after a session by retesting a previously weak muscle and showing that it is now strong or uninhibited. The functional test results are better used for exercise programming and require more time to assess because of the repetitions.

The cause of weakness in a muscle test is not always from the muscle being weak. It could be due to; 1) gross asymmetries that force the muscle to operate at a mechanical disadvantage, 2) corresponding nerve root dysfunctions, or 3) weakness in a stabilizer muscle that is more proximal than the muscle being tested. It is essential to keep all these factors in mind when analyzing results.

The following muscles and tests were chosen because they generally represent the most influential results regarding a LBD. However, always test the influential muscles that were most often indicated in the ROM and postural assessments, even if they are not mentioned below.

Unless mentioned otherwise, the tests are scored 0-5, just as described in Chapter 2.

Standing

- Gluteus medius (ability to stabilize body weight)

Supine

- Psoas
- Curl-ups
- Lower abdominals

- Neck flexors
- Q.L.

Prone

- PMAP for transverse abdominis
- PMAP for multifidus
- Trunk extension w/rotation against resistance
- PMAP for hip extension
- Gluteus maximus
- Hamstrings
- Piriformis

Side

- PMAP for hip abduction
- Gluteus medius (ability to abduct the leg)
- Lateral flexors

Standing

Gluteus medius

The gluteus medius one leg standing stabilization test described below evaluates the ability of the muscle to transfer weight and side-bend the pelvis to the ipsilateral side. The endurance aspect of the muscle is assessed in the Functional Strength Tests section on pg. 192 under endurance/proprioception.

Strength - utilize the Trendelenburg test.

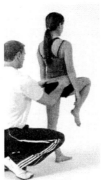

Fig. 12-81

Observe or palpate the sacral dimples (which should be level) while the person is standing.

When testing the right side, instruct the person to stand on the right leg with the arms relaxed at their side and the left hip flexed and knee bent so that the left foot is right beside the right knee.

The right sacral dimple should move inferiorly along with a slight shift in weight and side bending of the pelvis towards the right side.

This inferior movement of the sacral dimple indicates normal gluteus medius functioning. If the right sacral dimple does not move inferiorly, or other compensations occur, then the gluteus medius is thought to be weak or dysfunctional.

❖ Gross pelvic asymmetries can influence the outcome of the standing gluteus medius tests and should therefore be kept in mind when interpreting results.

Supine

Psoas[12,49]

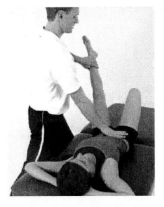

Fig. 12-82

Lying supine, the tested straight leg is placed into hip flexion, slight abduction, and slight external rotation. The opposite hip is stabilized by the examiner's hand reaching over the body (not done in this photo so that the entire body position could be seen). The pressure is against the lower leg in the direction of extension and slight abduction.

In order to save time, test the psoas muscle for strength before testing the abdominals; because a weak psoas muscle can cause the appearance of a weak abdominal test.

Curl-ups

Before testing abdominal strength it is important to understand the motions of the cervical, thoracic, and lumbar spines, as well as; the two phases of a sit-up, the intradiscal pressures involved, and which muscles are most activated in a given exercise or movement.

During flexion of the spine, the cervical and lumbar spines flatten (they don't actually flex much, if at all) while the thoracic spine flexes even more than its natural positioning. These relationships should be observed during a sit-up. Any deviation will point to dysfunction at one, two, or all three regions of the spine.

There are two main phases of a sit-up. The first is the curling of the trunk, which should mostly involve the abdominals, although the neck musculature also has to stabilize and flex the cervical spine in proportion to the trunk flexion. The second phase is flexion at the hip (rising up into a sitting position), which can occur only from activation of the hip flexor muscles.[49] Completing the second phase creates more intradiscal pressure[69] and compression forces[71] than simply doing the trunk curl.

Fig. 12-83 The photo on the left is phase I (curl-up), and on the right is phase II (sit-up).

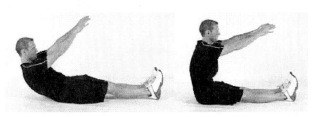

Completion of the fist phase is considered a curl-up, and completion of both phases is considered a sit-up. *The following studies encourage the avoidance of sit-ups as a regular exercise.*

McGill et all[72] showed in a small study (5 men and 3 women) that the "bent knee curl-ups" (feet on the floor) had less than half the psoas EMG activity of a sit-up (straight or bent leg), and that the "bent knee cross over curl up" (same as the curl-up but with rotation towards the opposite knee) had less than a third of the psoas activity compared to the sit-ups.

McGill[37] also showed that the curl-up exercise had over 1000N, 1300N, and 1500N less of lumbar compression than the cross knee curl-up (feet off the ground), bent leg sit-up, and straight leg sit-up respectively. The amount of compression (3350N and 3506N) caused by both types of sit-ups is associated with increased injury rates in workers when repeatedly loaded[37], which is how everyone does sit-ups, repeatedly!

Fig. 12-84 (bent leg curl-up)

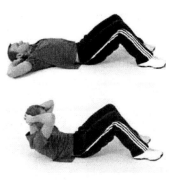

These two studies show that the bent leg curl-up is safer and isolates the abdominals from the psoas better than the sit-up (straight or bent leg). The next study shows that the straight leg approach eliminates the hip flexors even more than the bent leg position.

A small (5 subjects) study[68] saw no iliacus involvement during the first 30° of a straight leg sit up, but did detect activity in that range with a bent knee sit up.

These studies, albeit small studies, validate the utilization of the straight leg curl-up tests that will be used in this manual. The use of a pillow under the extended legs will allow for the back to be flatter and the legs more relaxed. The straight legs also make for an easier observation or feel of the gluteus maximus activation levels to see if it pushes the feet into the ground. This hip extensor contraction is undesirable because it will assist or dominate the abdominals in posteriorly tilting the pelvis, thereby relieving them of one of there most important duties.

Test # 1, the Forward Trunk Curl, is for upper abdominal flexion, # 2, the Anterior Oblique Trunk Curl, is for flexion with rotation, # 3, the Lateral Oblique Trunk Curl, is for flexion with side bending, and # 4, the Forward Trunk Curl into a Sit-up, is for hip flexor strength. Each utilize a straight leg testing position, unless the person has extreme lumbar lordosis and tight hip flexors, or the inability to posteriorly tilt the pelvis, which is usually in conjunction with weak lower abdominals.

In these latter cases, an alternate test position must be

used for all four tests in order to keep the low back flat. The position and test are the same with the modification of bending the knees and keeping the feet flat on the table or ground. The rest of test proceeds exactly as the straight leg tests, however, gluteus maximus involvement is much more difficult to evaluate with the knees bent, see test # 1.

A goal for this person is to be able to properly complete the straight leg tests. This can be done by starting with a bigger pillow under the knees and slowly reducing the size of it or by placing a wedge or wedge like object behind the person's back enabling them to be in increased flexion and utilize the abdominals with less strain. The main objective for this person is to keep their low back flat in order to reduce stress in that area.

While observing test #'s 1-4 (legs straight) for function, the flow and ease of the movements are the main signs of strength or weakness. A test is positive if:

1. The legs pop up.
2. The knees bend and heels push into the   ground.
3. The movement is jerky or shaky.
4. The abdomen protrudes outward (signifies an overactive R.A. and inhibited T.A.)
5. Extreme effort is needed to complete the curl-up.
6. The applied pressure cannot be matched.

The same signs are used for the bent leg test except for the knees bending and feet pushing into the floor.

To grade the strength of the abdominals during the tests, three variations of arm positions can be used. These have been modified from Kendall and McCreary[49], whose tests do not use a pillow under the legs, added resistance, or repetitions to grade for strength. They merely move into and hold the position.

Always start the person with their arms behind their head in the most difficult position, and then change positions only if they are unable to complete one repetition effortlessly at that level.

It is common for the cervical muscles to fatigue and strain the neck before the abdominals fatigue. This is likely due to overactive superficial neck flexors. In this case, the person can place their tongue on the roof of their mouth (in the same position as after swallowing); this will activate the supra and infrahyoid muscles and stabilize the cervical spine against the anterior shear forces caused by the strenocleidomastoid.[212]

The following grades are based on the person completing the test without any positive signs (the five mentioned above). If they cannot complete the test with the arms in the extended position, the abdominals are considered weak.

- Normal (100%) – hands behind the head
- Good (80%) – arms crossed on chest
- Fair (60%) – arms extended forward

Resistance by the examiner is applied at the end of the

curl-up after a 1-2 second hold for each test (#'s 1-4) in order to test for strength.

The ability to resist applied pressure is a gauge for maximum strength. The ability to complete ten reps is a gauge for fitness and endurance strength, which is tested in the Functional Strength Tests section.

1. Forward Trunk Curl

Lie supine with a pillow (about 4-5 inches thick) under the knees and thighs. The legs should be kept in neutral alignment and relaxed throughout the test, except for the slight tension needed to keep the legs in neutral.

Test # 1 Forward trunk Curl

Fig. 12-85

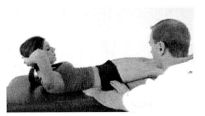

The examiner is beside the person with one hand or a pressure cuff underneath the low back to assess for lumbar movement and the other hand's fingers are on the lateral buttocks to check for gluteus maximus contraction, which should not occur. The practitioner's eyes are also watching for any movement in the legs and puffing out of the abdomen.

Before curling the trunk, instruct the person to posteriorly tilt the pelvis and flatten the back, using the lower abdominals and not the gluteus maximus. This may take some time to learn.

Ask them to slowly curl the trunk up as far as they can without using the legs, leading the movement by tucking the chin. The curl should start with a slow, smooth, and natural cervical and thoracic flexion.

Fig. 12-86
(faulty head positioning)

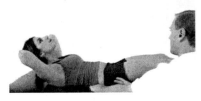

If the head protrudes instead of flexes it indicates a deep neck flexor weakness and dominance by the SCM, which will be addressed on pg. 181 in the neck flexion test.

The flexion should continue until the scapulas are a few inches off the ground. Everyone will be different regarding how high they can go, but everyone should be able to get the scapulas off the ground with little effort.

Fig. 12-87
(applied resistance)

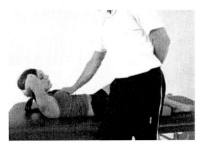

Once at the peak of the curl for 1-2 seconds, the examiner applies a moderate amount of pressure against the person's sternum (if the hands are behind the head or extended out) or forearms (if the arms are crossed) in the direction of pure extension. The pressure should be gradual, lasting 1-2 seconds and resisted without much movement. Weakness is noted if the person falls back or cannot resist strongly.

2. Anterior Oblique Trunk Curl

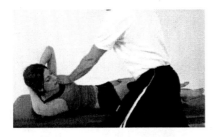

Fig. 12-88

This test starts at the peak of test # 1 and evaluates the strength of the anterior fibers of external oblique on the side of anterior rotation and the anterior fibers of internal oblique on the opposite side.

The examiner is again on the side of the individual with one hand or pressure cuff underneath the low back. Once the person is at the end position of test # 1, ask them to rotate about 45°.

If this position can be held for 1-2 seconds, then the examiner applies a moderate amount of pressure in the direction of derotation and slight extension to the shoulder that is anteriorly rotated. Weakness is noted if derotation or falling back occurs. Any falling back weakness should be differentiated from a rectus abdominis weakness.

3. Lateral Oblique Trunk Curl

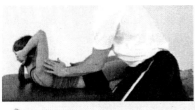

Fig. 12-89

The top photo is the test with resistance. The bottom photo is a better look at the motion.

This test again starts at the peak of test # 1 but evaluates the strength of the

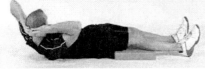

lateral fibers of the external and internal obliques on the same side as the lateral bending or side curl takes place.

Once the person is at the end position of test # 1, ask them to side bend and bring their shoulder (the side to be tested) towards the same hip.

If this position can be held with the scapulas off the ground for 1-2 seconds, then moderate pressure is applied to the armpit (if the hands are behind the head or extended out) or shoulder (if the arms are crossed) in the direction of extension and side bending away from the tested side. Weakness is noted if side bending and extension away from the pressure occurs.

4. Forward Trunk Curl into a Sit-up

Fig. 12-90

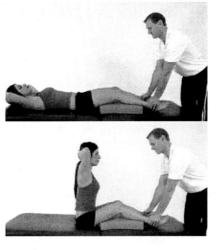

This is also a continuation of test # 1 and evaluates the strength and coordination of the hip flexors and abdominals. The examiner is located at the feet of the person instead of at their side.

Once the person is at the end position of test # 1, the examiner stabilizes their lower body by anchoring the feet downward. They should be able to pull themselves all the way up into to an upright sitting position, see Failure to do so indicates hip flexor weakness, usually in the iliacus, rectus femoris, and or psoas. A ten rep endurance test is not needed for the hip flexors unless they are thought to be weak and yet still pass the single rep strength test.

This test should not be attempted by those with LBP.

Lower abdominals

This test assesses the ability of the lower abdominals (mainly the external obliques and rectus abdominis) to stabilize the pelvis in a posterior tilt and keep the low back flat against the floor while resisting the progressively increasing weight of the legs, which are lowered towards the floor.

This test is commonly weak when the curl-up test is strong, indicating strong upper abdominals and weak lower abdominals. Results from this test are essential for learning the relationship between the hip flexors and lower abdominals. *Weakness and or pain in this test usually correspond with a hyperlordotic posture and tight or facilitated psoas muscles.*

Weak hip flexors can make this test difficult to assess because they are the prime movers of the legs. The abdominals cannot directly assist the hip flexors in raising the legs because they do not cross the hip joints.[49]

There are three ways in this manual to test the function of the lower abdominals; (1) strength test, (2) function test, and (3) endurance test. The strength and function tests are assessed here in the Muscle Testing section and the endurance test in the Functional Tests section.

All of these tests should be performed on a firm surface, not on a soft table, and a normal breathing pattern should be maintained with no holding of the breath.

1. Strength test[49]

This test (fig. 12-91) should not be done for those with LBP or injury because of the potential for lumbar soft tissue strains.

Lie in the supine position with the arms crossed on the chest (for the average person) or on top of the head (for athletes or physically active persons) and place a blood pressure cuff or the examiners hand under the lumbar curve. Pump the blood pressure cuff to about 40mmHg, ideal control results in minimal needle movement.

Assist the person in placing their legs pointing vertically towards the ceiling.

Have the person posteriorly tilt the pelvis and flatten their back against the floor, make sure that the abdominals are working and not the hip extensors.

Instruct them to keep the lumbar spine flat against the table and slowly lower the legs until they feel the low back *start* to come off the table. Reiterate the fact that lowering the legs past this point can aggravate the low back.

If the legs can be lowered to just above the floor and held for 2 seconds, have them lower the legs all the way to the floor and rest for 1 second, keeping the back flat. Then instruct them to raise the legs off the floor and up to the starting position while keeping the low back flat, this equals a 100% test. If the raising portion cannot be properly accomplished, even with the ability to completely lower the legs, the grade is only 90%.

The combination of raising and lowering the legs constitutes for a 100% strong lower abdominal test.

To grade the strength of the lower abdominals if they cannot lower all the way to the floor, take note of the angle (between the legs and table) where the low back starts to come off the table, as perceived by the examiner's hand or blood pressure cuff. With 90° being straight up towards the ceiling and 0% being legs straight and heals on the floor, the following angles correspond to percentages of strength.[49]

- 50% = 75°
- 60% = 60°
- 70% = 45°
- 80% = 30°
- 90% = 15°
- 100% = 0°

If the posterior pelvic tilt and flat lumbar spine cannot be held at 60°, then the lower abdominals can be considered weak, and likely inhibited from short psoas muscles.

2. Function test

This test is useful for determining the extent of hip flexor dominance during simple movements (fig. 12-92).

The person is supine with their hips flexed to 90°, knees bent, and the lower legs dangling.

Lower Abdominal Strength Test

Fig. 12-91

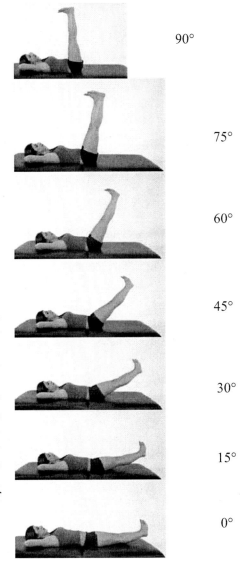

90°

75°

60°

45°

30°

15°

0°

Instruct them to slowly lower the feet to the floor while keeping the low back flat.

Then, maintaining a flat back, slowly slide the feet on the floor (shoes make this task nearly impossible) until the legs are fully extended.

Reverse this process and bring the legs back to the starting position.

If the low back cannot be held flat against the floor the entire time, then lower abdominal weakness or inhibition is present.

If *one leg at time* cannot be performed with the back flat the entire time, then extreme weakness or inhibition is present.

Fig. 12-92 (function test)

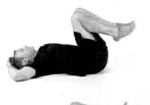

❖ When using a blood pressure cuff, slide it under the spine and pump it up enough to get a reading without interfering with the natural curve of the spine. This can usually be accomplished with about 30-40mmHg of pressure. The goal is to keep the needle on the gauge relatively still while moving the legs up and down.

N o t e   a n y movement of the needle and at what angle of leg flexion or extension it occurs.

The gauge is a very useful visual aid for the person to see their functioning.

Fig. 12-93 (Two legs at a time)

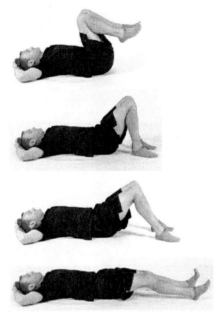

Neck flexors

This test is used to see if the deep neck flexors are weak and dominated by the superficial neck flexors, mainly the SCM.[52] Weakness in this group of muscles is associated with upper crossed syndrome, TMJ, shortness in the suboccipitals, headaches, and altered head/neck flexion.[41]

The person is supine and asked to tuck their chin and raise their head a few inches off the table. This position

Fig. 12-94 (neck flexors)

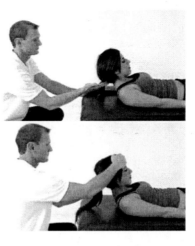

should be able to be easily maintained for three seconds (top picture), then able to resist pressure in the direction of neck extension from the examiner (bottom picture).

This is a pass or fail test, with failing including; (1) not being able to maintain the head off the table and chin tucked for three seconds, and (2) not being able to resist moderate pressure into extension while keeping the chin tucked (overactive SCM muscles will cause the chin to push out).

Q.L.

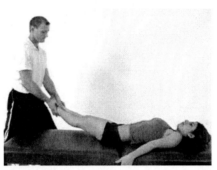

Fig. 12-95

The person is supine with their hands grabbing the side of the table on each respective side.

The examiner grabs the person's heels and brings both of their legs out laterally towards the side to be tested, about 20º.

Ask the person to maintain this position against moderate resistance (at the ankles) while activating their lateral trunk muscles, mainly the Q.L., and try to resist with both legs.

Weakness is noted on that side if moderate pressure cannot be resisted and or the opposite hip comes off of the table.

Prone

PMAP for Transverse Abdominis

Even though the T.A. and multifidus muscles are normally activated together, they should be assessed separately in order to improve the focus on the individual multifidus activation intensities at each vertebrae level.[138]

This assessment is beneficial to perform on everyone, not just those with LBP. Studies have demonstrated that T.A. weakness is quite common in non-LBP sufferers and is a good indicator of those with or who have had LBP.

One study[261] showed that only 13 of 30 people *without* LBP could optimally recruit the T.A. muscle. Another study correctly identified 90% of subjects with a history of LBP (only 54% of those studied had a history of LBP) by utilizing the results of T.A. activation tests.[262]

Richardson et al[138] recommends two tests for the T.A. muscle. The first is performed in the prone position with a pressure cuff and is ideal for obtaining biofeedback data that can be used to compare for improvement later on. The second is in the supine position (it will be tested here in the prone assessment so that the focus is not lost on the T.A.) and uses palpation to assess for symmetry of activation of the muscles of the abdominal wall.

1. Prone Test[138]

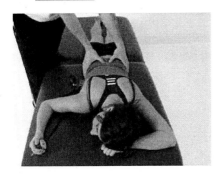

Fig. 12-96

This assessment is performed in the prone position with arms at side, head at midline, and a pressure cuff underneath the abdomen so that the naval is in the center of the cuff.

Inflate the cuff to 70mmHg and allow for a few moments to notice how breathing causes small deviations in the pressure that can alter results if they are not taken into account.

Instruct the person to fully relax their abdomen, then take a natural breath in and out and then, without breathing in, pull the lower abdomen in towards the spine without taking a breath or causing any other movement in the body other than the stomach drawing inward.

The evaluator should be monitoring four things; 1) the pressure gauge, 2) the body for movement, especially the pelvis and trunk, 3) both sides of the anterolateral abdominal wall for bulging, which signifies that the T.A. is not activating correctly, and 4) the control or smoothness of the contraction. Repeat this procedure a few times until the person understands what they are doing.

Once the person understands the procedure, have them perform the test and take note of the four things monitored above. It is imperative to have notes on all three categories of performance in order to keep track of improvement, which may come in one or all three forms. For example, it is common to improve in the ability to pull in the abdomen, but not improve in the ability to maintain a neutral body position throughout the contraction.

Ideal performance results in a *reduction* of pressure in the cuff by 4-10mmHg, no compensatory spinal or pelvic movement, and no bulging of the abdomen.[138] If the T.A. can be properly activated, then an endurance test may be

performed by holding the contraction for 10 seconds, and then repeating this up to 10 times.

There are two important compensations to be aware of that involve the global muscles being hyperactive. The first is a bulging of the abdomen (bad) but the ability to keep the spine immobile (good). This results in an *increased* pressure reading by the cuff. The second compensation is when the spine or pelvis moves and the stomach bulges, causing a *decrease* in the pressure cuff reading. This creates a false-positive test result if the spine and abdominal area are not monitored by palpation.

If the prone test did not yield satisfactory results, then the supine test is recommended for further evaluation.

2. Supine Test[138,263]

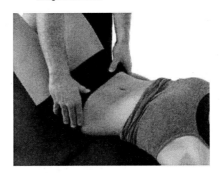

Fig. 12-97

The supine position is ideal for palpation assessment of the symmetry of activation of the muscles of the abdominal wall. It is also the position that most individuals find is easiest to activate the T.A. in.

The main tools for this test are the palpating fingers. According to Hides et al[263], the ideal position for palpation is medially and inferiorly to the anterior superior iliac spines and lateral to the rectus abdominis.

The thumbs are pressed gently but deeply into the abdominal wall in the location described above, while the rest of the fingers reach around the waist. The thumbs monitor anterior bulging and the fingers monitor lateral bulging.

Ideal activation patterns result in a slowly developing tension deep in the abdominal wall, including a narrowing of the waist and lateral abdomen.

A dysfunctional activation pattern causes one of four results.

1. No activity
2. Hyperactivity of the oblique muscles, resulting in a quick superficial contraction
3. Bulging of the anterior and or lateral abdominal wall (weak/inhibited T.A.)
4. Bulging asymmetrically, i.e. more on one side than the other (weak/inhibited T.A. on one side only)

In observing both the supine and prone tests, the quality of the activation must be taken into account. It is essential to be able to activate the T.A. in a slow, smooth, and controlled manner. Each person should also be able to hold this natural contraction for 10 seconds and maintain a normal breathing pattern.[138]

PMAP for Multifidus

This test is usually failed by those who have or have had chronic or acute LBP. Hides et al showed that these populations have inhibited multifidus muscles at and on the same side as the specific symptomatic vertebral segment.[146,147] These studies also concluded that the multifidus muscle does not return to normal functioning without the intervention of specific activation exercises.

Because no spinal movement is allowed during this test, the deep fibers of lumbar multifidus are being evaluated; as opposed to the more superficial fibers that create an extension torque and are virtually impossible to differentiate from the other extensor activation patterns.

Assessing these fibers requires experienced palpation skills. The professional can also take advantage of technology by utilizing ultrasound imaging to view the consistency of the multifidus muscle at each segment, as described by Richardson et al.[138]

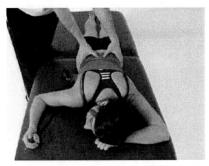

Fig. 12-98

The assessment begins in a relaxed prone position with the evaluator's fingers palpating the left and right side of two adjacent lumbar multifidus segments, starting at L1, the thumb and index finger of one hand monitor the left and right multifidus fibers of L-1, while the same fingers on the other hand monitor the left and right fibers of L2. This multi-segment observation allows for the comparison of left to right and segment to segment activation levels. Different variations in finger arrangement are possible.

Palpation of the multifidi muscles needs to be just lateral to each vertebra. Be aware of palpating too far laterally because the erector spinae muscles will cause false-positive tests with their activation patterns easily felt on the surface.

The fingers are pressed firmly but gently into the muscle belly along side the spine. As with the T.A. assessment, the person is asked to breathe in, then out, and to hold the breath out with the initial contraction. The following instructions are then given;

"Gently and slowly swell out your low back muscles underneath my fingers without moving or tensing your body. Hold this contraction and start to breathe normally. Focus on swelling the muscles underneath my fingers without moving your spine or tensing the rest of your body."

While the person is "swelling" out their muscles, it is important for the evaluator to ease up on the pressure into the muscles in order to allow the muscles to properly

expand and not inhibit them.

Things to look and feel for are; 1) anterior tilting of the pelvis and lumbar extension, due to the more superficial extensors activating, 2) quick, superficial contractions beneath the fingers, indicating global, not local, muscle activation, 3) the thoracic extensors activating and causing movement in the spine, and 4) the person pushing their low back into the evaluator's fingers, usually inducing a posterior pelvic tilt.

The quality (speed and control) of each contraction is noted for all levels (L1-L5) and sides (right and left) of the lumbar spine. Any inhibitions should correspond with past and present LBP locations.

It is important to realize that only small amounts of force are needed from the multifidus to stabilize the lumbar segments.[138] Therefore, the contractions felt by the evaluator are not going to be large or powerful, as would be the case with most other muscles palpated for activation levels.

The test is graded as follows.

0 pts = no contraction
1 pt = slight contraction, but no control (sporadic)
2 pts = good control, but only a slight contraction
3 pts = good control and contraction

Back extension w/rotation   **Fig. 12-99**

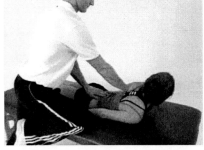

This test allows the examiner to evaluate the strength of each side of the erector spinae.

The person is prone with their hands on the table near their head (if the arms are extended or placed on the buttocks, it allows the latissimus dorsi to contribute a lot of strength).

Instruct the person to raise their chest and arms a few inches off the table and rotate towards the side to be tested, including the head.

Very firm and gradual pressure is applied to the rotated shoulder in the direction of flexion and derotation of the spine (trying to push the shoulder back into the table) while the examiner stabilizes the upper thighs against the table with the other arm. Watch for compensations in the hamstrings, such as lifting the legs off the table.

Weakness is noted on one side if strong pressure cannot be resisted for at least three seconds. Pain and S.I. joint dysfunctions can interfere with the test, as can stabilizing the lower back against the table instead of using the upper thighs.

This test allows the experienced evaluator to get a feel

for the individual's strength on each side of the erector spinae, as opposed to the strength and endurance test in the Functional Test section, which focuses on the endurance of both sides together.

It is easy to assume that strong results in this test will translate over to the endurance test and therefore the latter is not needed. This is, however, a common misjudgment. Always utilize both assessments to get an overall picture of strength and endurance in the erector spinae because people with LBP tend to have the same back extensor strength as the general population, but significantly less endurance strength.[138]

PMAP for hip extension

Fig. 12-100

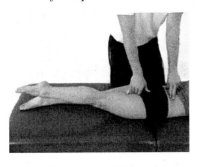

The purpose of this test is to assess the relationship between the muscle activation patterns during prone straight leg hip extension, which should occur in the following order; (1) hamstrings (synergist) and gluteus maximus (agonist), (2) contralateral lumbar erector spinae (stabilizer), (3) ipsilateral erector spinae (stabilizer).[41]

The firing patterns can be felt by placing one hand on the low back and the other on edge of the buttocks with the thumb on the gluteus maximus and the pinky on the hamstring. Then instruct the prone person to raise their straight leg into extension. The above pattern of activation should be palpable.

If the gluteus maximus strongly activates and the leg raises at least 10° without any lumbar extension, excessive or initial erector spinae involvement, shoulder girdle and thoracic musculature recruitment, or anterior pelvic tilting, the test is normal.

If any of these altered patterns occur, there is likely gluteus maximus *inhibition*, and erector spinae, hip flexor, and hamstring *facilitation*.

There is some disagreement whether or not the hamstrings or gluteus maximus should fire first or at the same time. The main observation to make is how strong the gluteus maximus is activated and if the erector spinae are activated before it, which would indicate weakness and or poor recruitment patterns.

The significance of hip extension coordination is that it is associated with lower crossed syndrome, LBP, buttock pain, hamstring pulls, decreased hip extension, and chronic or recurrent neck pain.[41] These all exaggerate and create wear and tear injuries on the lumbar spine.

Gluteus maximus

Before testing the gluteus maximus for strength, it is important to check for PMAP in hip extension, as in the prior test. This gives an idea of any compensations that might occur during the strength test.

Fig. 12-101

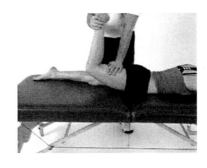

To test for gluteus maximus strength, the person should be prone with the tested knee bent to at least 90° and raised a few inches off the table by grabbing the ankle of the tested leg. The examiner then applies downward (towards the table into hip flexion) pressure on the lower part of the posterior thigh against the person's upward effort,[12] while the examiner's opposite hand is stabilizing the ipsilateral pelvis.[49,53]

The range of controlled hip extension in this test should be about 10° against moderate to strong pressure. If any pain is present during the test, check for S.I. joint or lumbar spine problems.

To test more specific fibers of the gluteus maximus during the above mentioned test, follow these modifications;

• Superior fibers – externally rotate the leg.
• Inferior fibers – internally rotate the leg.

If there is great restriction of hip extension due to hip flexion tightness, then an alternate testing position should be used, such as prone on the table with the lower body off of the table and the nontested side's foot flat on the floor with the tested leg suspended in the air resisting pressure into flexion.[49,53]

Hamstrings

Fig. 12-102

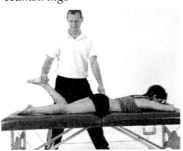

Bend the knee to be tested to 45° and ask the prone person to maintain this position while the examiner applies hard pressure to the ankle to straighten the leg.

Note any lumbar compensation, i.e. arching or twisting, which indicates weak hamstrings and or weak stabilizers in the lumbo-pelvic region.

Weakness and cramping during this test are common and likely due to the stretched position that the hamstrings are constantly in with an anteriorly tilted pelvis.

It is important to remind them that this is not a strength contest and to start the contraction gradually, otherwise cramping is likely.

Piriformis

Fig. 12-103

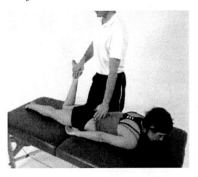

The tested knee is bent to 90º while lying prone. The examiner handles just above the ankle and places the leg into internal rotation until it is at the comfortable end range (internal rotation brings the legs away from the midline).

The examiner's gradual pressure is in the direction of hip internal rotation while the person resists by rotating the leg externally towards the midline of the body.

A moderate to strong pressure should be able to be resisted for at least three seconds without any compensation in the low back and pelvic area.

Side

PMAP for hip abduction

This test shows if the Q.L. and or TFL are dominant in the motion of hip abduction, as well as the strength of the gluteus medius and mimimus and flexibility of the adductors. Dysfunctional interactions here are; 1) short adductors that prevent the leg from rising to 45º, 2) overactive Q.L. (stabilizer) that hikes the hip excessively, 3) overactive TFL (synergist) that internally rotates and or flexes the thigh, 4) overactive pirformis that externally rotates the leg, and 5) inhibited hip abductors and superior fibers of gluteus maximus that force the entire pelvis to rotate posteriorly and utilize the hip flexors.

Altered activation patterns in this movement are associated with lower crossed syndrome, hip hiking during gait, low back and buttock pain, pseudo-sciatica, and lateral knee pain[41], as well as IT band syndrome, chronic hamstring and groin tightness and soreness (due to the hamstrings and adductors intimate connection through the fascia), decreased lateral stabilization and ROM, and sprained ankles on the ipsilateral side.

To test for PMAP in hip abduction, the bottom leg and hip are flexed and the top leg is straight. The examiner stands in front and towards the head of the person to best observe the movement.

Instruct the person to slowly raise the leg into hip abduction. Ideally, it should abduct to 45º without any rotation, flexion, excessive hip hiking, shaking, or other compensations mentioned above. If any compensation occurs, then the test is failed.

Palpation can be used to monitor when the TFL and Q.L. activate by placing fingers on them. They should fire after the gluteals. This palpation takes a keen sense;

(PMAP for hip abduction)

Fig. 12-104

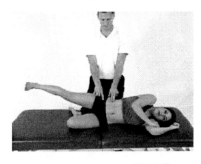

fortunately, pure visual observation is usually good enough to notice any compensation.

This test, or slight variations of it, are used by many well known practitioners[4,11,43,52] to test the function of hip abduction.

Gluteus medius

Fig. 12-105

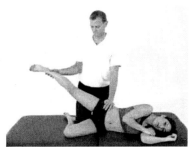

If the PMAP test for hip abduction was failed, then this test is unnecessary because it would only test the strength of compensations.

Start at the end of the hip abduction PMAP test, with the leg in the air at about 45º of pure abduction. Have the person hold this position for 10 seconds. If this can be done without much shaking or wobbling, then a strong pressure is applied against the ankle in the direction of adduction for 1-2 seconds.

Weakness is noted if both steps cannot be completed successfully. Watch for any compensations such as hip hiking or pelvic or femur rotation during the resistance test.

Lateral flexors

Fig. 12-106

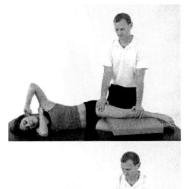

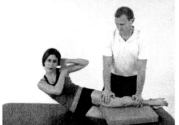

This test involves strength from the lateral flexors and hip abductors of the tested side. It is difficult and usually unadvisable to assess obese individuals using this test.

To test for strength, start in the side-lying position with side to be tested facing up. The person has their bottom hand on top of the opposite shoulder and the top arm pointing towards the feet. The knees are slightly flexed and in a relatively straight line compared to the rest of the body. A pillow is optional between the knees.

The examiner is behind the person and stabilizes the legs by placing the cephalad forearm along the lateral thigh of the individual and placing strong downward pressure on the ankles with the other hand. Leverage is required by the evaluator for this stabilization.

The stabilization on the lateral thigh should "give" with the movement to allow for the natural downward displacement of the pelvis on that side, otherwise it will be pinned down and not allowed to move, giving a false weak test result.[49]

The movement should be pure side flexion with no rotation to either side. Rotation would show an imbalance in the oblique muscles. If the person does not have full normal ROM for side flexion then 100% ability in this test will be hidden.

Kendall and McCreary[49] grade the test as follows, and Chaitow[12] grades it almost identically as well (within an inch).

- Normal (100%) – ability to raise the trunk to a point of maximum lateral flexion
- Good (80%) – ability to raise the bottom shoulder about four inches from the ground
- Fair (50%) – ability to raise the bottom shoulder slightly, one or two inches

Functional Strength Tests

The functional tests are more demanding than the muscle tests because numerous reps and prolonged holding of a contraction are required here, which leads to an accumulating fatigue affect throughout the body. Therefore, if an individual cannot pass a specific test towards the end of this section it could signify a lack of overall fitness instead of weakness in just that particular test.

The tests have been spaced out so that the same muscle groups are not tested in immediate succession of one another, and thus positions (standing, sitting, etc.) will need to be changed a lot more often than in the rest of the assessment. Those who are fit should have no problem passing the tests, but those with poor fitness levels will be affected by the accumulating efforts. In fact, for someone who has been sedentary for the last couple of years, it can be assumed that they will score poorly and performing the functional tests is unnecessary. However, performing poorly in these tests provides a baseline for improvement and can motivate some individual's to try harder than they previously thought would be necessary.

The tests here challenge many of the important muscles and directions of movement needed to perform simple and complex tasks. They can be made more intense by performing them in sequence without any rest, therefore creating a more work or sport like environment.

This strategy is only for those who participate in intense activity on a frequent basis. Individual results are harder to analyze this way because overall fatigue and lack of fitness can be more of a factor than the muscles being tested. In this case, completion of the entire sequence can also be a goal of training and mark of improvement for stamina and fitness.

Functional Strength Tests

Squats	Lunges
Push-ups	Oblique curl-ups
Lower Abs	Push-pull
Trunk extension	Curl-ups (endurance)
Side Plank	Proprioception
Toe Raises	Cardio

Squats

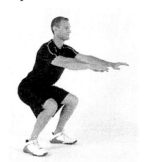

Fig. 12-107

This is the most functional and endurance based assessment possible for the quadriceps. It also challenges the entire kinetic chain. Lack of endurance in the quadriceps is associated with losing lordosis and stooping during lifting.[73,80]

Proper form consists of standing with the feet shoulder width apart and squatting down so that the thighs are close to or equal to parallel with the floor. The arms should reach outward and slightly upward on the way down and lumbar lordosis should remain throughout the entire test.

The knees should not move anterior to toes and should be aligned between the big toe and the next toe. A chair or any knee high square object is useful to place in front of the feet in order to prevent the knees from going past the toes.

The chest should remain pushed out and the entire spine extended proportionally.

It is helpful to instruct the person to "pretend like your going to sit back into a chair." This encourages them to properly stick their hips out backwards, which is not a natural or comfortable act for many people.

It will take at least a few repetitions for each person to learn the proper form. Inform them to continue squatting as you, the evaluator, keep giving them advice on how to improve their form.

The squats should be performed with little to no rest and should be at a moderate pace. Signs of weakness and compensation are;

1. The lumbar spine or torso flexes = short hip flexors and or weak erector spinae
2. The heels rise off the floor = short soleus or tight Achilles tendon.
3. The feet point outward more than 15º = short lateral hip rotators and or gastocsoleus complex, and or weak medial gastrocnemius
4. The knees sway inwardly = pronation or weak hip stabilizers are likely and short adductors are possible
5. Poor balance = proprioception system is not efficient
6. The abdomen protrudes outward = T.A. cannot stabilize so the R.A. kicks in and creates lumbar instability

For most people the squats are performed without weight, but for those who are very active or engage in daily strenuous activity, holding a medicine ball or weight of 10-20 pounds at the chest can be added.

The following grading system is flexible according to the needs of the individual. For example, someone who sits at a computer the majority of the day probably does not need the same strength and endurance that an athlete or manual labor worker needs. A mother who has to constantly bend down and pick up their baby, clothes, toys, groceries, etc. is considered a manual labor worker.

For simplicity, the former group will be labeled sedentary and the latter active. The grading system for a *sedentary population* is as follows.

- Normal (100%) – 50 squats, easily
- Good (80%) – 50 squats, moderate to hard
- Fair (60%) – 50 squats, very difficult
- Weak (50%) – Less than 50 squats

This population may need to be graded as in the active population if they are sedentary during the day but play sports or are very active other times. It is up to the clinical wisdom of the examiner to know where to place each person.

The grading system for an *active population* is as follows.

- Normal (100%) – 100 squats, easily
- Weak (50%) – Less than 50 squats, easily

There is no middle grade, i.e. 60-80% because the normal (100%) grade can only be given if it is achieved with relative ease, meaning that many more reps could be performed. It is common for athletes to be able to perform 200-250 squats in a row without ever training to do so. It is up to the examiner to decide if a maximum number of squats should be assessed. One hundred reps are used here, along with the observation of effort exerted, to grade the abilities of the person and save time by not having to perform hundreds of reps.

Push-ups

This test does not only assess the strength of the chest and triceps, but also the CORE muscles and most of the kinetic

chain. There are many compensations to be seen with this test, including scapulas winging, head pushing forward, stomach sagging, back arching, buttocks pushes up into the air, and more. These compensations show weakness somewhere in the body and it is the examiner's duty to figure out where and strengthen those areas before incorporating push-ups into a workout regimen that would then encourage these compensations.

In the absence of serious disc or spine pathology, any pain noted in this test is often due to short and facilitated psoas muscles. Normal psoas activity during a push-up is over 25% MVC (maximum voluntary contraction), which is enough to produce over 225 N of compression and 175 N of shear force on the lumbosacral junction.[72] These numbers would surely rise in a facilitated psoas muscle.

If pain occurs during the test, then try stretching the psoas before performing the push-ups. If this reduces pain, then the psoas are suspected as being facilitated. If no difference in pain is noted, then a more detailed investigation (weak abdominals can cause instability pain as well) is needed and the push-up test should not continue.

Fig. 12-108 (men's test)

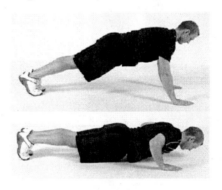

The positions used in this push-up test include on the knees for women and straight legs for men. The arms are not allowed to flare out; instead, they are kept in close to the body (the elbows point backwards toward the feet). The movement should be slow and controlled going up and down while the chest barely or almost touches the ground. No rest is allowed at the top by locking the elbows; the reps should be continuous and fluid.

Fig. 12-109 (women's test)

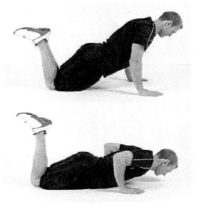

*Notice the elbows in close on both tests. The test is graded as follows.

Normal (100%) – 12 reps

Good (80%) – 10 reps

Fair (60%) – 5-8 reps

Weak (50%) – Less than 5 reps

These numbers are for men and women. To earn a grade, no compensations can occur, such as the head pushing forward or the low back dropping. The number of reps at which compensation begins is the number graded.

Lower Abdominals

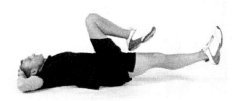

Fig. 12-110

This test assesses endurance and is easier on the low back than the strength test. It should, however, still be performed with caution for those with LBP.

The test begins in the supine position with the arms on top of the head, hips flexed to 90°, knees bent, and the lower legs dangling.

A blood pressure or special cuff device, or the examiner's hand is placed underneath the lumbar spine (however for this picture that is kept out so the entire view can be seen).

Instruct the person to alternate straightening each leg to about 20° off the floor, keeping the low back flat against the floor. The legs should continue alternating at a moderate pace, somewhat resembling riding a bike.

To pass the test with 100%, the legs must be fully extending each time and the low back kept flat for at least *30 continuous seconds* with a regular breathing pattern maintained.

It should be relatively easy for the person to perform. Anything less than this is considered unfit for endurance levels. The pressure reading on the cuff device should not deviate much at all, especially not quickly.

Trunk Extension Strength and Endurance Test[41]

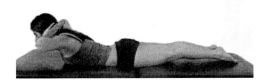

Fig. 12-111

Lying prone with their hands behind their head and elbows horizontal, instruct the person to lift their chest about 2 inches off the table and repeat this motion 15 times, each with a 2 second pause at the top. Hold the final repetition for 30 seconds.

Signs of weakness and compensation are shaking or twisting, feet or legs rising off the table, and an inability to raise the trunk two inches of the table. This is a great test for the isolated strength and endurance functioning of the spinal erectors.

The test is graded as follows.

0 pts = unable to lift trunk off floor
1 pt = unable to complete 15 reps
2 pts = able to do 15 reps, but not easy 30 sec hold
3 pts = 15 reps + 30 sec hold (easily)

Side plank (lateral core endurance)

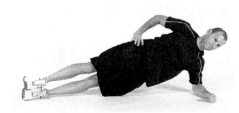

Fig. 12-112

Those with shoulder problems or extreme obesity should skip this test.

Start by side lying with the bottom forearm and elbow resting on a pillow or pad. The top leg should be in front of the bottom leg with the feet lying one in front of the other on their sides. The top arm can support the bottom shoulder by cupping it with the hand.

Instruct the person to lift their body up sideways using the lateral flexors so that only the bottom forearm and two feet are touching the ground. Have them hold this position isometrically for the appropriate amount of time listed below. Then test the other side.

The body should be straight as a board with no sagging of the hips.

The *side plank* test is graded as follows.

0 pts = Less than 10 seconds
1 pt = 1x 10 sec w/3 sec rest
2 pts = 2x 10 sec w/3 sec rest
3 pts = 3x 10 sec w/3 sec rest
4 pts = 4x 10 sec w/3 sec rest
5 pts = 5x 10 sec w/3 sec rest

As with all the tests, a certain grade should not be given if it is a struggle to obtain it. In order to earn a grade, the result should be well within the abilities of the person and therefore seem relatively easy or at most moderately difficult.

Toe raises

The strength and endurance of the gastrocnemius and planter flexor muscles is tested here by simply standing and rising up onto the balls of the feet and repeating up and down thirty times.

The test is done one leg at a time with the other knee bent and the foot off the floor. *One finger* can be used from each hand to help balance against a wall or stationary object. The goal is to have the strength and balance to do 30 toe raises on one leg without much assistance.

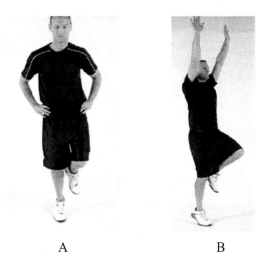

A   B

Fig. 12-113   A shows a regular toe raise, with no external help for balancing. B shows a more advanced version with the arms above the head. This is ideal for athletes.

The *30 reps* should be broken down into two groups. The first 15 proceed up and down slowly, each time having the heels touch the ground. The last 15 should immediately follow and be faster with the heel avoiding the ground the entire time. These two methods work the fast and slow twitch fibers of the muscle. If no compensations are used, this exercise helps to develop hip stability and proprioception.

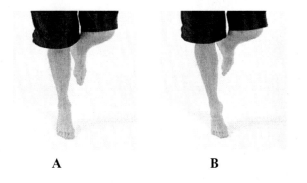

A   B

Fig. 12-114   A shows normal foot position. B shows the foot plantar flexing up onto the lateral side of the foot; usually indicating weakness in the medial gastrocnemius.

Common compensations are; 1) external rotation of the lower leg during the test; this often indicates a weakness in the medial gastrocnemius and or tightness in the lateral gastrocnemius and piriformis, 2) a protruding abdomen, i.e. T.A. inhibition, 3) wobbling all over the place or leaning into the wall; this is a sign of weak gluteals and poor proprioception, and 4) the foot plantar flexes up onto the lateral side of the foot, placing little weight onto the big toe area; this indicates a weak medial gastrocnemius.

The test is graded as follows.

0 pts = unable to lift heel off floor w/one leg
1 pt = unable to complete 15 reps w/help
2 pts = 15 reps before compensating or needing help
OR
2 pts = 30 reps using assistance/help
3 pts = 30 reps w/out assistance/help or compensations

Lunges

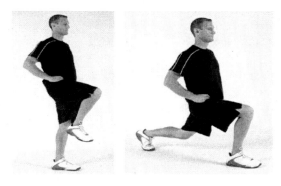

Fig. 12-115

Start by standing with the feet about shoulder width apart and arms relaxed by sides or on the hips.

Instruct the person to step forward with one leg far enough to allow the knee to be directly above the ankle upon flexing the knee to 90º. The back knee should almost touch the ground and the spine and pelvis should remain in proper alignment without flexing. The arms should remain where they are and the front knee should also be relatively still and not sway to one side.

After pausing for a second in the down portion of the lunge, instruct the person to controllably push back up to the starting position without any jerking movements. Then perform the same on the other side.

This test is usually best demonstrated and explained before having the person try it themselves.

The inability to control the movement, presence of wobbling at the knees, arms reaching out for balance, or jerky movements are signs of quadriceps and or hip stabilizer weakness. Sometimes it will take the person a few tries to get the movement right, so don't rush to judge on the first few reps if they are poor. Give them another chance or two to learn the movement.

Most people should be able to perform *10 total reps* with good coordination, alternating each side. Those with knee pain or who are obese often cannot and should not perform this test.

Anterior Oblique Curl-ups

After completing the straight leg anterior oblique curl-up, just as in the Muscle Testing section (without resistance at the top), ask the person to rotate back to neutral and slowly roll back onto the table, one vertebrae at a time. Then instruct them to perform nine more reps, or *10 total reps* on that side. Follow up by testing the other side.

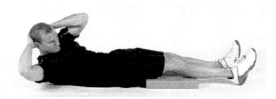

Fig. 12-116

Weakness in the anterior oblique abdominals is noted if the entire movement cannot be repeated equally ten times, using a slow motion with a 1-2 second pause at the top. Note if the height of the curl-up starts to diminish, this could be a sign of rectus abdominis fatigue instead of the obliques, either way, the weakness should be noted. Another common weakness is in the lower abdominals, which results in the inability to keep the lumbar spine flat against the floor. Lower abdominal weakness can also make this test painful on the low back if it allows the lumbar spine to arch on the way up.

This test is pass or fail.

Push-Pull

These exercises are unique because they simultaneously challenge the stabilizing system in two alternating directions. The first assessment focuses on stabilizing against straight pushing and pulling in the frontal plane with two arms at the same time. The second test focuses on the same motion but with only one arm and resistance at a time, thus challenging the spine with a rotational pushing and pulling force (transverse and frontal planes).

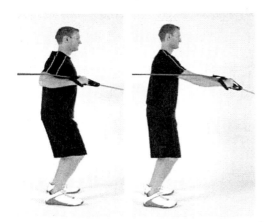

Fig. 12-117
(Test # 1 - two arm push-pull)

1. Stand with good posture and the feet shoulder width apart. Grab an exercise band from behind, as if to perform a chest press. The hands also simultaneously hold onto handles from a pulling machine, or another exercise band wrapped around a stationary object in front of the person.

Once the exercise is set up properly, a rowing motion against resistance (coming from the front) is performed and smoothly transitioned into a pushing movement against resistance (tubing from behind). This tests the ability to keep a neutral spine and utilize the stabilizing mechanism of the core while the arms move against resistance.

Proper form and stability are the goals and failure consists of arching the low back, twisting, protruding the abdomen, or flexing the spine while performing the movements. The resistance used should be moderate, about 15-30% (women-men) of body weight for the pulling and a moderately strong tubing for the pushing.

1.5 min of continuous pulling and pushing without loosing a stable spine position or balance is required for a passing grade.

This exercise <u>and</u> test is very important for transference of stability strength and coordination for daily activities, such as vacuuming, mowing the lawn, pushing the kids in a stroller, etc.

This test is pass or fail. If the person can do the action properly, but only for a short amount of time, it means that they need to work on endurance more than coordination.

2. Stand in a mini-squat position with one arm holding onto a tube that is anchored behind the person, and the other arm holding tubing that is anchored in front.

Maintain the squat position with spinal stability, then push one arm while pulling the other arm. Once this can be performed smoothly, a rhythm should be kept as long as they have stability or for the appropriate amount of time, no jerky movements.

The goal is to be able to perform continuous pulling and pushing for 45 seconds in each direction (change feet and arm positions) without loosing a stable spine position or balance. Use about the same resistance as the first test.

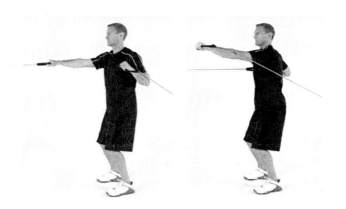

Fig. 12-118
(Test # 2)

This test is pass or fail. It is common to be able to perform this test better on one side; the dominant arm pushing is usually the strongest because of the external oblique and pectoral strength on that side. Therefore, there is often a need to strengthen one side more than the other. A 3:1 ratio between weak and strong is a good start.

Curl-ups

After completing the curl-up, just as in the Muscle Testing section (without resistance at the top), ask the person to slowly roll back onto the table, one vertebrae at a time, exactly opposite as the curl-up, including keeping the low back flat. The head should touch the table before starting each curl-up.

Fig. 12-119

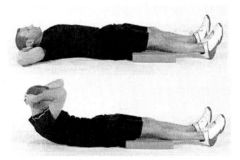

Weakness in the upper fibers of the rectus abdominis muscle is noted if the entire movement cannot be repeated equally *ten times,* using a slow motion with a 1-2 second pause at the top. Weakness includes kicking the legs up or having to use jerky motions. Lower abdominal weakness can also make this test painful on the low back if it allows the lumbar spine to arch on the way up.

This test is pass or fail.

Proprioception

- Foam roll
- One leg balance

Foam Roll

An approximately 6″ in diameter foam roll, the length of the spine and head, is needed for this assessment.

The person lies supine on the foam roll with their entire spine, including the head and sacrum, supported by each end. The knees are flexed with both feet flat on the floor and pointing straight, about shoulder width apart. Both arms are extended out perpendicular to the body with the hands on the floor for stability.
Instruct the person to raise one leg off the floor so that the hip is flexed about 90° and the lower leg is relaxed and dangling.

Then instruct them to slowly raise both arms from the floor, *allow them a few minutes to get the feel of this test.*

Fig. 12-120

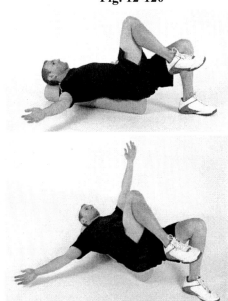

Once ready, ask them to move one arm up towards the ceiling, and slowly back down to where it was. Repeat this on the other side for a total of ten times, then switch to the other leg and arm for ten total reps.

This test mostly challenges the oblique abdominals and the proprioception system.

The grading system is for completion of each side and is as follows.

- Normal (100%) – 10 reps, no assistance (feet or hands)
- Good (80%) – 10 reps, some assistance but in control
- Fair (60%) – 10 reps, some assistance but very shaky and jerky
- Weak (50%) – Can't stay on the roll unless both hands are on the floor

It is common to have one side 100% and the other only 60%. This is a great indicator of muscle imbalance and where and why injuries occur in the person; it is also related to CORE instability on one side.

One leg balance – (endurance/proprioception)

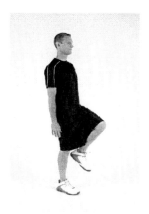

Fig. 12-121

This test assesses hip stabilization strength and endurance, as well as the ability of the proprioception system to coordinate reflexes throughout the kinetic chain.

Utilize the same stance as in the standing gluteus medius strength test in the Muscle Testing section. Instruct the person to maintain the one

192

legged position for as long as they can while keeping steady, up to 30 seconds. The test is over once the person; 1) touches the floor with the raised foot, 2) moves the grounded foot, 3) drops the "floating" hip and can't keep it up, or 4) has to use the arms for balance. Perform each side once with the eyes open and once with them closed if they passed the first test.

The following normative data can be used as a standard for varying ages.

Box 12-6

Age (years)	Eyes open (seconds)	Eyes closed (seconds)
20-59	29-30	21-28.8/25avg
60-69	22.5	10
70-79	14.2	4.3

Byl NN, Sinnot PL. Variations in balance and body sway. *Spine* 16:325-330. 1991

This test and its timed results are also used by Craig Liebenson and Scott Chapman in their lumbar spine rehabilitation video series.[73]

In addition to time observations, this author has made the following interpretations of the one leg balance and endurance/proprioception test.

If, during the test of the right side (standing on the right leg), the pelvis drops towards the left and pushes the right hip out laterally without excessive leaning of the trunk towards the right side, then the gluteus medius is simply weak. But, if that same scenario exists and the trunk leans excessively towards the weight bearing leg, it indicates a weak gluteus medius *and* an overactive Q.L., which should be double checked with the PMAP test for hip abduction.

The test is graded as follows and is based on the normative date by age group in Box 12-6.

0 pts = Less than 5 seconds w/eyes open
1 pt = Needs assistance at about ½ the avg. time
2 pts = Completes avg. time only w/eyes open
3 pts = Completes avg. time w/eyes open and closed

Cardiovascular system

Choose a mode of workout (walking, biking, or cardio machine) that best suites each person. Follow the guidelines below for each type of individual.

Beginner – 20 min @ 50% HRR

Intermediate – 30 min @ 65% HRR

Advanced – 30 min @ 75% HRR

The numbers for beginner and intermediate populations meet the average requirement of duration and intensity standardized by ACSM[33] guidelines. Athletes and advanced populations require a much more detailed assessment. For example, elite sprinters probably cannot and do not even need to perform at 75% HRR for durations longer than ten minutes. Instead, testing them at higher intensities for shorter durations may be more beneficial for assessing their ability to perform in their specific activity.

See Chapter 3 for the formula used to derive HRR.

Note if it is easy or difficult for each person to complete their appropriate level and create a cardiovascular training program from these observations and the individual needs of the participant. Depending on the time available for the assessment, this test can be done on the same day as the rest of the assessments or on the first day of weight training.

This is a pass or fail test.

Keeping Notes

The following three pages are good ways to learn the system, keep notes for future reference, and hand the client something that they can look at and get an idea of the type of program you will create for them.

It takes many trials to get a feel for the flow of a good assessment. It is good practice to perform the full assessment on as many people as possible so that you can get an idea of how normal and dysfunctional people score on each test. The more people you assess, the more experience and references you have to relate to every new person you encounter.

POSTURE   (pts = ___/48)

Anterior View

Feet - N/pronated/supinated
Feet - N/toeing in/toeing out
Knees - N/bowlegged/knock-kneed
Femur rotation - L/R = N/ext/int

Structural Pelvic Tests

Stork Test - N/R/L dysfunction
Standing Flexion - N/R/L
Seated Flexion - N/R/L

ASIS height - N/L↓/R↓
Iliac crest levels - N/L↓/R↓
Pelvic rotation - N/L/R = anterior
Torso rotation - N/L/R = anterior
Shoulder elevation – N/L↓/R↓
Arm rotation – L/R = N/int/ext
Head tilt – N/L/R
Head rotation – N/L/R

Posterior View

Feet - N/pronated/supinated
Gluteal folds – L/R = N/deeper/↓
PSIS – N/L/R = ↑/↓/ant/post/med/lat
Iliac crest level - N/L↓/R↓
Rib cage level - N/L↓/R↓
Full spine curvature - N/apex R/L
Lumbar scoliosis - N/apex R/L
Thoracic scoliosis - N/apex R/L
Scapula rotation - L/R = N/sup/inf
Scapula ab/add - R/L = N/ab/add
Scapula elevation - R/L =N/↑/↓
Shoulder elevation - R/L =N/↑/↓
Head tilt – N/L/R
Head rotation – N/L/R

Side view

Knees - R/L = N/flx/ext
Pelvic tilt - N/ant/post (sway/flat)
          - R/L Ilium = ant/post rot
Thoracic curvature - N/kyphosis
Shoulder - R/L = N/ant/post
Head – N/anterior/posterior
Head tilt – N/up/down

ROM   (pts = ___/65)

Standing

Lumbar flexion - N/↑/↓ = _____ °
Lumbar extension - N/↑/↓ = _____ °

Lumbar ext w/rot - N/↑/↓ = __°/__°
Lumbar side flex - N/↑/↓ =___°/___°

Sitting

Lumbar flex on floor - N/↑/↓ ____°
Lumbar flex (legs bent, off table) -
                    N/↑/↓ ____°
Sitting torso rot - N/↑/↓ = ___°/___°
Neck ROM
Flexion - N/↑/↓ = _____°
o Extension - N/↑/↓ = _____°
o Lateral flex - N/↑/↓ = ____°/____°
o Rotation - N/↑/↓ = _____°/_____°

Supine

Leg length -N/L/R = longer/shorter
Pelvic assessment
o ASIS height - N/L/R = sup/inf
o Pelvic rotation - N/L/R
o ASIS flare - L/R = N/in/out
o Hemipelvis -L/R=N/up/down slip
Hip flexion - N/↑/↓ = ____°/____°
Hamstring - N/↑/↓ = ____°/____°
Piriformis
1. Femur rot - N/↑/↓ = ____°/____°
2. Leg cross - N/↑/↓ = ____°/____°
3. Straight leg - N/↑/↓ = ___°/____
4. Passive observation – L___/R___
Hip abduction
1. Figure 4 - N/↑/↓ = ____°/____°
2. 45° flx/abd - N/↑/↓ = ____°/____°
3. 45° flx/60°abd - N/↑/↓ = ___°/____
4. 30° flx/60°abd - N/↑/↓ = ___°/____
Hip adduction - N/↑/↓ =____°/____
Psoas - N/↑/↓ =____°/____°
Rectus femoris - N/↑/↓ = ___°/____°
Gastocnemius - N/↑/↓ = ___°/____°
Soleus - N/↑/↓ = ___°/____°
Pec minor - L/R = N/TT
Latissimus dorsi - N/↑/↓ =___°/___°
Pec major - L/R = N/TT
TFL - inches from table N/L___ R__
Torso twist - ″ from table N/L__ R__

Prone

                (int / ext) - (int / ext)
Femur rot - N/↑/↓=___/___-___/___
Quadriceps - ″ from butt - N/L__ R__

MUSCLE TESTING
(pts = ___/178)

Standing

Gluteus Medius - N/L↓/R↓

Supine

Psoas – L/R = ___/___
Curl-ups
1. Forward - _____
2. Oblique - L/R = ____/____
3. Lateral - L/R = ____/____
4. Sit-up - _____
Lower abs - S = _____% Funct = P/F
Neck flexors - N/____
Q.L. - L = _____ R = _____

Prone

PMAP for T.A.
          (mmHg / M / bulge / control)
o Prone = ___/___/___/___
o Supine - L = N/↓   R = N/↓
PMAP for multifidus (score 0-3)
(L) = L₁___L₂___ L ₃___ L ₄___ L₅___
(R) = L₁___L₂___ L ₃___ L ₄___ L₅___
Trunk ext w/rot - L = ____ R = ____
PMAP (hip ext) - L = P/F - R = P/F
Gluteus maximus - L = ___ R = ___
Hamstrings - L = _____ R = _____
Piriformis - L = _____   R = _____

Side

PMAP (hip abd) - L = P/F - R = P/F
Gluteus medius - L = _____ R = ____
Lateral flex - L = ____% R = ___%

FUNCTIONAL TESTS
(pts = ___/74)

Squats - ____% ____reps
Push-ups - ____% ____reps
Lower Abs – P/F ____sec
Trunk ext - ___pts(0-3)___reps___sec
Side Plank - L___ R___ (0-5 pts)
Toe Raises - L___ R___ (0-3 pts)
Lunges - knee/abs/reps - P/F/P/F/P/F
Oblique curl-ups - L = P/F - R = P/F
Push-pull - P/F wt.= ____-____
Curl-ups - P/F ____reps   (0-3 pts)
Proprio - FR = __/__% 1 leg = __/__
Cardio - P/F - ___min @ ___%HRR

---

0 points for each abnormal test; 1 point for each normal test; 0-5 points for each appropriate muscle test (5 points = normal/0 points = no ROM or contraction)
A number or letter that is followed by an * signifies that pain was present / ↓ = weak or deficient / ↑ = excessive / mmHg = pressure change / R = right / L = left / N = normal
flx = flexion / ext = extension / ant = anterior / post = posterior / rot = rotation / sup = superior / inf = inferior / med = medial / lat = lateral / int = internal / ext = external
TT = too tight / S = strength / Funct = functional / P = pass / F = fail/ % pts; 100% = 10pts, 70% = 7pts, 50% = 5pts, etc /

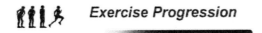 *Exercise Progression*

EVALUATION

Name _____ Date _____

Red Flags	Priorities	Faulty Postures
Tight/Facilitated Muscles	**Weak/Inhibited Muscles**	**Functional Deficiencies**
Strengthening Exercises	**Stretching Exercises**	**Functional Exercises**

Notes _____

_____

_____

_____

_____

_____

_____

_____

_____

_____

Personal Profile

Name_____ Date_____

Areas of Concern

Goals

Recommendations

Program Plan

Chapter 13   Corrective Actions

It can be argued that low back post-rehabilitation time is best spent restoring function instead of correcting imbalances, because there is no way to be sure of which dysfunctions are the main cause of low back symptoms. This may be true in a setting where time and assessments are limited, but in an ideal situation, correcting as many key factors as soon as possible is most beneficial for long term results.

It is difficult for the body to function properly as a whole if its pieces are not balanced. Therefore, if time permits, it is more important to correct a lordotic posture and faulty recruitment patterns for hip extension than it is to practice specific activities or exercises; otherwise, these activities and exercises will be performed with an unstable spine and improper muscle coordination.

It is not always possible or necessary to correct all major imbalances. It is up to the examiner to find "key links" and decide which imbalances are most important and which have the greatest chance of improving in the time that each person is willing to spend doing the exercises. Sometimes the focus will change throughout an individual's routine, depending on what is working and what is not. That's ok, trial and error is better than stubbornness towards an ineffective program, as long as the errors are not serious or traumatic.

Figuring out how often a person should come in and workout under supervision is highly dependent upon each individual's motivation and understanding of exercise and personal limits. Utilizing exercise handout sheets is cost effective for the self motivated individual because they would only need guidance about once every four weeks to learn the new exercises. But, for those who have difficulty performing the exercises properly and pushing themselves enough to improve, it can take up to four times per week under professional supervision in order to improve.

The goal is of course to educate and motivate everyone to want and know how to workout for the good of their body. This can be done with a knack of knowing what to say and how to talk to people, because everyone has at least one button that if pushed will cause an internal chain reaction of perception shifts and habitual changes. These can be more powerful than any exercise or manual therapy technique and is an invaluable tool for any trainer or practitioner.

This chapter deals with corrective exercising and is the perfect compliment to a post-rehabilitation program that involves corrective soft tissue manual therapy.

In general, manual therapy and bodywork ideally accompanies corrective exercising, although it is not for everybody.

Please note: This chapter deals mostly with the specific corrections of assessment findings and not the entire exercise routine or philosophy of how to progress the different stages of recovery (acute, subacute, chronic, and traumatic injuries); these are in Chapters 2, 9, and 10.

Many of the corrective actions in this chapter involve exercises or actions that may be too difficult for a novice or someone in pain. In these cases it's best to start with Stage I exercises and begin the more advanced corrective actions once the body is more efficient.

Low Back Corrective Actions Categories

Neurological	Palpation
Structural	ROM
Posture/Gait	Muscle testing
Breathing	Functional Tests

Neurological

Peripheral nerve involvement

Follow guidelines in chapter 2.

Nerve root compression and Disc pathology

In general, finding the positions that cause and relieve pain, and then utilizing them effectively is the best approach to centralizing nerve root compressions, such as in the McKenzie techniques.

Rehabilitation of a disc syndrome must not begin until conservative care has taken place and decreased the irritability or compression of the nerve root, once this occurs exercise is very beneficial.[41] See Box 13-1 for details on exercise contraindications and guidelines for LBD's.

Sciatica

The following guidelines are from Bigos et all[77] and the Clinical Standards Advisory Group of Back Pain, London.[78] The exercise portion of the active-care phase would utilize the same guidelines as above if the cause was a nerve root compression or disc pathology.

A true sciatica or nerve root cause should first be treated by a licensed practitioner with conservative care, i.e. up to seven days of rest, Mckenzie methods, light stretching and aerobic activity, manual therapy, and medication if needed. This protocol continues for up to six weeks if it is yielding favorable results and is then followed by a more active care program. However, if the person is unresponsive, then a more active approach can be implemented by the second week, but no later than four weeks, although strengthening exercises should be avoided until week three.

Once a more active-care regimen of strengthening, stretching, proprioception training, and cardio has begun, a temporary increase in pain is acceptable and often expected from the exercise.[77,78] If the person is unresponsive to active care after six weeks, a biopsychosocial assessment is indicated. See Box 13-1 for more on sciatica guidelines in the active care phase.

Sciatica Management[77,78]

Conservative care (2-6 weeks)
Active care (at least 6 weeks)
Biopsychosocial assessment (12-16 weeks)

Structural

Spondylolisthesis

If neurological signs accompany a spondylolisthesis (slipping of one vertebrae on top of another) then referral to a specialist for possible surgery is necessary. Otherwise, see Box 13-1 for guidelines.

Facet Joint Dysfunction

Facet joint dysfunction is related to all other dysfunctions of the three joint complex. It is unlikely that a disc injury will occur without some sort of dysfunction in the facet joints.[84,91]

Spinal Segment Instability

In Phase II of the degenerative process of a 3-jt. complex (see pg. 87, Box 11-1), hypermobility and weakening of the facet capsule are present, along with the loss of nuclear matter and annular bulging.[213]

This is not a time for joint movement or extreme stress. Exercise and manual therapy strategies should be aimed at stabilizing the joint(s) and balancing the surrounding soft tissue tension. X-rays and MRI's can be helpful for finding out what type of issue is present.

Releasing tension surrounding vertebral instability is acting with disregard for the body's protective mechanisms and can create even more instability.

Degenerative Joint Disease (arthritic changes)

Stenosis (central or lateral) is a common result of repeated injury or simply living a long and physically demanding life. The vertebral segments of the spine go through three phases of degeneration[213] (see Box 11-1). Phase III involves the forming of osteophytes that often intrude on the spinal canal and nerves and cause symptoms.

There are other methods that can cause stenosis, such as structural abnormalities, but these will not be discussed here because they can have very unique conditions that require special guidelines. Therefore, stenosis will be the main focus of the Degenerative Joint Disease section, along with the awareness that there are other forms of degeneration.

S.I. Joint Dysfunction

S.I joint dysfunction is best treated with manual therapy prior to participating in an exercise program. Unfortunately these techniques are out of the scope of this text.

General exercise guidelines include; 1) balance tension around the joint, especially the T.A., piriformis, erector spinae, hamstrings, hip ad/abductors, and pronated feet, and 2) avoid impact exercise and excessive local ROM until the joint is normalized.

Spine Surgery

Exercise approval from a specialist is required for all of the surgeries mentioned in Box 13-1.

Lumbo-Pelvic-Hip Dysfunctions

The standing flexion and stork tests only demonstrate which side of the pelvis is most dysfunctional. They do not show what type of dysfunction is present. These two tests need to be compared to the posture assessment of ASIS symmetry. Whichever side was dysfunctional for the standing flexion and stork tests will dictate which side is considered out of alignment if there is a faulty pelvic posture.[4]

For instance, if the *right* ilium is viewed as dysfunctional by the standing flexion and stork tests, and the right ASIS is inferior to the left during posture evaluation, then the *right* ilium is thought to be rotated anteriorly, not the left rotated posteriorly. This also applies to the findings in the supine ROM pelvic evaluation, which should reinforce the findings and strategies of the rest of the assessment.

Strategies for improving each dysfunction (innominate tilt, inflare, etc.) will not be discussed here because they require advanced manual therapy techniques. Instead, the dysfunctions are used to validate other findings and provide progress reports.

Posture

Before describing each individual correction, it is important to mention an integrative posture exercise that is useful for combining all or most of the individual corrections listed below into one exercise. This allows the neuromuscular system to integrate the isolated corrections into dynamic actions. Otherwise, individual corrections will only be useful in the static and independent situations they are trained in. The exercise is as follows, see pg. 200.

Exercise Contraindications and Guidelines For LBD's

BOX 13-1

Condition	Goals	Contraindications
Non-Specific LBP (mainly myofascial origin)	1. Establish PMAP for the CORE muscles 2. Balance tension in the kinetic chain 3. ↑ leg and abdominal strength/endurance 4. Improve functional capabilities 5. Improve cardio 6. Improve overall flexibility, esp. hamstrings, lumbar spine, hip flexors and adductors 7. Apply manual therapy	• Prolonged or repetitive trunk bending or twisting • Prolonged or repetitive sitting exercises or activities • Prolonged rest or inactivity • Complex or intense activity (applies to all conditions)
Back Surgery (fusion, laminectomy, or discectomy)	1. Learn neutral and safety positions for spine[5] 2. Establish PMAP for the CORE muscles 3. Emphasize spine stability[5] 4. Improve cardio[5] and leg and trunk strength 5. Improve strength and flexibility slowly	• Prolonged or repetitive trunk bending or twisting • Prolonged rest or inactivity • Extreme ROM[5]
Spondylolisthesis	1. ↑ lumbar stability 2. Limit spinal extension movements and appropriately utilize flexed postures[5] 3. Emphasize cardio, abdominal and leg strength, and CORE stability training[4,5] 4. Stretch and apply manual therapy to short psoas[4], hamstring, and erector muscles[5]	• Hyperextending the lumbar spine • Prolonged extension postures[5] • Prolonged rest or inactivity • Extending the spine against high loads
Nerve Root Compression and Disc Pathology	1. Utilize postures throughout the day that relieve pain and posterior disc stress, i.e. extension[41] 2. Non-weight bearing and aerobic exercises[41] 3. Practice neutral spine position and proper lifting techniques 4. CORE stabilization[5], minimize IAP and lumbar vertebral movements, i.e. isometric 5. Increase leg strength 6. Stretch hip flexors, pirifromis, and spinal erectors without excessive lumbar motion 7. Utilize daily anti-gravity postures[41] 8. Be aware of the likelihood of facet syndrome	• Bending and twisting • Exercises with a lot of motion, impact, or load • Lifting heavy objects, especially after prolonged sitting or laying • ↑ IAP intentionally • Attempting to correct a leaning posture if it relieves the pressure on the nerve • Prolonged rest or inactivity • Placing high loads on the spine in any position
Sciatica (active care)	1. Improve flexibility of hamstrings, gastrocnemius, and piriformis 2. Gentle massage and ice therapy along the pain path of the posterior thigh and leg 3. Improve overall fitness	• Strengthening local muscles when nerve is irritated • Prolonged or repetitive sitting exercises or activities • Over-stretching the hamstrings
Spinal Segment Instability	1. Learn PMAP for CORE muscles 2. Practice neutral spine position 3. CORE stabilization training[4] 4. CORE endurance training 5. Cardiovascular training	• Self manipulation, i.e. cracking own back • Repetitive or prolonged bending or twisting • Prolonged rest or inactivity

Exercise Contraindications and Guidelines For LBD's

BOX 13-1…..continued

Condition	Goals	Contraindications
Facet Syndrome	1. Rest[4] 2. PMAP for hip extension and abduction, and flexion and sit-up movements 3. Normalize the multifidus muscle 4. Stretch erector spinae, hamstrings, and hip flexors[41] 5. Strengthen the gluteus maximus[41] 6. Improve hyperlordosis, usually by stretching and or applying manual therapy to the hip flexors and erectors 7. Utilize flexed postures (tilt pelvis posteriorly) during stressful extension activities, i.e. reaching overhead or simply prolonged standing (place a small stool under one foot during cooking, ironing, washing dishes, etc. to flex spine) 8. Be aware of the likelihood of a disc syndrome	• Rotation exercises • Repetitive or prolonged bending or twisting[4] • Hyperextension • High impact exercises • Prolonged unsupported sitting
Degenerative Joint Disease (spinal stenosis)	1. ↑ leg and trunk strength and stability[5] 2. Improve cardio and endurance[5] 3. Slowly improve flexibility in the hip and spine 4. Reduce lordosis[4] 5. Find positions of comfort (most often slightly flexed[4,5]) and emphasize them during exercise and daily routine	• Exercises with a lot of motion, impact, or load • Attempting to correct a leaning posture if it relieves the pressure on the nerve. • Prolonged rest or inactivity

Some of the above goals do not include the obvious; learning PMAP for CORE muscles, balancing posture, reducing pain, improving nutrition and daily habits, education about low back health and exercise, and adopting exercise as a required lifestyle change in order to deal with and prevent future LBP. The conditions listed should only be dealt with by a licensed professional; otherwise, exercise clearance is required from the treating physician.

Integrated Posture Correction Exercise

Stand with the feet about 3-5 inches apart and point them straight or slightly rotated outward, 10° maximum. Assume the "short foot" position described on pg. 47 and adopt a relaxed knee position (neither straight nor bent). Make sure that the entire body is not leaning forward onto the balls of the feet. There should be a great amount of weight distributed onto the heels; this is however very difficult for many people as it makes them feel like they are going to fall backwards.

Rotate the thighs so that the knees point straight forward (squeeze the buttocks slightly to externally rotate, or push the heels outward to medially rotate).

For the pelvis, adopt a neutral position and lumbar curve by either posteriorly tilting the pelvis (sucking in the lower abdominals and "tucking in the tail") or anteriorly tilting the pelvis (sticking buttocks out), depending on which posture fault is present.

Next, place the shoulders, chest, and head into proper alignment. This usually involves slightly squeezing the shoulders backwards and downwards to externally rotate the arms so that only the thumb, index finger, and half of the middle fingers' knuckles are showing (from an anterior view point), and standing as tall as possible without looking up.

Now hold this position for at least one minute while learning to relax and breathe comfortably.

The key is learning to relax without letting go of the proper alignment. If done correctly, a deeper set of muscles, the postural muscles, will be felt slowly taking over the duties of holding proper posture. Once this position is held for at least one minute, begin walking around while maintaining this "ideal" alignment and trying to keep it as natural and relaxed as possible.

This exercise is great for everyday use; the more it is practiced, the more permanent the results will become. In a society where sitting and poor ergonomics are prevalent, good posture will hardly become automatic. It must be constantly trained with conscious awareness of positioning and incorporated into the daily routine, not just into an exercise program.

Common Postural Faults

The following boxes show important factors for combined interrelated dysfunctions that are frequently seen together, as described in Chapter 12. They are meant to compliment and condense the numerous assessment findings.

Desk Jockey Syndrome

This is a combination of the common faulty postural patterns (lower and upper crossed syndrome and layered syndrome), which are described individually by Chaitow and Delaney[4], Janda[60], and Liebenson.[41]

These patterns, pictured and described on pg's. 153-154, can occur separately or together, both are common. For simplicity, each dysfunction will be described by itself, but corrective actions can be combined for those who have two or more of the following syndromes.

Flat Back Posture

This is a less common posture fault and does not have as many constant findings as the other faults do. An attitude or accident seem to play a role in this fault often. Here some common findings.

Short/Tight Muscles:	**Long/Weak Muscles:**
Hamstrings	Paraspinals
Gluteus maximus	Hip flexors
Anterior abdominals

Corrective Actions
- Stretch/strengthen appropriate areas
- Focus on creating lumbar lordosis

Sway Back Posture

This is a common fault and is associated with poor breathing patterns, a desk job, poor or lazy body awareness, and increased stress in the low back, hips, and knees. Care should be taken to improve this posture slowly due to the chronic stress in the key areas mentioned above.

Right Handedness Posture

Postural Distortions	**Muscle Group Imbalances**	**Causes**
Slight C curve of thoracolumbar spine, concave right Depressed right shoulder Elevated right ilium (R) = right side	Short latissimus dorsi (R) Short erector spinae (R) Short Q.L. (R) Short lateral obliques (R) Short adductors (R) Short psoas (L) Short lateral thigh muscles and fascia (L) Weak hip abductors (R) Weak psoas (R)	Being right handed, especially athletes and manual laborers Frequently holding baby on right hip Carrying heavy bags on left shoulder Driving and leaning to the right Standing with most of weight on right leg

Corrective Actions	**Consequences**
It is not possible to fully correct an adult who has been a right handed athlete for most of their life, but the following actions will improve structure, performance, and aches and pains. Start with Stage I of Exercise Progression Improve any causes (listed upper right of this box) Apply manual therapy to and or stretch the short muscles on the right and left Strengthen the weak muscles on the left at least twice as often as the dominant ones on the right. Try doing as many daily activities as possible using the left side, i.e. opening doors, cleaning windows, vacuuming, etc.	• Left upper trapezius can become overactive from trying to keep the head level and consequently develops TP's • Altered spine mechanics, especially lumbar spine • Altered shoulder mechanics • Tendency to sprain right ankle • Decreased lateral stability • Altered hip abduction patterns on right and therefore increased low back tension

Short/Tight Muscles:

Upper anterior abdominals
Hip extensors

Long/Weak Muscles:

Lower anterior abdominals
Hip flexors

Corrective Actions
- Stretch/strengthen appropriate areas
- Focus on strengthening the lower abdominals slowly.

Lazy Posture

This posture epitomizes the new generation of people who live sitting down. Their gravity muscles have little to no endurance and prefer to rest, as they do when sitting. The muscles involved here vary as do the corrective actions. But the main thing to focus on is gradual endurance and awareness of the postural muscles.

Individual Posture Corrections

The following tables and text have each low back postural assessment along with their possible faults and corrective actions. Some of the assessments overlap in the anterior and posterior views, and thus will only be described in the anterior view section. The muscles listed directly under

Lower Crossed Syndrome

Postural Distortions	Muscle Group Imbalances	Consequences
Anterior pelvic tilt Protruding abdomen Lumbar hyperlordosis	Inhibited gluteus maximus Inhibited lower abdominals Short/facilitated hip flexors Short/facilitated lumbar erectors Tight/overactive hamstrings *and* Inhibited gluteus medius	• Altered hip extension patterns • Altered hip abduction patterns • Altered trunk flexion (curl-up test) • Chronic or recurrent neck, low back, and buttock pain • Hamstring strains • Pseudo-sciatica • Decreased hip extension/abduction • Lateral knee pain/IT band syndrome • TP's in many areas • Joint dysfunctions throughout spine • Lumbo-pelvic rhythm dysfunction
Groove in IT band Foot externally rotated	Short and facilitated TFL Short and facilitated Q.L. Short adductors Short piriformis	

Corrective Actions	Causes

Start with Stage I of Exercise Progression
Stretch and or apply manual therapy to the appropriate muscles in the following order:
   Supine – lower and upper abdominals, psoas, hip flexors, and adductors
   Prone – myofascial connections of back and hip hamstrings, and gastrocnemius
   Side – quadratus lumborum, lumbar erectors, piriformis, gluteus maximus, TFL, gluteus, medius and minimus, and the IT band
   Prone – hamstrings, and gastrocsoleus complex
Correct any detrimental habits, i.e. the causes mentioned in the box on the right.
Sit towards the back of the chair with the buttocks and low back up against the back of the chair, this forces the lumbar spine into a more natural lordosis.
	Upper crossed syndrome
	Acute LBP
	Prolonged sitting, especially without a back rest (bleachers), or slouching
	Frequent walking or running on treadmill (the leg is thrown into extension by the momentum of the treadmill, thus relieving the gluteus maximus of the duty and forcing the psoas to work double time by having to decelerate leg extension)
	Predominantly hip flexor oriented exercises coupled with little stretching
	Not enough hip stabilization exercises relative to larger muscle strengthening
	Excessive foot pronation

Upper Crossed Syndrome

Postural Distortions	Muscle Group Imbalances	Causes
Elevation of shoulders	Inhibited lower/middle trapezuis Short/facilitated upper trapezius Short levator scapula *and* Inhibited deep neck flexors Short and facilitated SCM	Lower crossed syndrome Prolonged sitting or standing, especially slouching, looking down at a desk, resting the chin on a hand, or reclining backwards in a chair while looking straight ahead or down.
Forward head and C0-C1 hyperextension	Short suboccipitals *and* Inhibited serratus anterior Facilitated rhomboids, upper traps, pec major and minor, and levator scapula	Improper exercise habits, i.e. lat pulls behind the head, sit-ups while pushing the chin forward, too much chest and not enough upper back strengthening, lack of stretching the appropriate areas, lifting too heavy and improper breathing techniques.
Scapula winging		
Thoracic kyphosis Rounded shoulders and forward head	Inhibited thoracic erectors Short/facilitated pectoralis major *and* Overactive scalenes Overactive upper trapezius Overactive intercostals	Heavy backpacks worn low on the back Sleeping, watching T.V., or reading supine with too tall a pillow behind the head Being tall and always looking down
Improper breathing rhythm		

Corrective Actions

Stretch and apply manual therapy to the appropriate muscles in the following order:

Side – pectorals, serratus anterior, and intercostals

Sitting – upper trapezius, levator scapula, occipitals, and cervical extensors

Supine – cervical mobilization, scalenes, SCM, and sternum

Prone – rhomboids, middle and lower trapezius, intercostals, erector spinae, fascia from head to sacrum, and rotator cuff tendons

Correct any individual posture faults as described in the posture section.

Correct any detrimental habits, i.e. the causes mentioned in the box on the upper right

Sit towards the back of the chair with the buttocks and low back up against the back of the chair, this forces a more natural lordosis.

Start with Stage I of Exercise Progression

Consequences

- Neck and shoulder pain
- Headaches
- Cervical joint dysfunctions
- Altered scapulahumeral rhythm
- TMJ
- Altered neck flexion patterns
- Thoracic outlet syndrome
- Cervical strains
- Pseudo-carpal tunnel syndrome
- TP's in many areas
- Difficulty relaxing due to impaired breathing
- Rotator cuff strains or tears

each fault, i.e. pronation or supination, are responsible for that particular movement or positioning and are commonly tight if that fault is present, unless mentioned as otherwise.

For example if someone has a pronated foot, the peroneus longus, brevis and tertius and extensor digitorum longus are probably tight and short. The muscles will be in order from top to bottom of which are the most likely and influential for that fault.

Although the weak muscles are not often listed below, *it is also possible that the contralateral partner of a short muscle is weak and requires strengthening or activation* in conjunction with or instead of stretching the short side.

There are certain muscles listed in this section that are to be tested for strength or ROM, i.e. the peroneus longus and the sartorius, yet their individual tests are not described. These muscles that do not have individual tests are the less often involved muscles and will usually improve on there own once the other corrections are applied.

The following lists of muscle actions and functions (pronation, bowlegs, etc.) throughout the chapter are a compilation from various authors: Travell and Simmons[7,8], Kendall and McCreary[49], Chaitow and DeLany[4] Vasilyeva and Lewit[55], Hislop and Montgomery[53], and Henry Gray.[54]

Anterior View

Feet

Pronation (Eversion)	Supination (Inversion)
Peroneus longus	Tibialis posterior
Peroneus brevis	Tibialis anterior
Peroneus tertius	Extensor hallucis
Extensor digitorum longus	longus
	Flexor hallucis longus
	Flexor digitorum longus
	Plantaris

There are no muscles with the exact function of pronation or supination, so the muscles that perform eversion and inversion are used because these movements include a combination of pronation with forefoot abduction (eversion) and supination with forefoot adduction (inversion).

Pronation is a common fault and can be caused by; *genetics, obesity, lax ligaments in the arch of the foot, excessive lumbar lordosis, forward sway of the body with weight distribution mainly on the ball of the foot, weak leg muscles, and other factors.* An important relationship that influences pronation and supination is the balance between the myofascial connections of tibialis anterior and TFL/IT band and the peroneus longus and biceps femoris.

As mentioned by Thomas Myers in Anatomy Trains[63], the tibialis anterior and peroneus longus form a "stirrup" under the arch of the foot that can rock it back and forth between pronation and supination depending on which side is short (a short tibialis anterior encourages supination and a short peroneus longus encourages pronation).

Due to our habits and tendencies, the tibialis anterior is prone to lengthening, peroneus longus to shortening, and the pelvis to anterior tilting. This relationship is essential to foot positioning because the stirrup mentioned above continues upward by way of the myofascial lines of the biceps femoris and IT band/TFL and anchors into the posterior and anterior aspects of the pelvis, making a sling-like loop that connects the arch of the foot to the pelvis.

An anteriorly tilted pelvis will pull the biceps femoris into a state of elongated tension, which can reinforce an already short peroneus longus (by way of the myofascia), thereby creating a tendency for pronation or a fallen medial arch. The anteriorly tilted pelvis will also slacken the upper tensional support to the tibialis anterior and reinforce its elongation that also leads to pronation. The reverse is of course possible with a posteriorly tilted pelvis and supinated feet, but it is much less common.

On the other hand, it is possible to have the opposite situations, such as an anteriorly tilted pelvis and supinated feet or posterior pelvis and pronated feet, or even a tilted pelvis (in either direction) and normal feet.

In the most common posture of an anteriorly tilted pelvis and pronated feet, the peroneus longus is short not because it is overactive but because it is pulled into this position by the short and facilitated gastrocsoleus complex. The peroneus longus is actually short and inhibited due to the synergistic dominance of the gastrocsoleus complex, which also causes reciprocal inhibition in the tibialis anterior that adds to the tendency for pronation.

Therefore, the peroneus longus shortness is a symptom, not a cause of the myofascial imbalance that leads to pronation. The main cause in this instance is the anterior tilt of the pelvis and a facilitated gastrocsoleus complex that results from the tendency to plantar flex the foot, such as when sleeping or lounging with the feet plantar flexed.

Supination is less frequent but still occurs in some individuals. A weakness in the gastrocsoleus complex can cause planter flexion synergistic dominance by the tibialis posterior and facilitation of the main dorsi flexor, tibialis anterior. This combination can lead to excessive supination.

Corrective Actions

Pronation

1. Improve any lumbar lordosis and anterior pelvic tilting.
2. Check the peroneuls, extensor digitorum longus, soleus, and gastrocnemius for shortness or tightness and stretch or apply manual therapy where appropriate. In regards to manual therapy for foot pronation, Thomas Myers[63] recommends that "the fascia of the tibialis anterior needs to be lifted and that of the peroneus lengthened inferiorly."
3. Focus weight distribution of the body onto the heels more than the ball of the foot. For example, lining up the entire body directly over the anterior portion of the lateral malleolus, as in the ideal side view posture position, pictured in Chapter 12.
4. If the person stands with their feet more than about six inches apart, have them position the feet closer together. Somewhere between 4-6 inches will provide the strongest foundation for the rest of the body as well as place it in a position of most relative ease. This of course has to be modified for those with large legs.
5. Practice making a "small" or "short" foot and performing different tasks in that position, especially standing posture and other daily activities that the person performs. See pg. 47 for details on "short" foot positioning..
6. Test the muscles for strength that perform inversion and strengthen if necessary (usually the tibialis anterior), including foot circles and dorsi flexion.
7. Orthotics may be necessary.

- Supination

1. Improve any posterior tilting of the pelvis, flat back or lack of lumbar curvature.
2. Check the muscles that perform inversion for shortness or tightness and stretch or apply manual therapy if appropriate.
3. Test the muscles for strength that perform eversion, as well as gastrocnemius and soleus, and strengthen if necessary.
4. Practice making a "small" or "short" foot and performing different tasks in that position, see pg. 47 for details.
5. Orthotics may be necessary.

Feet

Toeing in	Toeing Out
Medial hip rotators	Lateral hip rotators
Associated with medial hip rotation, supination, and weak lateral hip rotators	Associated with lateral hip rotation, prona-tion, and weak medial hip rotators

These are secondary postural faults in the sense that it

takes another postural abnormality to create a toeing in or out. Therefore, the corrective actions should follow those of lateral or medial hip rotation.

It is possible to have foot abnormalities that cause a toeing in or out, but they are not common or conducive to corrective exercise and require advance manual therapy techniques or surgery.

Corrective Actions

Knees

Bowlegged	Knock-Knees
Sartorius	TFL
Gracilis	Lateral hamstrings
Medial hamstrings	Weak gluteus maximus

- Postural Bowlegs

1. Check the sartorius, gracilis, and medial hamstrings for tightness and stretch if necessary.
2. Check for pronation, hyperextended or flexed knees, and medially or laterally rotated femurs. Correct each as specified in their appropriate sections on the previous and following pages.

- Knock-Knees

1. Check the TFL and lateral hamstrings for tightness and stretch if necessary.
2. Check for hyperextended or flexed knees, and medially or laterally rotated femurs. Correct each as specified in their appropriate sections on the following pages.

Femur/Hip Rotation

Medial	Lateral
TFL	Piriformis
Gluteus medius (anterior)	Obturator externus
Gluteus minimus (anterior)	Quadratus femoris
Medial hamstrings	Gemellus superior
Adductor longus	Gemelles inferior
Adductor brevis	Obturator internus
Aduductor magnus (anterior two parts)	Gluteus maximus
Gracilis (when the knee is flexed)	Sartorius
	Biceps femoris (long head)
	Gluteus medius (posterior)
	Gluteus minimus (posterior)
	Psoas major
	Iliacus

Hip rotation is a very important factor in effectively

stabilizing the body over its center of gravity, especially while on one leg. It doesn't matter if the imbalance is too much medial or lateral rotation, both indicate a weakness in some aspect of hip stabilization.   The deep six hip external rotators are also involved with stabilizing the sacrum to the pelvis and femur (see Ch. 11 for details), and because the sacrum is the base of the spine, these muscles also stabilize the entire spine via connecting it to the pelvis and lower body. So an imbalance at the hip equals instability somewhere in the pelvis and spine, depending on the specific imbalance and position of the body.

Strengthening weaknesses in the hip rotators is commonly done while sitting or lying, which is good for building a strong foundation, but in the long run will not build functional strength because for their role in stabilizing the pelvis and body while standing.

For example, while one side is assisting a movement (kicking a ball), the other side is stabilizing the body over the grounded leg. If this relationship is not trained, then practical or functional strength will not result, unless of course there is a need to externally rotate the leg while sitting or lying down.

Corrective Actions

- Medial Rotation

1. Correct any foot pronation and correct if indicated.
2. Check all of the medial rotators for tightness and stretch if necessary.
3. Strengthen any weak external hip rotators, especially in the standing position, i.e. squeezing the buttocks, or standing on one leg while twisting at the hips, rotating the ungrounded knee away the body, keeping the raised foot at the height of the opposite knee. Progress by adding cable resistance and or performing step up and overs, see fig. 13-1.
4. Strengthen the lateral fibers of the gluteus maximus and hamstrings if necessary, see pg. 232.
5. One leg balancing, emphasizing proper body alignment over the foot and leg. Progress to unstable surfaces.

- Lateral Rotation

1 Check all of the lateral rotators for tightness and stretch if necessary.
2. Strengthen any weak internal hip rotators, especially in the standing position, i.e. on one leg and twisting at the hips, rotating the opposite knee across the body, keeping the raised foot at the height of the opposite knee. Progress by adding cable resistance and or performing step up and overs, fig. 13-1.
3. Strengthen the medial fibers of the gluteus maximus and hamstrings if necessary.
4. One leg balancing, emphasizing proper body alignment over the foot and leg. Progress to unstable surfaces.

5. Lateral rotation of both thighs is commonly linked to an uptight attitude or being a "tight-ass". This obviously takes more than corrective exercising to improve the posture.

Fig. 13-1

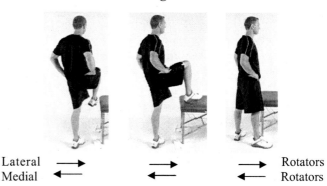

Lateral →   →   → Rotators
Medial ←   ←   ← Rotators

This exercise strengthens the hip rotators (lateral & medial) of the grounded, depending on the direction. Only use a height that promotes function, not compensation. A string tied to or bar lied on two objects also works as the apparatus. Focus on contracting the hip posterior hip muscles of the grounded leg.

Fig. 13-2

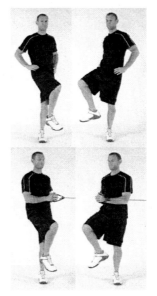

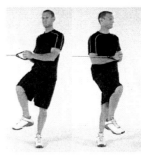

These exercises also strengthen the hip rotators (lateral & medial) of the grounded, depending on the direction.
Top left picture shows strengthening of the left lateral rotators. To strengthen the medial rotators, rotate back the other way.
Bottom picture shows strengthening of the left lateral rotators, no matter which direction because of the necessary eccentric/ deceleration contractions on the way back.
Top right picture shows strengthening of the left medial rotators, no matter which direction because of the necessary eccentric/ deceleration contractions on the way back.

➤ It is appropriate and often necessary to only rotate in one direction, or with a 3 to 1 ratio to improve imbalances.
➤ Strengthening the rotators in the prone position by using a tube wrapped around the ankle of the bent leg or manual resistance at the ankle from an assistant can be useful for those who cannot activate the proper muscles.

However, it is important to eventually strengthen these muscles in a standing position due to their influence on weightbearing hip and femur positions, especially in ballistic actions such as sports or simply jumping and landing on one foot with a little bit of rotation.

ASIS Height

Superior	**Inferior**
(Posterior tilted ilium)	(Anterior tilted ilium)
Abdominals	Lumbar extensors
Hamstrings	Rectus femoris
Gluteus maximus	Psoas
Piriformis	Iliacus
Other hip extensors	Sartorius
to a small degree	Latissimus dorsi
Longer leg	Other hip flexors to
	a small degree
	Shorter leg

The assessment here is for the rotation of an individual ilium, or innominate, as opposed to the tilt of the entire pelvis, which is assessed in the side view. These results should be compared to those in the supine ROM ASIS assessment for clarification of results.

The side that is actually rotated (superior or inferior) is the side that is dysfunctional in the standing flexion and or stork test[4], which is assessed in the structural evaluation.

Corrective Actions

• Superior

1. Check all of the superior rotators for tightness and stretch if necessary.
2. Strengthen any weak inferior rotators.
3. Manual therapy techniques are often required to relieve chronic or severe tightness.

• Inferior

1. Check all of the inferior rotators for tightness and stretch if necessary. Take care not to anteriorly rotate the pelvis while stretching the hip flexors.
2. Strengthen any weak superior rotators.
3. Manual therapy techniques are often required to relieve chronic or severe tightness.

Iliac Crest Level

Elevated	**Depressed**
Q.L. (ipsilateral)	Q.L. (contralateral)
Internal oblique lateral fibers (ipsilateral)	Internal oblique lateral fibers (contralateral)
External oblique laterl fibers (ipsilateral)	External oblique lateral fibers (contralateral)
Iliocostalis Lumbothoracis (ipsilateral)	Iliocostalis Lumbothoracis (contralateral)
TFL (contralateral)	TFL (ipsilateral)
Rectus abdominis (ipsilateral)	Rectus abdominis (contralateral)
Adductors (ipsilateral)	Adductors (contralateral)
Gluteus maximus (weak contralateral)	Gluteus maximus (weak ipsilateral)
Latissimus dorsi (ipsilateral)	Latissimus dorsi (contralateral)
Gluteus medius (weak ipsilateral)	Gluteus medius (weak contralateral)
Longer leg	Shorter leg
Small contralateral hemipelvis	Small ipsilateral hemipelvis

It is imperative to locate the key contributing factors (those which come up most often throughout the assessment or that will create a chain reaction of improvements) here so that time is not wasted trying to correct the many possible muscles involved. An elevated right side is a common posture with right hand dominant people.

Often times correcting faulty postural habits and stretching the Q.L. will improve an iliac crest level imbalance, although chronic tension usually requires manual therapy on the Q.L. and other main contributors. Improving muscle tension surrounding the area will be of little long term benefit if the person continues to carry a heavy bag or child on the same side everyday.

A lumbar compensatory scoliosis usually results from an elevated ilium. In this case, corrective actions are usually recommended unless neutralizing imbalances exist, such as a permanently angulated (crooked) L5 vertebrae on top of an uneven pelvis, which can result in no compensatory spinal curvature, but yet an elevated ilium.[8]

In this situation, correcting the pelvic imbalance would increase the spinal curve and therefore be contraindicated, especially in an asymptomatic individual. *Always think twice before correcting an elevated or depressed ilium in the absence of a compensatory lumbar curve or the presence of a structural (fixed) scoliosis.*

When postural faults are to blame for pelvic asymmetries, correcting them is as simple as stopping the bad postures, introducing proper postures, stretching short muscles, strengthening lengthened muscles, and applying manual therapy to the chronically tight areas. This is a difficult task if the imbalances have had time (many years) to create osteoarthritic changes in the pelvis and spine.

On the other hand, when structural influences are to blame for the asymmetries, then unique corrections to each specific abnormality must be made, i.e. lifts under the buttocks during sitting and or feet when standing. Once structural balance is more stable, stretching and manual therapy are useful in long term relief of symptoms.

➢ Make sure to compare results of the standing assessment to the supine iliac crest level assessment, it is possible for one of the innominates to be sheared upward or downward (usually upward), thus giving the illusion of an elevated side.

Corrective Actions

- Elevated/Depressed

1. Because it is difficult to be sure of structural abnormalities without the use of X-rays, start by correcting the key muscular imbalances with stretches, exercises, and manual therapy.

Common key factors are 1) releasing tension on the elevated side in the lateral trunk muscles and hip adductors, and on the depressed side in the lateral thigh muscles 2) strengthening the lateral trunk flexors and gluteus maximus on the depressed side and gluteus medius on the raised side 3) manipulating pelvic dysfunctions (if properly licensed) 4) improving faulty postural habits, i.e. standing with weight predominantly on one leg or holding a child on that side every day.

Fig. 13-3

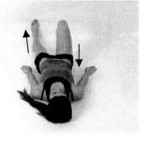

The elevated side is pushed downward while the other side is pulled/hiked upwards. Maintain a neutral spine, proper breathing, and tensed abdominals during the process. Repeat 10 seconds on, 10 seconds off for several minutes.

2. Utilize the pelvic correction exercise mentioned below for correcting any pelvic rotation.

If this approach (steps 1 and 2) fails after attempting four weeks of correction, then reassess and employ one of the appropriate corrections listed below (#'s 3-5), or change the corrective strategy that was used for the initial four weeks.

3. *Shear dysfunction.* If one of the innominates is more superior than the other (ASIS, PSIS, and pubic ramus are all higher[4]), muscle energy techniques (MET) should be applied to release the structure. MET techniques are out of the scope of this text.

4. *Small Hemipelvis.* Correct compensations from a small hemipelvis by placing a lift under the ischium of the smaller side during sitting (for a vertically small side) and lying supine (for an anterioposterior small side). Also,

crossing the thigh of the short leg over the opposite knee while sitting can level out the pelvis.

5. *Leg length inequalities;* When, Why, and How to correct.

<u>When</u> (both conditions must be met)
- It must produce an asymmetry that requires compensations.[6]
- It must create TP's or vulnerability to TP's in the affected muscles.[8]

<u>Why</u>
Correcting major inequalities decreases the chance of osteoarthritis in the hip joint of the longer limb and in the lumbar spine[8]

<u>How</u>
Have a special lift made for the shoe of the short leg, if present. When a substantial difference is present, add half of the height to the short side and take half out of the long side.[8] This avoids an unstable shoe or heel. Only correct with shoe alterations once all other possibilities have been exhausted.

6. *Short upper arms.* Create support for the elbows by either altering the chair or using a pad under the elbows.

Pelvic Rotation

<u>Anterior</u>	<u>Posterior</u>
External oblique (contralateral)	External oblique (ipsilateral)
Internal oblique (ipsilateral)	Internal oblique (contralateral)
Pronated foot (ipsilateral)	Pronated foot (contrateral)
Supinated foot (contralateral)	Supinated foot (ipsilateral)

These results should be compared to the supine findings in order to clarify the findings. For instance, anterior pelvic rotation during standing that evens out when lying supine is indicative of a lower extremity influence more than a pelvic imbalance. But if the pelvis remains anterior when supine, it points to an abdominal imbalance or a structural abnormality, possibly in conjunction with lower body influences.

If the pelvis *and* torso are rotated anteriorly on the right side while standing, then the external and internal obliques are probably short on the right side. But if the pelvis is rotated anteriorly on the right and the torso anteriorly on the left (posteriorly on the right), then the internal oblique is probably short on the right while the external oblique is short on the left; these relationships are more common than oblique weaknesses causing the rotation imbalance, but both are possible.

Balance among the opposing external and internal obliques is very important to spinal stability due to the locking force they produce on the torso and pelvis. If one quadrant is comparatively weak to another, it will allow rotation to occur in the spine and thus reduce stability; this is a common imbalance when there is one side of the body that is predominantly used, i.e. sports or job.

Corrective Actions

• Anterior/Posterior

1. Correct any contributing postures or habits, i.e. foot pronation, keyboard or monitor off to one side, sports or job that involve twisting to one side (counterbalance this by doing exercises that twist the other way), etc.
2. Stretch and strengthen the appropriate internal and external obliques if necessary, sometimes simply correcting faulty habits and postures is good enough to correct the imbalance.
3. ***Pelvic correction exercise***. This exercise is not to be done if there is a fixed structural abnormality that is not being corrected by lifts in the shoes.

   Lie supine and tilt the pelvis (posteriorly or anteriorly) to obtain a neutral position. Place each hand over its ipsilateral ASIS and note the difference in height between the two hands. Try to level the pelvis by contracting the abdominals (not the gluteus maximus) to rotate the pelvis appropriately, make sure not to press the heels into the floor.

   If there is also an iliac crest level difference, it can be corrected during this exercise simultaneously by contracting the appropriate side to elevate the depressed ilium.

   This exercise can be done in sets and reps, or as an isometric hold. If done in sets and reps, then resistance from one hand against the ASIS can be added once the proper activation patterns are obtained. If done isometrically, then a natural and relaxed breathing pattern should occur.

   Once the correct position can be maintained by utilizing the appropriate muscles, begin practicing this position in sitting and standing postures, as well as exercises, especially in other abdominal exercises.

   This exercise is essential for the safety zone spine position, see pg. 81.

Fig. 13-4

4. In extreme cases, a wedge or even a shoe can be placed under iliac crest of the posteriorly rotated side and another wedge under the femoral head of the anterior side just enough so that the two ASIS's are level while lying supine. Lie in this position for up to 15 minutes twice a day. Stop if

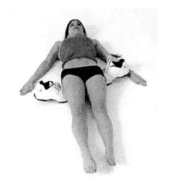

any pain is felt. This position can relax chronic ligament tension and help realign the rigid structure.
5. Structural manipulation is often necessary.

➢ **Special note on pelvic corrective actions.**

Corrective actions for individual hemipelvis tilts and rotations can require complex strategies involving muscle energy techniques (MET) and manipulations which are beyond the scope of this text. The corrective actions presented here are exercises and stretches that can be beneficial, but long standing or complex abnormalities often require manual therapy techniques in addition to the corrections mentioned here.

Torso Rotation

Anterior	**Posterior**
Spiral and Front Functional myofascial lines	Spiral and Back Functional myofascial lines
External oblique (ipsilateral)	External oblique (contralateral)
Internal oblique (contralateral)	Internal oblique (ipsilateral)
Iliocostalis lumbothoracis (contralateral)	Iliocostalis lumbothoracis (ipsilateral)
External intercostalis (ipsilateral)	External intercostalis (contralateral)
Internal costalis (contralateral)	Internal costalis (ipsilateral)
Multifidi (ipsilateral)	Multifidi (contralateral)
Spinal rotatores (ipsilateral)	Spinal rotatores (contralateral)
Latissimus dorsi (contralateral)	Latissimus dorsi (ipsilateral)
Rectus abdominis (ipsilateral)	Rectus abdominis (contralateral)

Torso rotation is mainly accomplished by the shortening of the external and internal abdominal obliques, which if chronic will create restrictions along the related myofascia lines. See volume II for muscles involved with the myofascia lines.

The other muscles listed assist in varying degrees, and some depend upon the position of the torso on the hips.

Corrective Actions

• Anterior/Posterior

1. Eliminate poor postural habits by constantly being aware of alignment while talking to others, waiting in line,

watching television, cooking, etc.

2. Correct any faulty ergonomics, i.e. keyboard, computer monitor, or television set off to one side.

3. Place a pillow between the arms and knees while sleeping on a side.

4. Implement torso twist stretches in the opposite direction of the faulty rotation.

Fig. 13-5 (torso twists)

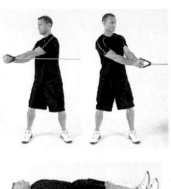

5. Chronic compensations will usually demand more attention, such as manual therapy on the tight muscles and fascia and manipulation of the restricted joints.

6. If the imbalance is do to an overuse of a dominant side, such as in sports or a manual labor job, then strengthening exercises are necessary for the weaker side to "catch up" in strength. Although the weaker side may never match the strength of the dominant side and correct the imbalance as long as the sport or job are continued, the exercises will improve overall strength and stability in the body and thus reduce the risk of future injuries.

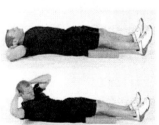

Fig. 13-6

The strengthening exercises are torso rotations toward the side of limitation, against resistance or gravity. In other words, if there is limited torso rotation to the left, then rotate the leading shoulder to the left.

Low, middle, and or high attachments can be used for the cables. It can be one or two arms. The amount of exercise needed depends on the frequency and intensity of the sport or job, as well as the severity of the imbalance.

Shoulder Elevation

Elevated	Depressed
Upper trapezius (ipsilateral)	Upper trapezius (contralateral)
Latissimus dorsi (contralateral)	Latissimus dorsi (ipsilateral)

A LLI or pelvic level imbalance is another cause of shoulder asymmetry, but is tricky because a longer limb or uneven pelvis can induce either an elevated shoulder on the same side by compensating with an "S" curve, or an elevated shoulder on the opposite side by compensating with a "C" curve, see pg. 113 for drawings.

The lateral flexors of the trunk are also tricky because they can be in a shortened position and cause either the pelvis to be tilted without effecting asymmetry above, or they can tilt the pelvis in addition to pulling the torso and shoulder downward.

These three exceptions (LLI, pelvic level asymmetry, and lateral flexor imbalance) are not mentioned as main factors because it takes additional compensations for the asymmetry to occur. But they should always be ruled out before trying to correct a shoulder elevation discrepancy.

Many times a shoulder imbalance will be corrected indirectly by balancing the hips, so it is important to find the root of the uneven shoulders if time is not to be wasted on unnecessary exercises.

Corrective Actions

• Elevated

1. Check the iliac crest and 12th rib levels to rule out other causes, if this area is asymmetric, then correct as mentioned in the appropriate section.

2. Change any faulty habits, i.e. leaning to one side while working on the computer or driving.

3. Stretch ipsilateral upper trapezius and contralateral latissimus dorsi if appropriate.

4. Strengthen the ipsilateral latissimus dorsi if necessary, especially if it is the non-dominant side (usually a 3 to 1 ratio of non-dominant vs. dominant side). Contralateral upper trapezius strengthening is only necessary if that scapula is rotated inferiorly.

Arm Rotation

This may seem to be an unrelated imbalance to LBP, but

Medial	Lateral
Latissimus dorsi	Infraspinatus
Pectoralis major (both divisions)	Teres minor
	Posterior deltoid
Subscapularis	
Teres major	
Anterior deltoid	

enough medial arm rotation will draw the shoulders forward and eventually cause the head to follow, forcing the low back to carry more weight, not to mention all of the shoulder problems it creates.

Corrective Actions

- Medial

1. Correct any head or shoulder asymmetries as well.
2. Stretch the tight medial rotators.
3. Strengthen the lateral rotators, they can almost always use more strength.
4. Practice awareness of shoulder position while sitting and standing.

- Lateral

1. This imbalance is not likely, but if it is present, then the activity or habits causing the posture must be found and improved.
2. Test the medial rotators for weakness and strengthen where appropriate.
3. Palpate the posterior shoulder for adhesions and tightness and stretch or apply manual therapy where appropriate.
4. A military posture (shoulders held backwards and chest upwards) can pull the arms into lateral rotation if the shoulders are pulled back far enough. In this case, stretching the upper back and scapula adductors will help.

Head Tilt

Left Tilt	Right Tilt
Upper trapezius	Upper trapezius
SCM	SCM
Scalenes	Scalenes
All left	**All right**

There are at least ten other muscles in the neck that also latterly flex the head, including deep neck flexors and extensors, but they will be left out here due to the dominance of the three muscles listed above.

The other muscles should be kept in mind when applying manual therapy, as should the following guidelines for exercising; stretch away from the tightness, including any rotation, flexion, or extension, and strengthen into the weakness, including any rotation, flexion, or extension.

Be aware of overexertion or too much resistance during neck strengthening exercises, it is easy to overload these small muscles and even smaller ligaments of the cervical spine.

Corrective Actions
- Left/Right tilt

1. Check for any pelvic or lower body asymmetries (even pronation) that could tilt the head, and correct as described previously.
2. Correct any faulty postural habits, i.e. squeezing the phone between the shoulder and ear, incorrect pillow size, etc.
3. Stretch away from the tilted side.
4. Strengthening the contralateral muscles is only necessary when all else fails, extreme weakness is present (prolonged immobility), or extreme strength is required (a wrestler), and can be done isometrically against hand resistance and then progressed to lateral bends while side lying and hanging the head off a table.

Head Rotation

Left Rotation	Right Rotation
Upper Trapezius (right)	Upper Trapezius (left)
Levator scapula (left)	Levator scapula (right)
SCM (right)	SCM (left)
Scalenes (right)	Scalenes (left)

As with the head tilt, there are many other muscles involved with rotation of the head, up to seventeen total depending on the resource, and again they will be left out due to the dominance of the muscles listed above.

Strengthening the cervical rotators against resistance should not be done past 45° of rotation.

There are two main types of posture rotation distortions; one is when the head is actually rotated to one side of the body, and the other is when the torso is rotated to one side while the head rotates to the opposite side in order to keep face pointing forward. The latter imbalance may be improved by correcting the torso rotation, but some stretching of the neck is usually helpful. The cause of the former imbalance is most likely a faulty postural habit or activity, instead of a distant asymmetry elsewhere in the body, and therefore finding and correcting the faulty habits is the goal.

Be aware of overexertion or too much resistance during neck strengthening exercises, it is easy to overload these small muscles and even smaller ligaments of the cervical spine.

Corrective Actions

- Left Rotation

1. Correct any faulty habits or activities, i.e. reading with the book off to one side, computer or TV set off to one side, constantly talking to people without turning the *entire body* to face them, swimming and only breathing to one side, etc.

2. Correct any torso rotation.
3. Stretch the left levator scapulae, and right SCM, scalenes, and upper trapezius muscles.
4. Strengthen any weak rotators only in special cases, see strengthening for head tilt. Use only hand resistance exercises.

- Right Rotation

1. Apply same corrections as for the left side, but on the opposite side.

Posterior View

Feet

See anterior view corrections.

Gluteal Fold

Use the clues in the assessment section to figure out the cause of any discrepancies and apply the appropriate corrective action from that section.

PSIS

If these findings agree with the ASIS results, then follow the corrective actions for ASIS asymmetry. If not, then make sure the person is standing properly and reassess in standing and lying postures.

Iliac crest level

See anterior view corrections.

Rib Cage Level

Lower	**Higher**
Q.L.	Q.L.
External oblique lateral fibers	External oblique lateral fibers
Internal oblique lateral fibers	Internal oblique lateral fibers
Iliocostalis lumbothoracis	Iliocostalis lumbothoracis
Latissimus dorsi	Latissimus dorsi
Rectus abdominis	Rectus abdominis
All ipsilateral	**All contralateral**

An asymmetry of the rib cage level is usually in conjunction with other nearby asymmetries, such as iliac crest levels or scoliosis. If the rib cage is the lone asymmetry, then utilize the following corrective actions. If other abnormalities exist, then follow the corrective actions for those abnormalities, and the rib cage asymmetry should then improve.

Corrective Actions

- Lower/Higher

1. Correct any influential habits, such as leaning to one side while sitting, carrying a heavy bag on only one shoulder, carrying children, etc.
2. Manual therapy is often necessary to relieve adhesions and chronic tightness in the lower side.
3. Stretch the muscles on the lower side that test tight.
4. Strengthen the muscles on the higher side that test weak.

Scoliosis

Corrective exercise for scoliosis should only be attempted with the approval of the treating physician. General exercise is beneficial for uncomplicated cases because it keeps the tissues and bones healthy while improving cardiovascular functioning. Surgery, bracing, and other techniques are out of the scope of this text, although they are usually the best option for severe cases.

Exercise rehabilitation for scoliosis has not proven to be very effective, especially in the absence of bracing, manual therapy, and a home program. This is likely due to the fact that most cases of scoliosis are of unknown origin. Everything from birth defects and nutritional deficiencies to emotional factors and childhood accidents has been thought to cause scoliosis.

Interesting conclusions have come from studies linking virus-like particles to idiopathic (unknown cause) scoliosis.[264,265] These studies showed that certain microorganisms can end up near the spinal cord and encourage deformities. These intruders can also cause spine pain and inflammation, occasionally leading to sciatica.[266]

Although the use of applying essential oils with massage is out of the scope of this text, it is worthwhile mentioning that Gary Young (founder of Young Living Essential Oils) has had tremendous success treating scoliosis and other spinal deformities with specific and pure essential oils. The reasoning being that the essential oils have bacteria fighting properties as well as the knack for penetrating deep into the body and bloodstream.

A scoliosis treatment program should focus on the back and spine asymmetries along with the effects of the fascia system throughout the entire body. The following lists of muscles and corrective actions are only concerned with the spinal curvature; other corrective actions (as determined from findings in the rest of the assessment) are often needed in order to pull the body into a more even overall tension. A keen sense of palpation is useful for finding rigid areas that require stretching.

Because scoliosis seems to be very individual in terms of the origin of cause, keeping an open mind about the source and studying the many different treatment plans available is the best way to learn the proper corrective actions for the individual in question.

Corrective actions for <u>*asymptomatic*</u> *individuals with structural scoliosis should be very conservative, if at all.*

Adolescents with scoliosis should be monitored closely during growth spurts because of the increased progressive potential of the scoliosis.

The following corrective actions are more successful with functional scolioses than structural scolioses, but results are possible with any type as long as a total body approach is taken.

Note that there are many different distortions and abnormalities that when combined cause opposite effects on the spine. For example, someone with a higher iliac crest on the right may have a left convex lumbar curve while another person has the same high iliac crest on the right but their L5 is crooked (permanently) and causing a right convex lumbar curve.

The above example is one reason that the following corrective actions should be thought of more as guidelines or possibilities instead of actual corrective actions.

Lumbar Scoliosis

A *functional* lumbar scoliosis is most often caused by a LLI[8], but can also be caused by numerous muscular imbalances or faulty habits. The complexity of interactions involved in a lumbar curve include the following; pelvic asymmetry, angulated (crooked) vertebrae, LLI, different fibers in the Q.L. muscle can cause concavity away from the short muscle *or* towards it, the apex of the curve can be towards the elevated pelvis or away from it[55], and more.

Due to these complexities, there are no muscles listed as contributors to lumbar scoliosis. Important muscles to keep mind however are; psoas (pulls lumbar spine towards it when short) and Q.L. (can pull lumbar spine into convex or concave curve, depending on which fibers are short).

Although impossible to be sure of the key factors, it is helpful to know which muscles can be involved. If a lumbar scoliosis is in conjunction with an un-level pelvis, then follow the corrective actions mentioned previously for that abnormality. Otherwise, stretch and strengthen any influential muscles that were found to be dysfunctional in the assessment.

Also be aware that a lumbar scoliosis in the presence of a level pelvic girdle is indicative of a structural abnormality in the spine and should not be "corrected" in asymptomatic individuals.

Remember, it is more important to function efficiently then to be straight. Some people will straighten out, others won't.

Thoracic Scoliosis

<u>Convex Left</u>	<u>Concave Left</u>
Thoracic paraspinal muscles (right)	Thoracic paraspinal muscles (left)
Rhomboids (left)	Rhomboids (right)
Middle trapezius (left)	Middle trapezius (right)
Lower trapezius (left)	Lower trapezius (right)
Intercostal muscles (right)	Intercostal muscles (left)

Corrective Actions

• Thoracic scoliosis

1. Bracing or surgery for severe cases.
2. Correct any faulty contributing habits or postures, i.e. a LLI, leaning to one side while sitting, etc.
3. Stretch or apply manual therapy (including essential oils onto the spine) on any of the indicated muscles that tested tight. Include side bending away from the concavity, especially over an exercise ball).
4. Strengthen any of the indicated muscles that tested weak.

Fig. 13-7

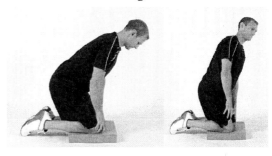

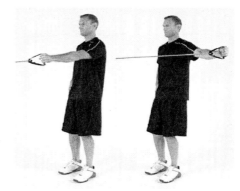

The *top photo* shows how to activate one side of the thoracic erectors. Keep the abdominals and lumbar spine locked in neutral while the thoracic spine extends, relaxes, and repeats for 10x 10 seconds.

The *bottom photo* shows strengthening of the middle traps. Palm facing away. To strengthen lower traps, palms up. Rhomboids, palms down.

"C" Curve Scoliosis (full spine)
Corrective Actions

Convex Left	**Concave Left**
Shorter leg (left)	Shorter leg (right)
Oblique abdominals (right)	Oblique abdominals (left)
Q.L. (right)	Q.L. (left)
Psoas (left)	Psoas (right)
Rectus abdominis (weak on left)	Rectus abdominis (weak on right)
Intercostal muscles (right)	Intercostal muscles (left)

"C" Curve

Bracing or surgery for severe cases.
Correct any faulty contributing habits or postures, i.e. a LLI, routinely carrying a heavy bag on one side only, playing an instrument that requires uneven pelvic postures, etc.
Stretch or apply manual therapy on any of the indicated muscles that tested tight. Include side bending away from the concavity.
Strengthen any of the indicated muscles that tested weak.

"S" Curve Scoliosis (full spine)

Corrective actions for an "S" curve full-spine scoliosis usually involve combining the corrections for opposite (right and left) thoracic and lumbar scolioses.

Scapula Rotation

Inferior	**Superior**
Levator scapulae	Upper trapezius
Rhomboids	Lower trapezius
Pectoralis minor	Serratus anterior
Latissimus dorsi	

Scapula rotation is not directly related to LBD but it is important to neutralize it for long term results because of the compensation the low back has to make due to the altered shoulder mechanics caused by scapula imbalances.

Corrective Actions

- Inferior rotation

1. Stretch any of the inferior rotators that test tight.
2. Strengthen any of the superior rotators that test weak.

- Superior rotation

1. Correct any habits or postures that may influence scapula rotation, i.e. holding the phone between the shoulder and ear, tense and shrugged shoulders, wrong pillow size, etc.
2. Stretch any of the indicated muscles that test tight.
3. Strengthening in the neck is usually unnecessary unless prolonged disuse occurred, such as in severe injuries or neck braces, but the rhomboids and serratus anterior are often in need of strengthening.

Fig. 13-8 Serratus anterior strength exercises.

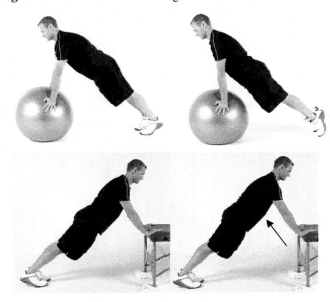

Scapula Ab/Adduction

Abduction	**Adduction**
Serratus anterior	Rhomboids
Pectoralis minor	Upper trapezius (all divisions)
Pectoralis major*	

* Even though the pectoralis major doesn't directly abduct the scapula, its shortness will round the shoulder and cause the scapula to follow.

Scapula abduction and adduction are important to the weight distribution on the lower back. It is common for people to have rounded shoulders and abducted scapulas, this pulls the upper torso forward and creates a larger moment force in the lumbar spine.

Corrective Actions

- Abducted

1. Correct habits and postures that encourage rounded shoulders, such as slouching while sitting or standing, prolonged sitting at a desk without a break, etc.
2. Stretch any of the abductors that test tight.
3. Strengthen any of the adductors that test weak.

- Adducted

1. Stretch the adductors.
2. Strengthen the abductors that test weak, utilize protraction exercises.

Scapula Elevation

Elevated	Depressed
Upper trapezius	Lower trapezius
Levator scapulae	Serratus anterior
Rhomboids	(lower fibers)
Serratus anterior	Latissimus dorsi
(upper fibers)	Pectoralis minor

Corrective Actions

- Elevated

1. If stress is a cause, practice breathing and relaxation exercises.
2. Correct any faulty ergonomics or habits, i.e. too high of arm rests on chair, keyboard too high, chair too low, etc.
3. Stretch the elevators that test tight.
4. Strengthen the depressors that test weak.

- Depressed

1. Strengthen the elevators that test weak, especially the upper trapezius.
2. Stretch any depressors that test tight.

Shoulder Elevation

See anterior corrective section.

Head Tilt

See anterior corrective section.

Head Rotation

See anterior corrective section.

Side View

Knees

Hyperextended	Flexed
Quadriceps	Hamstrings
Soleus	Popliteus
	Gastrocnemius
	Longer leg

A posture with hyperextended knees is typical in individuals who lack overall postural strength. Their entire postural musculature can be similar to jackets on a coat rack; the spine and leg bones are the coat rack and the muscles (jackets) are just hanging on without giving much resistance to gravity.

It is also seen as a lazy posture because the muscles don't do much work, and it is commonly in conjunction with rounded shoulders and a forward head, such as in sway back and forward leaning postures.

Although the quadriceps are in a lengthened position with flexed knees, they are constantly contracting to hold the position, which can in turn be caused by tight hip flexors.[49] If the hip flexors are tight, there will be compensations in the knee and or low back.[49]

Corrective Actions

- Hyperextended

1. If a "lazy" posture is suspected, then education about the effects of poor posture is usually beneficial, along with practice on being aware of not hyperextending the knees when standing.
2. Stretch the quadriceps and soleus if appropriate.
3. Strengthen the flexors as needed.

- Flexed

1. Correct any LLI and pelvic asymmetries, especially lordosis.
2. Stretch the appropriate knee flexors.
3. Strengthen the quadriceps and soleus if needed.

Pelvic Tilt

Anterior	Posterior
Lumbar extensors	Abdominals
Rectus femoris	(especially lower fibers)
Psoas	Hamstrings
Iliacus	Gluteus maximus
Sartorius	Piriformis
Other hip flexors to	Other hip extensors
a small degree	to a small degree
Pronated feet	

Correcting pelvic tilt, especially an anterior tilt, is an integral part to improving posture throughout the entire body. Abnormal pelvic tilting is usually present with upper body distortions that need to be corrected as well in order to gain long term improvements.

Corrective Actions

- Anterior

1. Correct any faulty habits or postures that contribute to the problem, i.e. wearing high heel shoes, sit-ups with feet

anchored, pronated feet, prolonged sitting without standing up and stretching into extension, too many hip flexor oriented exercises compared to hip extensor exercises, etc.
2. Stretch the hip flexors and any other muscles that test tight (utilize active stretching whenever possible).
3. Strengthen any weak posterior pelvic tilters, especially with isometric postural exercises; such as the sitting and standing (see fig. 13-9) pelvic tilts. These two exercises should be performed as a workout and then repeated throughout the day in a normal sitting and standing position whenever necessary in order to retrain posture.
4. Practice different exercises and activities while maintaining the new and improved posture so that new patterns of muscle recruitment replace the old faulty ones.

- Posterior

1. Practice postural awareness of proper alignment over the feet, especially in regards to softening the knees if they are extended.
2. Differentiate between a flat and a sway back see pg. 154. They have similar corrective actions with the main difference being that a flat back needs to focus on creating a lumbar curve by strengthening the hip flexors and a sway back needs to focus on strengthening the lower abdominals.
3. Stretch the hamstrings and upper abdominals if appropriate.
4. Strengthen the lumbar erectors and hip flexors if appropriate
This posture is often in conjunction with the anterior

Thoracic Curvature

Kyphosis

Pectorals (major and minor)
Internal oblique
Rectus abdominis (upper portion)
Intercostals
Inhibited thoracic spine extensors
Weak middle and lower trapezius

shoulder and anterior head postural faults, as well as lumbar lordosis and foot pronation. Therefore, these distortions should be corrected along with the kyphosis. It is possible to correct kyphosis, forward head posture, and forward shoulders by correcting imbalances in the lower body, such as foot pronation, lumbar lordosis, and forward leaning posture. This of course only works if the imbalances in the upper body have not had time to settle in and create serious changes in the musculoskeletal system. Chronic imbalances here will require exercises for all areas.

Corrective Actions

- Kyphosis

1. Practice awareness of faulty posture habits (slouching) and correct any ergonomical errors.
2. Stretch and or apply manual therapy to the pectorals, internal oblique (upper and lateral fibers), and intercostals, if short, and apply manual therapy to areas that have adhesions or chronic tension. Deep breathing exercises are useful in stretching the intercostals and internal oblique.
3. Strengthen the thoracic extensors with isolated movements and the middle and lower trapezius muscles.
4. Practice the standing pelvic tilt against the wall (see below).

Fig. 13-9 The wall stand

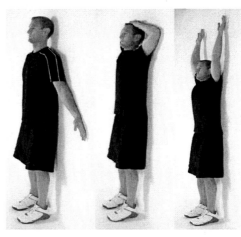

Standing with feet about 3inches from wall, use the lower abdominals to flatten the lumbar spine against the wall (do not use the glutes or bend the knees). The entire spine and back of head should be resting against the wall, without leaning the head backwards. Hold for as long as comfortable up to a few minutes. Take breaks if necessary because spasms in the thoracic and neck muscles are common due to their sedentary habits. Progress from arms down (photo on left) to arms up.

Fig. 13-10 Isolated thoracic extensions.

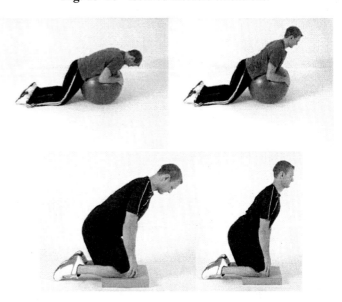

Either exercise (previous page) is good, but sometimes the ball makes it easier to isolate the thoracic muscles. Keep the abdominals and lumbar spine locked in neutral while the thoracic spine extends, relaxes, and repeats for 10x 10 seconds. Keep the head in line with the spine so that the neck extensors do not take over.

The most important aspect of this exercise, and any posture exercise, is to incorporate into daily life. Once this motion is learned, because it is difficult at first, it should be a motion that is practiced throughout the day, waiting in line, at the desk, etc. This way the exercise does not have to be practiced at the gym or even thought of as an exercise. Rather a way of life, or posture.

Shoulder

Anterior	**Posterior**
Pectorals	Posterior deltoid
(major and minor)	Middle trapezius
Serraus anterior	Lower trapezius
Anterior deltoid	Rhomboids
Upper trapezius*	
Levator scapulae*	

* Levator scapulae and upper trapezius tightness that elevates the scapula is commonly involved with, but not responsible for, a forward shoulder posture.

It is most common for the shoulders to be anterior rather than posterior, and also in conjunction with thoracic kyphosis, abducted and elevated scapulas, forward head, and lower body distortions, such as a lower cross syndrome. A total body approach should be taken in order to achieve long term improvements of an anterior shoulder.

Corrective Actions

• Anterior

1. Practice proper posture alignment during sitting and standing postures.
2. Stretch any of the indicated anterior muscles that test tight. Active stretching is ideal for a forward shoulder because it is easy and safe to activate the weaker posterior muscles and place the short anterior muscles in a lengthened position.
3. Strengthen any of the indicated posterior muscles that test weak. Utilize isometric exercises (active stretching as mentioned above) and high reps in order to build endurance in these muscles and activate postural mechanisms.

• Posterior

1. Figure out why this posture has occurred. It is rare and must be due to something unusual.

Head

Anterior

Upper trapezius
Levator scapule
SCM
Weak deep cervical spine flexors

Corrective Actions

• Anterior

1. Practice awareness of faulty posture habits (slouching) and correct ergonomical errors.
2. Stretch the upper trapezius, levator scapula, and the SCM (mostly the upper fibers) if tight.
3. Strengthen the deep cervical flexors if weak - start with fig. 13-11 and progress to fig. 13-12.
4. Make sure to correct any faulty shoulder, lumbar, or thoracic spine postures.
5. Practice the standing pelvic tilt against the wall, pg. 216 (wall stand).

Fig. 13-11 Assist in holding up their head, then slowly release pressure until they are holding up the weight of the head. Not everyone can tolerate the entire weight so greater assistance is often necessary. Progress to 6x 10 sec holds with 3-5 seconds rest in between each hold.

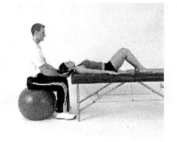 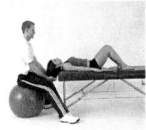

Fig. 13-12   Deep cervical neck flexor strength exercise. Perform sit-ups on a ball with the head being the focus of movement, moving it from extension to flexion as the torso curls up. Stop when the neck gets tired or starts to push forward instead of curl into flexion. Keep the lower abdominals tensed and lumbar spine protected from excessive bending.

When the tongue is pushed to the top of the mouth during this exercise it activates the deep stabilizers of the neck and helps maintain stability throughout this motion.

Dizziness, lightheadedness, and other similar symptoms can be caused by trigger points in the anterior neck muscles or even more complex issues.

Progress to 25 reps.

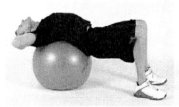 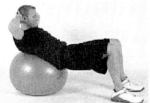

Head

Chin Up	Chin Down
Upper trapezius	SCM
Neck extensors	Scalenes
SCM	

Pain or discomfort associated with the chin up posture can come from facet joint irritation and will require a gentle recovery with limited ROM until the pain subsides.

The SCM muscle can flex or extend the head, depending on the position of the cervical vertebrae. If the cervical spine is flattened by the smaller neck muscles, then the SCM will flex the head and spine, but if the cervical spine is extended, the SCM will increase the amount of spinal extension (lordosis) in the neck and head, as well as flex the cervical column on the thoracic column.[11] This is very similar to how the psoas act on the lumbar spine.

Corrective Actions

- Chin up

1. Correct any postures or habits that involve looking up for prolonged periods of time.
2. Stretch the upper trapezius, neck extensors, and SCM.
3. Strengthen the SCM and scalenes with flexion exercises.

- Chin down

1. Correct any postures or habits that involve looking down for prolonged periods of time.
2. Stretch the SCM and scalenes if tight.
3. Strengthen the upper trapezius and neck extensors.

Gait

Observations from gait analysis give results that are already described and have corrective actions for in their appropriate sections. Therefore only a brief description of the results will be mentioned here, and any individual corrective actions should be looked up in the proper section.

There is however one overall corrective exercise for gait dysfunctions, and that is simply practicing walking in a relaxed manner while focusing on the following ideals, especially the ones that are dysfunctional.

Level head and shoulders

If either of these deviates abnormally upward and downward, it can be a sign of a LLI or pelvic imbalance.

Arms swing opposite of the legs

People who have had strokes or brain injuries can have a hard time alternating the arms and legs during the gait cycle. These are unique cases that require specialized attention. Cross-crawl pattern exercises are helpful for this dysfunction.

In general, if one arm swings more freely and with greater ROM, it is usually on the side of a shorter leg or more inferior hip.

Torso rotates opposite of the hip

This is along the lines of the previous pattern (cross-crawl). This is a good relationship to visualize while walking in order to loosen up the pelvis and spine. Restrictions of this movement can be from tight fascia and or muscle in the latissimus dorsi, thoracolumbar fascia, and contralateral gluteus maximus connection. Thomas Myers[63] includes this connection in his "Back Functional Line", which describes the fascial interconnectedness from the humerous to the latissimus dorsi, LDF, and contralateral sacral fascia, sacrum, gluteus maximus, femur, vastus lateralis, patella, subpatellar tendon, and tibial tuberosity. Myofascial release of this soft tissue link can dramatically improve limited torso rotation.

Hip extends and toes push off

The hip flexors can be so dominant that they take over as the prime movers during walking, along with the arm flexors. This pattern neglects the important posterior muscles that help propel us forward. It is beneficial to experience walking by utilizing predominantly the posterior muscles of the body; gluteus maximus, hamstrings, gastrocnemius, and the posterior rotators of the spine. One will notice that the stance is more upright and there is more of a bounce or spring in the step, which is usually associated with health or happiness.

This brings up an important issue in posture and gait corrective actions. One can stretch the hip flexors and strengthen the posterior muscles all day, but if the person is unhappy or depressed, their posture will most often mimic their feelings and attitude.

If hip extension and toe off movements are limited, then utilize the corrective actions for altered PMAP of hip extension, and strengthen the gastrocnemius. Also check the dorsiflexion of the big toe (it should be 20 degrees), because it can cause postural and gait dysfunctions throughout the entire body.[4]

Knees point forward without rotating

A common imbalance is when a knee rotates or falls inwardly. This can be from a pronated foot or weakness in the hip.

Feet pointing forward

The feet should point slightly outward or straight. Any

deviations should be further assessed in the hip evaluation.

Fig. 13-13

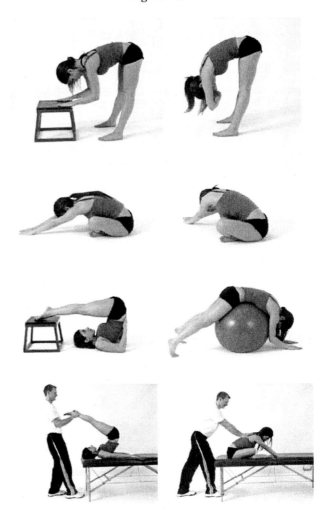

Time spent on each foot should be equal

The side of the longer leg or more superior hemipelvis will be the side that more time is spent on the foot, unless there is pain on that side, which will cause a noticeable limp with more time spent on the short leg, away from the pain.

The torso rotation should initiate the arm swing

A tight and rigid torso can induce excessive effort by the shoulder and arm muscles to produce a rotation momentum force to make up for the lack of movement in the spine and torso. Stretching for the spine and torso are indicated by this and other tests (torso rotation, forward bending, seated rotation, etc.) throughout the assessment.

The lumbar spine should be naturally curved

If the spine is straight or flat, then assess further with the pelvic and spine evaluation. Include the assessment of the big toe for dorsiflexion (should be 20°) and palpation tenderness because it is known to create compensations such as a reduced lumbar curve.[4]

Leaning to one side

Leaning to one side during the stance phase can indicate ipsilateral hip abductor weakness, inferior hemipelvis, or a short leg.

ROM

See the stretching chapter for pictures of all the stretches for each muscle.

STANDING

Standing flexion

The inability to bend at the hips requires practice of the forward flexion exercise, which involves sucking in the stomach and then bending at the hips, not the low back.

Excessive thoracic curvature requires the same corrective actions as are mentioned for kyphosis, see pg. 216. This alone will not help the thoracic hypermobility as long as there is tightness elsewhere in the posterior myofascial system causing the thoracic spine to compensate with more movement.

If a lack of a lumbar curve is verified by the sitting flexion tests, then low back stretching is indicated , as well as manual therapy on the erector spinae. Also check the tightness of the hamstring and gastrocnemius muscles.

⇒ All of the stretches in fig. 13-13 target the low back. Not all are appropriate for someone with a low back disorder.

Standing extension

If there is pain, the results should be compared to the structural pathology section in order to rule out any serious dysfunctions. Pain in the low back on this test can also be from TP's in the abdominals, iliacus, or psoas muscles.

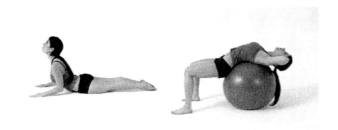

Fig. 13-14 Spinal extension stretches. Also try psoas stretches.

Limited spinal extension without pain points to tightness in the abdominals and or hip flexors that should be confirmed by the other assessments, especially the ROM tests for these muscles. Once confirmed, the appropriate areas should be stretched, and if needed, practice of PMAP for hip extension.

Excessive spinal extension is conducive to facet joint problems, arthritis, and instability, and is associated with weak abdominals and or hip flexors and participating in hypermobile sports (dancing, gymnastics, diving, etc.) at a young age. Corrective actions for these people should focus on core stability, not mobility exercises.

Standing lumbar extension with rotation

If restriction is noticed without pain, then the psoas stretches shown are indicated.

If pain is present on the opposite side of the rotation, then the psoas, lateral abdominals, and Q.L. muscles should be further assessed.

If pain is felt on the same side as the rotation, then the S.I. and facet joints and ipsilateral Q.L. and deep paraspinal muscles should be furthered assessed.

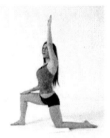

Fig. 13-15

This stretches the psoas, anterior hip joints, oblique fascia, and lumbar spine. Squeezing the buttocks of the posterior leg will stabilize the low back and prevent excessive motion in the hips and spine.

Standing lumbar side flexion (L/R)

If limited side flexion on one side is in conjunction with a short leg or inferior hemipelvis on the opposite side, then corrective actions should follow those already mentioned in the posture section to correct the imbalance.

If there is limited side flexion with a level pelvis, then stretching of the Q.L. and lateral abdominals on the side opposite of the reaching is indicated. The psoas and latissimus dorsi can also limit side flexion and should be evaluated for shortness.

Fig. 13-16 Lateral stretches (cont. on next page)

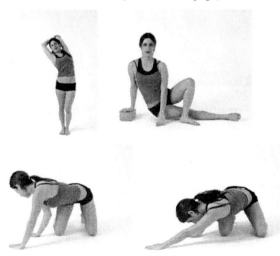

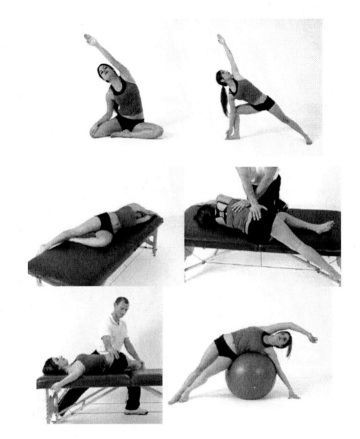

Neck Flexion

If the chin cannot touch the sternum, then stretching of the neck extensors is indicated. This restriction could be due to faulty postures, such as rounded shoulders, kyphosis, and a forward head.

Fig. 13-17 Neck extensor stretches

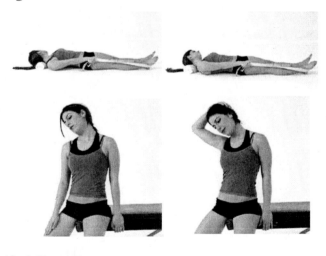

Neck Extension

If this ROM is limited in the absence of pain, then stretching the neck flexors is indicated. If the cervical spine doesn't seem to move, even though the head is moving, then manual therapy and joint manipulation are indicated.

Fig. 13-18 Neck flexor stretch. Rotate chin upward to increase the stretch.

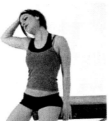

Neck Lateral Flexion

Lateral flexion that is limited by muscle requires stretching of those muscles (upper trapezius, SCM, and scalenes) and correction of any influencing postures, such as; an elevated shoulder or scapula, uneven pelvis, forward shoulder, functional scoliosis, and more.

Lateral flexion that is limited by a restricted cervical spine requires mobilization techniques and joint manipulations, along with stretching of the upper trapezius.

The stretches for lateral flexion are just like the previous two but with an emphasis on side bending.

Neck Rotation

Limited neck rotation to the *right* (in the absence of pain) points to tightness in the left levator scapula, and right upper trapezius, SCM, and scalenes. Stretch the muscles that correlate to the person's restriction. Apply the stretches from the previous corrective actions.

SITTING

Sitting lumbar flexion (straight legs)

Determine which imbalances, if any, are present by comparing the person's form to that of the standing test.

Stretch the appropriate areas according to the correlating muscle tightness stated in the assessment section for this test. Manual therapy is indicated for chronically tight muscles.

Instruct upon the proper way to activate the T.A. during this stretch in order to protect the lumbar spine from unprotected anterior shearing forces.

Apply the stretches from the standing flexion and hamstring corrective actions.

Sitting lumbar flexion (legs bent, off table)

If there is more trunk ROM in this test than the previous test, hamstring shortness is probable.[4] This test should confirm and narrow down the results from the other two forward flexion tests. Utilize the corrective actions from those tests to incorporate the findings from this test.

Sitting torso rotation

Corrective actions for restricted torso rotation require stretching of any tight muscles; see the posterior rotators of the torso in the posture section for possible tight muscles.

The oblique abdominals may also be weak in one direction from overuse by a sport or job; this dysfunction should be noticed in the posture section and its correction is mentioned in that section.

Other influences such as pelvic asymmetries can influence torso ROM and should thus be assessed and corrected if appropriate.

Fig. 13-19   Also use the stretches from the torso rotation posture section.

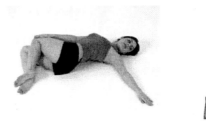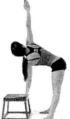

SUPINE

ASIS height

Once the side and origin of displacement are known, utilize the corrective actions for the appropriate fault (inferior or superior), which are already mentioned in the anterior posture corrective actions section for ASIS height.

Pelvic rotation

Make sure the results are the same for standing and supine positions, if so, follow the corrective actions mentioned in the posture section for ASIS rotation.

ASIS flare

This distortion requires manual therapy and muscle energy techniques (MET).

ASIS, PSIS, and pubic ramus

This type of distortion is corrected with manual therapy and MET.

Leg length test

If the LLI is structural, then correcting it is not the goal, but tension can be eased by using the corrective actions for iliac crest height and looking into shoe lifts and the like. If the LLI is functional, then look for asymmetry in the pelvis and correct appropriately.

Hip flexion

Limited hip flexion is rarely because of a tight gluteus maximus, it is more likely due to myofascial tension in the low back; the gluteus maximus, biceps femoris, and sacrotuberous ligament are all attached myofascialy to the ipsilateral multifidi and erector spinae aponeurosis, and the contralateral latissimus dorsi, LDF, and iliocostalis thoracis[64], and can therefore restrict the motion of hip flexion.

This indicates that stretching the low back and hamstrings and applying the appropriate manual therapy would improve limited hip flexion. See those specific anatomy sections for individual corrective actions.

Hamstrings

Tight hamstrings can often be relieved by stretching the hip flexors and balancing the muscles surrounding the lumbo-pelvic-hip area. *Rarely is it beneficial to only stretch the hamstrings in order to improve their flexibility.* All influential assessment findings and corrections must be utilized to relax the hamstrings. Any restrictions in the posterior myofascial system can limit hamstring ROM and therefore must be corrected as well. Look for posterior lower leg, foot, and lumbar tightness to interfere with hamstring length.

Because the hamstrings are usually stressed from battling the hip flexors over pelvic positioning, stretching should be gentle, not forceful. Appropriate manual therapy (myofascial and TP release) is also very helpful in relieving hamstring stress, but results are short lived if the surrounding muscles are imbalanced.

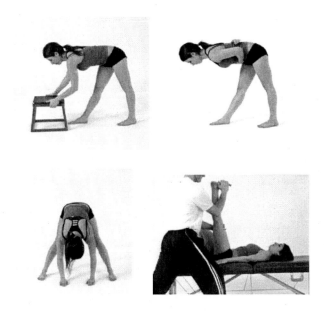

Fig. 13-20   Hamstring stretches (8)

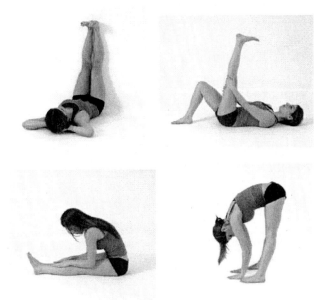

Piriformis

If the piriformis tests short or tight in the absence of pain, then simple stretching of the muscle is indicated, along with balancing any influential postural faults (pronation, pelvic asymmetry, LLI, and more) and ROM deficiencies.

If the piriformis is tight and painful when stretched or palpated, it is likely due to chronic tension and requires manual therapy (to it and nearby muscles and structures), stretching, and habitual posture changes, such as; placing a pillow between the knees while sleeping, not crossing the legs, avoiding prolonged sitting (especially driving with the leg externally rotated), and not wearing high heel shoes.

If the area is hypersensitive and there are sciatica like symptoms, care should be taken to avoid overstretching or palpating the region due to the possibility of irritating the sciatic nerve, which can travel through or around the piriformis.[4,8] Utilize neurological assessments to clarify a sciatic nerve involvement and follow the corrective actions in the neurological section if appropriate.

If the piriformis also tests weak in the muscle testing section, additional exercises are needed, see pg. 233.

Fig. 13-21

Piriformis stretches

Hip abduction

Whichever test(s) the adductors test short in is the position (s) they should be stretched in. Manual therapy in this area can be very sensitive but provide relief from chronic adhesions and tightness.

Tight adductors will influence the movement of the hip and activation patterns of related muscles, see pg. 233 for details on interactions and corrections.

If the adductors are elongated there is likely a corresponding hypermobility of the hip joint that is related to gymnastics, dancing, or other sports and will require stabilization exercises of the hip, especially the lateral and medial rotators.

Any involvement of the medial hamstrings, gracilis, or myofascia should be taken into account when stretching and applying manual therapy.

Fig. 13-22 Adductor stretches

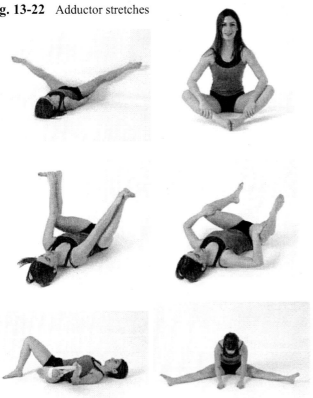

It is very important to activate the gluteus medius during these stretches whenever possible. A weak gluteus medius/minimus is common and requires strengthening to ensure long term adductor stretching results. Utilize the strengthening exercises mentioned in the muscle testing section for gluteus medius (fig.'s 13-?).

Hip adduction

Any restriction in this test indicates tightness in the TFL, gluteus medius or minimus, and or the lateral fascia of the leg or hip. Clarification of which muscles are most involved can be had by utilizing the results from the TFL ROM test and muscle tests from TFL and gluteus medius and minimus. Then stretching and manual therapy techniques can be applied to the appropriate areas.

Psoas

If the psoas was the main muscle indicated for shortness, then stretching it is indicated, as well as utilizing results from the other assessments in order to correct influential postures and habits. See corrective actions for lordosis (anterior pelvic tilt) in the posture section.

If the other hip flexors are short along with the psoas, continue testing in order to validate the tightness in the TFL and rectus femoris.

Fig. 13-23 Psoas stretches. Gluteus maxmius strengthening is also imperative for long term results (see pg. 232).

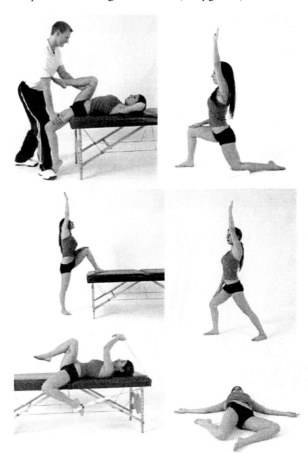

Rectus femoris

Stretching the rectus femoris should be distinguished from stretching the rest of the quadriceps by adding hip extension into the movement. This can be done by placing a pillow or pad underneath the knee while lying prone and placing that knee into flexion until the resistance barrier is met.

A more intense stretch is possible by placing the nontested leg off the side of the table with the foot on the floor directly under the hip. Then apply the same stretch mentioned above, see fig. 13-24.

The table should be at a height that allows for a good stretch but keeps the pelvis aligned. If the table is too high it will not provide a very good stretch, and if the table is too low it will cause too much torque in the pelvis and make for an extreme stretch.

Any weakness in the rectus femoris is usually from general deconditioning or an injury and should be strengthened with general cardio, squats, lunges, and the like.

Fig. 13-24

Rectus femoris stretches. Focus on tightening the gluteus maximus so the pelvis stays stable.

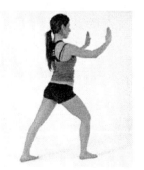
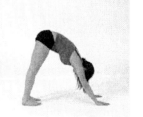

Gastrocnemius

If the gastrocnemius tests short, then stretching it is indicated, along with strengthening the dorsi flexors if weak and correcting any faulty habits or postures, i.e. wearing high heel shoes or sleeping with tight sheets or heavy blankets that force the ankles into plantar flexion.

Check for any related tightness in the posterior fascia system, foot, hamstrings, erector spinae, and neck

Fig. 13-25 Gastrocnemius stretches

extensors.

Apply manual therapy to adhesions and TP's in the above mentioned areas if the tightness persists.

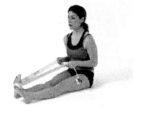

Soleus

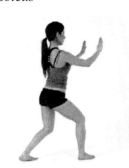
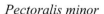

Fig. 13-26

See gastrocnemius corrective actions, but apply the bent knee soleus stretch.

Pectoralis minor

Stretching this muscle will not improve its shortness as much as correcting the faulty habits associated with the shortness, such as poor work station ergonomics (the keyboard or mouse being too far from the body), frequently holding a baby while rounding the shoulders, improper breathing patterns, etc.

Stretching is beneficial for the relief of discomfort from this muscle, but should be in conjunction with actions that correct the problem, not the symptom, if long term improvements are desired.

Fig. 13-27 Pectoralis minor stretches

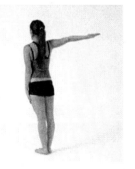
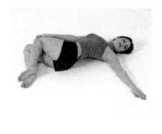

Latissimus dorsi

If the latissimus dorsi (lat's) tests short, then stretching it is indicated, as well as utilizing the corrective actions for uneven shoulders (if appropriate).

Myofascial and TP release are very effective at lengthening the latissimus dorsi.

If the lat's test weak, then pull downs, pull ups, etc. are necessary.

Fig. 13-28 Latissiumus dorsi stretches

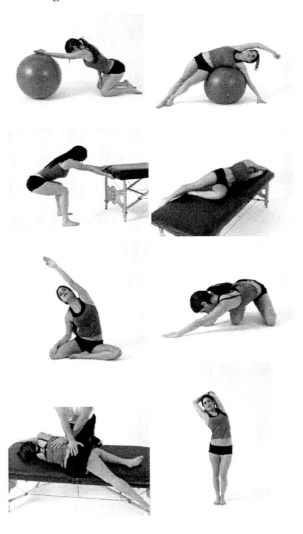

Pectoralis major

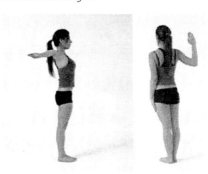

Fig. 13-29

Pectoralis major stretches. It is very important to contract the rhomboids and middle traps to encourage stability in the shoulder joint. The pec minor stretches are usually appropriate here also.

If the pectoralis major is short, the associated postural distortions (forward head and shoulders and kyphosis) should be corrected, if appropriate, as mentioned in the posture section. Along with stretching the muscle in the direction it tested short in. Active stretching is a great way to lengthen this muscle by activating its antagonists, which subsequently improves the balance between the anterior and posterior shoulder.

Myofascial and TP release along the "front functional line" (a term used by Thomas Myers in Anatomy Trains[63] to describe the myofascial connection between the anterior proximal humerus and linea aspera of the contralateral femur, basically a diagonal line across the front of the body) are very effective at lengthening the pectoralis major and its surrounding soft tissue structures.

TFL

Stretch the TFL if the test shows it to be tight. Also compare results from the latissimus dorsi, Q.L., and torso twist ROM tests in order to see if the tightness goes beyond the TFL and into the lateral myofascial network.

PMAP for hip abduction may be necessary, see muscle testing section.

Fig. 13-30 Tensor fascial lata (TFL) stretches

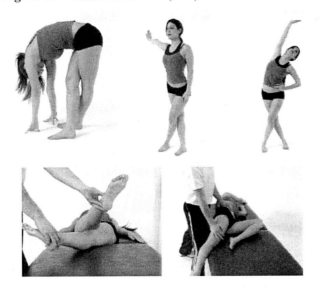

Torso twist

Stretch in the same position as the assessment test (torso twist stretch) and stretch the pectoralis minor to improve limited ROM in this test. Also use the same stretches as in the Pectorals minor corrective actions above.

Myofascial release of the "front functional line", as mentioned in the pectoralis major ROM section, and TP release of the pectoralis minor are recommended for relieving a restricted torso twist.

PRONE

Femur rotation

Limited internal rotation in this test points to tightness in the deep six external rotators, especially the piriformis, while limited external rotation points to tightness mainly in the adductor complex. Limited external rotation is rare in the absence of hip degeneration or adhesions.

Apply the corrective actions below for *limited*

225

internal rotation.

Fig. 13-31 External rotator stretches

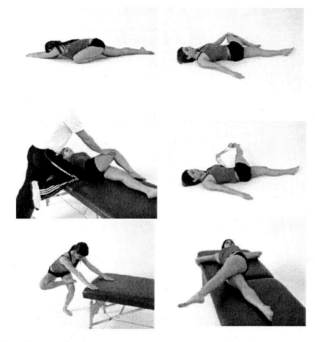

Quadriceps

Stretch the quadriceps if indicated by a failed test. Use the same stretches as in the Rectus Femoris corrective actions section. Also, utilize lateral and medial rotation of the femur to incorporate all four sections of the quadriceps.

Palpation

The findings for the palpation assessment will be grouped together as lipomas, tight, TP's, adhesions, inflammation, sharp pain, and swelling. Use the following guidelines to combine with the other assessment findings to help create a more specific corrective exercise program. An in depth palpation corrective actions section will be utilized in the next volume along with their manual therapy techniques.

Lipomas

A lipoma is subcutaneous and can be found all over the body[36] and better described as a "lumbar fascial fat herniation".[35] Lipomas feel very similar to trigger points, except they lack an accompanying taught band and they don't improve with applied compression, they can actually become aggravated. Applied pressure on the nodules can elicit pain, tenderness, and radiation into the sacrum and hip.[36] Treatment strategies for tender episacral lipomas are described by David Bond[36] as the following;

1. Avoid applying deep pressure directly on the lipomas. Focus any manual therapy on the surrounding tissues. Fascial stretching can be done on the thoraco-dorsal fascia.
2. Avoid stretching the low back, especially forward bending and twisting. Stretching can begin once the pain improves about 50 percent.
3. Avoid exercise until symptoms improve 50 percent. Then start with mild exercising such as tai chi, qigong, or swimming.
4. Apply ice.
5. Avoid lying on hard surfaces.
6. Avoid prolonged sitting.

Tight

This is a very general finding that can indicate a primary or compensatory tightness. The rest of the assessment will help clarify the reasons for the tightness. The reduction of a palpable tightness is a powerful sign of improvement.

TP's

Correcting TP's is done mostly by manual therapy techniques, although stretching can also improve TP's. Their existence points to muscular imbalance and dysfunction and therefore help to narrow down which muscles are compensating the most. Knowledge of the hierarchy of trigger point chains is necessary in determining the root of the TP's.

Adhesions

Adhesions are usually a result of chronic tension or injuries. The tissues can feel stuck together like old gum, and usually cause compensatory tightening along their fascia and stress lines. Adhesions require manual therapy and then stretching to improve flexibility and mobility.

Inflammation and Swelling

These are red flags that contraindicate exercise and require referral to a specialist to learn the reason of the irritation. Exercise with either one of these symptoms requires referral from a specialist and is usually not recommended near the site of the symptoms.

Sharp pain

Sharp pain elicited by palpation should have its origin known and treatment approved by a specialist before starting an exercise program.

Breathing

The corrective actions for breathing utilize the same position as in the assessment, with the addition of practicing breathing whenever possible. To begin, practice in quiet places so the rhythm can be felt and heard. Once this rhythm (explained in the assessment section) is achieved, start practicing it whenever and wherever possible, especially in stressful situations.

In order to really make a difference, breathing must

be incorporated into all facets of life, not just exercise.

It is possible to improve blood pressure, aches and pains, stiffness, anxiety, etc., simply by improving breathing. The easier (although not easy) part is breathing properly. The harder part is remembering to do it, especially in stressful situations.

Muscle Testing

STANDING

Gluteus medius

If the gluteus medius tests weak for strength or endurance while standing, then 1) one leg balancing (progress to eyes closed and then to unstable surfaces) 2) one leg minisquats focusing on keeping grounded hip stable 3) jumping exercises that land on one leg and focus on hip stability should be practiced and progressed along with the stages of Exercise Progression.

If the tendency to lean was noticed in either test, apply the same corrections as above with the addition of practicing PMAP for hip abduction. It is often necessary to first begin with PMAP for the gluteus medius in order to get it to activate during the standing exercises.

Focus on strength and or stamina depending on the results.

Fig. 13-32 Gluteus medius standing strength exercises

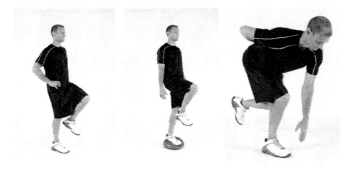

PMAP for Multifidus

If the person cannot properly activate the multifidus, then activation exercises are necessary. See pg. 183 for details on multifidus activation techniques.

SUPINE

Psoas

If the psoas is weak and short, then the cause of weakness must be found before correcting the weakness. For example, if a nerve disorder is causing the weakness, it is best to find out and improve the cause of the nerve problem first.

If the psoas is weak and of normal length or elongated, then general deconditioning can be assumed and strengthening can be performed in the way of cardio/hip flexor exercises like squats, lunges, stair climbing, etc.

The muscle test position (supine straight leg raise) can also be used as a strength exercise, especially with ankle weights.

Another exercise resembles marching in place and could be called "standing one leg bent knee raises with resistance." To perform, stand with tubing tied around the ankle to be strengthened and raise the leg against the resistance as if marching in place. The tubing should be anchored to the ground somewhere, a bed or couch leg works well. Perform one side at a time and switch after 10-15 reps, unless only one side is weak. Make sure to maintain good spinal alignment and balance. Extra support such as a hand rail can be used if balance is poor.

This exercise can also be performed by simply pressing against the raised thigh with the person's hands, making it more of an isometric exercise.

Sit-up tests

Before utilizing sit-ups, crunches, supine leg raises, hanging leg raises, or even curl-ups as abdominal strengthening exercises, it is essential to know if each individual can handle the risks associated with repetitively flexing the spine.

If a person has a history of lumbar disc or vertebral problems, then the risks usually outweigh the rewards, unless the person is an athlete and needs to perform at high levels, and even then the repeated flexion can cause reaggravation of the tissues which will perpetuate the injury cycle, build more scar tissue, and contribute to altered joint mechanics that can eventually become permanent.

Therefore, this injured, or previously injured population, along with those whose goal is health and not esthetics, should incorporate exercises that utilize the abdominals in more functional ways. Keep in mind that a lot of remedial exercises are needed to "wake up" weak or inhibited abdominal muscles before functional tasks can be performed.

Generally, if an individual's goal is simply to be healthy and perform the activities of daily living with greater ease, then *curl-ups should be done regularly only if the person lacks the strength to pass the tests in the assessment section.* 100's of reps are unnecessary and even harmful in most cases. The abdominals should be trained just like any other muscle in the sense that they need resistance and 2-4 sets of 10-15 reps for each muscle to increase their strength.

Endurance training for the abdominals comes mostly from circuit training that utilizes CORE exercises alternated with other functional exercises, not 100's of sit-ups.

In this manual the straight leg curl-ups (straight and twisting, with a pillow under the knees) are the only recommended type of "crunches" for the non-athlete or injured person (because of their low compression loads on the lumbar spine) and should be performed no more than three times a week.

Once the person has the "normal" ability of these motions (as described in the assessment section) it is no longer necessary to practice them more than once a week, if that much, because the newly acquired strength, and more importantly activation in these muscles will translate over into other activities where it was previously lacking and thus maintain strength through daily movements.

For instance, if the abdominals are weak, then they will not be utilized very much during daily movements such as twisting, bending, and lifting, instead, the paraspinal muscles will be overactive. This creates an imbalance that continues to overload the back and underutilize the abdominals, both of which can be improved if imbalances are corrected and the abdominals learn to function again, thereby *keeping* the abdominals strong by using them throughout the day for routine movements.

Athletes and other extremely active people have a unique need for abdominal strength that requires their training to test the limits of many high compression movements. To best do that, the environment in which the person performs in should be mimicked as much as possible, along with stabilizing exercises and as many safe variations of abdominal exercises as imaginable in order to prevent injuries from all angles. See the Stages III and IV for advanced abdominal exercises and techniques.

It has been shown that using unstable surfaces under the back during curl-up exercises will increase abdominal muscle activity from 21% to 34% in the rectus abdominis and from 5% to 10% in the external obliques, as well as elevate spine loads.[70] This confirms the muscular benefits of training on unstable surfaces, especially for the external obliques which had twice the activation levels, but introduces some concern about the load placed on the low back.

An important side note to abdominal strengthening is the fact that certain tight muscles can inhibit the flexion activation of the abdominals, most commonly the erector spinae and hip flexor muscles. Janda[48] found that during a curl-up exercise, tight erector spinae were active during the flexion movement, and that *stretching the erector spinae before performing the curl-up actually increased the EMG activity of the rectus abdominis* and relaxed the firing of the erectors.

This is exactly the goal of reversing reciprocal inhibition by stretching and is made possible by analyzing the results of a detailed evaluation. *Stretching the hip flexors before strengthening the abdominals can also be very beneficial.*

With all that being said and kept in mind, here are some ways to progress abdominal curl-up strength for specific populations.

Health Goals

1. Curl-ups (straight and both oblique angles)
   10 straight, 10 obliqueR/L, 10 obliqueR/L =50
   3x wk until strong, then 1 x wk

Fig. 13-33 Curl-ups

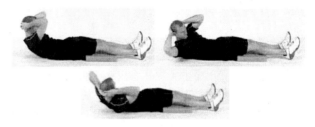

Fitness Goals

1. Curl-ups (straight and both oblique angles)
2. Curl-ups on unstable surfaces
3. Sit-ups
4. Hanging or supine straight leg raises
5. Curl-ups and or sit-ups with weight added*
6. Curl-ups and or sit-ups with med ball toss*
* Progress these to unstable surfaces.

Fig. 13-34 A few of many options for curl-up strength. The exercises above are also appropriate.

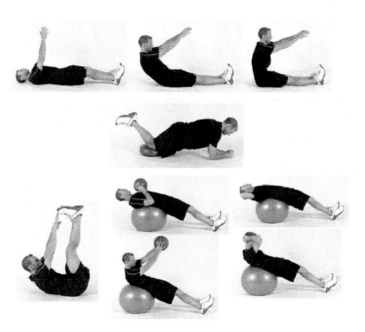

Lower abdominals

Care should be taken to not push past the limits of a posteriorly tilted pelvis (flat back), otherwise anterior shearing occurs in the lumbar spine from the activation of the psoas muscles, with the weight of the legs adding to the shearing force. This can cause pain and recurrence of low back symptoms. It also has no benefit for the lower abdominals because once anterior tilting occurs it indicates that the hip flexors have taken over and the abdominals are not strong enough to resist the weight of the legs.

It is beneficial to *stretch the hip flexors immediately before strengthening the lower abdominals* in order to inhibit their dominance during the exercise.

The low back can be spared by raising the legs higher and increasing knee flexion.

If the function test (pg. 181) was failed or very difficult, then progress with the standing pelvic tilt followed by bicycle kicks before starting the strengthening exercises (fig.'s 13-37 to 13-39). The function test (1 or 2 legs) can also be used as an initial strengthening exercise.

1. Begin by practicing the standing pelvic tilt exercise as described on pg. 216 and shown below.

Fig. 13-35 Standing pelvic tilt progression (left to right)

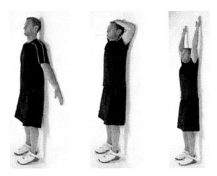

2. Once the standing pelvic tilt can be performed with the hands on the head and elbows against the wall, perform the same exercise as in the functional test on pg. 189 and shown below. *2-3x 30 sec, 3-4x wk*

Fig. 13-36 Bicycle kicks (lower abdominal strengthening)

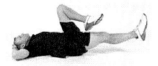

Once bicycle kicks can be performed easily, begin the strength exercises below for the lower abdominals, starting with # 3.

The following exercises are appropriate for improving strength or endurance, depending on the number of reps and intensity (angled bench, ankle weights, etc.) used, and can use either a blood pressure cuff or hands under the lumbar spine to monitor the arching of the low back.

It is common to have one ability (strength or endurance) without the other; maximizing training time is then done by using the appropriate amount of reps and resistance.

Many athletes will not like the remedial versions of the lower abdominal exercises because they don't feel challenged. It must be made clear to them that if they cannot keep the back flat during the easy exercises then their hip flexors are working and not their abdominals and this will eventually injure their low back.

If the strength test was around 80% then the person probably does not need any additional training, unless they are an athlete or physical active person. Then the training can begin on the declined bench as mentioned below.

If the strength test was at or below 70%, progress according to the following. All exercises should be performed with the hands on the head or underneath the low back to monitor the arching.

3. This exercise should not start until bicycle kicks can be performed with the legs about 5 degrees off the floor and the low back flat for 30 continuous seconds.

Start supine with the hips flexed about 90 degrees and lower legs dangling. Straighten and lower the legs as far as possible while keeping the low back flat, then bend the knees and curl the legs back up towards the chest like a reverse crunch, lifting the hips off the floor if possible, this is one rep.

Utilize all angles of the oblique abdominals on the way up by bringing the knees towards the opposite shoulder.

Fig. 13-37 Double leg kick & tucks (lower abdominals)

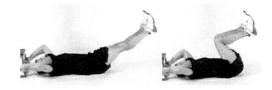

4. Raise and lower two legs at a time, trying to keep them as straight as possible while the back stays flat. This exercise can cause unnecessary strain on the lumbar spine for individuals who do not need advanced strength in this area.

Fig. 13-38 Straight leg swings (lower abdominals)

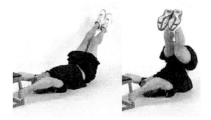

5. Once the previous exercises can be done properly with no compensations or pain, then they can be performed on a declined bench or on an exercise ball, see fig. 13-39.

This exercise (fig. 13-39) however is only for those with extreme needs, such as athletes.

Fig. 13-39 Lower abdominal curls on ball

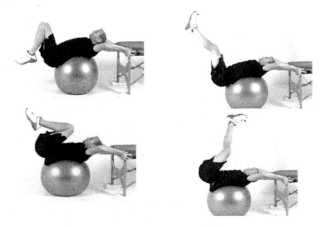

Neck flexors

Start with stretching the SCM and any other short or tight neck muscles as well as correcting any faulty posture tendencies and signs of upper or lower crossed syndrome.

If the curl-up test was also weak, then the curl-up exercises will also strengthen the neck flexors.

Once the curl-up exercises can be handled by the neck, at least 50 reps, then the following exercises can be used to add strength and stability to the cervical spine and neck flexors.

1. Lying supine, have the person move towards the head of the table so that their head is off of the table. This exercise is best done with assistance, but is still beneficial if the person is alone. The following directions are with assistance, if alone, then place the hands behind the head and rest after each rep. When alone, the feeling of when the head is level should be practiced and learned in the presence of a trained eye before attempting alone.

The assistant supports the underside of the head and maintains it at a horizontal level with the rest of the body. The person is asked to maintain the head in this position while the assistant slowly releases the head, keeping the hand near the head. Once the head starts to shake, the person becomes uncomfortable, or the chin pushes forward (SCM dominance), the hand should support the head again for a few seconds and then repeat the process of support and no support for up to 10 reps.

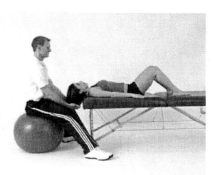

Fig. 13-40

Isometric head holds off table

10 reps of 5-6 second holds, 3-4x wk*

If cervical issues are present then less reps should be performed at the beginning. This exercise can aggravate sensitive conditions in the neck and should be performed with caution for these people.

The goal is to be able to easily hold the level position, chin is neither up nor down, for 30 seconds straight.

2. This exercise can be alternated with the previous exercise by days or weeks.

Lying supine with the head on the table, ask the person to tuck their chin and lift the head off the table a few inches. Moderate resistance is applied by the person or the practitioner in the direction of cervical extension, do not press straight down into the table. The individual should be able to resist without pushing the chin forward, otherwise the pressure is too great.

The head can stay in the same position throughout the exercise or it can move into different angles of flexion in order to locate the areas of the greatest weakness. The head can also return to the table after each rep if full ROM is desirable.

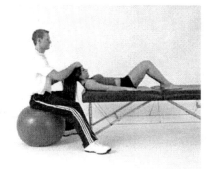

Fig. 13-41

Supine head flexion against resistance

10 reps of 2-3 second holds, 3-4x wk*

* The number of times listed per week is for both exercises combined. Therefore, these exercises should not be performed every day, even if they are alternated. Ideally, one exercise is performed one day and the other is performed after a day or two of rest and they are alternated in this manner until normal strength and function is present. Once this is established, they can be performed less frequently.

A good rule is that however many times per week the larger muscles are trained is the same amount that these and other smaller muscles should be trained.

Q.L.

Before strengthening the Q.L. check the results of the postural exam for iliac crest and rib cage levels. If a major imbalance exists it should be taken onto account so that more reps are performed on the appropriate side.

The Q.L. should not be strengthened until PMAP is had for hip abduction.

1. Side-lie with straight legs on the opposite side that is to be strengthened, with the top arm resting on the top leg and a pillow underneath the area directly above pelvis (the

230

love handles).

Ask the person to sit-up side ways and slightly backwards, reaching down towards the feet but behind the body.

Resistance can be added in the form of tubing or a cable machine, which is anchored in front of the body and up beyond the head, about where the outstretched bottom arm ends.

Fig. 13-42 Side bends (Q.L.)   *3x 10-15 reps*

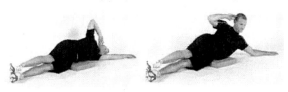

2.   Standing side bends. Start with light weight and progress according to the needs of the individual.

Start with the weight in the opposite hand of the side to be strengthened, side bend down towards the knee on that side until a comfortable limit is reached. Then using the Q.L. on the opposite side, pull the body up sideways until the next comfortable limit is reached, hold for 1-2 seconds and return back to neutral, this is one rep.

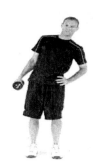

Emphasis on the Q.L. by side bending slightly backwards as in the previous exercise is avoided here because it reinforces a bad habit of picking things (a suitcase) up awkwardly.

Fig. 13-43

Standing side bends (Q.L.)

3x 10-15 reps

The two previous exercises can be alternated weekly or by days and should not surpass three times per week combined if done properly.

3.   Once the previous two exercises seem relatively easy, these exercises can be started.

Using a ball or 45° slant machine, perform side bends with the feet anchored. Progress to holding a weight.

Fig. 13-44 Side bends over ball (Q.L.) *3x 10-15 reps*

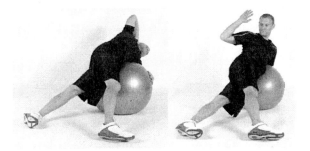

Athletes such as skate boarders, surfers, hurdlers, pole vaulters, martial artists, and others will need a similar but different function of the Q.L. that comes from the opposite origin and insertion action, which is hip hiking.

This exercise is best done closely resembling what the individual athlete needs. For example, a martial artist may need Q.L. strength for high side kicks and thus should train the Q.L. in positions similar to this activity instead of the simple hip hikes with one leg hanging off a stool. No individual hip hiking exercises will be given here, an imagination is the best tool.

PRONE

Back extension w/rotation

If only one side is weak, then perform up to 4 times as many reps on the weak side. If both sides are weak, still perform the one sided extensions with rotation, as opposed to coming straight up without rotating, but perform an equal amount on both sides.

The exercise is the same as in the test (pg. 184) with the exclusion of external resistance and the addition of some progressions. Make sure the movement is not excessive, only a few inches off the ground is necessary.

Start as in the assessment test and progress to;

1.   Ipsilateral arm reaching overhead.
2.   A pillow added under the hips and the arm back by the head.
3.   Same as above but with arm extended.
4.   A small weight can be added to the hand.
5.   All the above can be performed on an exercise ball

3-4x 10-15 reps, 3-4x wk

PMAP for hip extension

Stretch and or apply manual therapy to the hip flexors, erector spinae, and hamstrings where appropriate.

To properly activate the gluteus maximus, lie prone and place one hand on the buttocks and hamstrings and the other hand across the low back. Align the fingers (on the side to be tested) over the buttocks and hamstrings; these feel for the ideal firing pattern of gluteus maximus first and hamstrings second. The other hand (on the low back) feels for when the erectors are activated. The contralateral lumbar erector spinae (stabilizer) should activate before the ipsilateral erector spinae (stabilizer).[41]

For best results, correct any signs of upper or lower crossed syndrome, see box on pg.'s 202 and 203.

Fig. 13-45

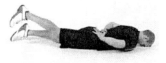

PMAP for hip extension. Utilize the gluteus maximus, not the hamstrings.

Gluteus maximus

If the muscle tests weak and there is a dysfunction in the hip extension PMAP, then practice PMAP according to the directions given above. If PMAP is present, then follow the corrections described below.

Whatever type (endurance, strength, or power) and direction (inferior, superior, or no rotation of the thigh) of weakness is present should be the method chosen for training the muscle.

Progress in the following order;

1. The person is prone with a pillow under their hips and the leg to be strengthened flexed to 90 degrees. Instruct them to squeeze their buttocks and lift the leg without arching the low back.

Fig. 13-46 Gluteus maximus strength exercise

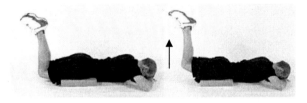

3x 10-15 reps, 2-3 second holds

2. Once exercise # 1 is easy, start the following exercise.

This exercise is called "supine one legged push-ups." The leg to be strengthened is bent with the foot flat on the floor (pointed in the direction of weakness) and the other leg is up in the air.

Instruct the person to tighten the abdominals and squeeze the buttocks on the side of the grounded foot and raise the pelvis off the floor and the other leg towards the ceiling. Hold for 2-3 seconds and slowly lower the pelvis to the floor. Watch for those who recruit the hamstrings by raising the pelvis off the ground too high and arching the low back.

Good form   Bad form (too high)

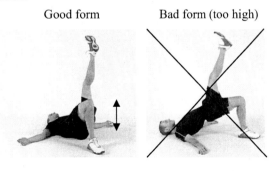

Fig. 13-47

One legged push-ups (Gmax)
Progress to unstable surface under foot

*3x 10-15 reps,
2-3 second holds*

3. Once exercise # 2 is easy, start this exercise.

This is the same movement and positioning as the previous exercise with the addition of placing the person's head and shoulders on an exercise ball.

With the head and shoulders resting on the ball, stabilize the body by placing the hands on the floor. Only one foot will be on the floor while the other is up in the air, knee flexed and lower leg dangling. *If this is too difficult, then both feet can start on the ground.*

Instruct the person to raise and lower their pelvis only by squeezing the buttocks and keeping the abdominals tight. The pelvis should move straight up and down like an elevator, no swaying.

Position the body on the ball so that the cervical spine does not look out of place, which can happen if the head and shoulders are too far up on the ball.

Fig. 13-48 One leg push-ups w/head on ball (Gmax)

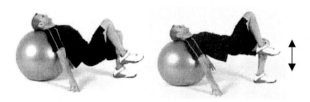

3x 10-15 reps, 2-3 second holds

Hamstrings

If the hamstrings are weak but no pelvic tilt is apparent, then assume it is of normal strength compared to the rest of the surrounding musculature. In this case all of the related muscles should be strengthened along with the hamstrings.

If the hamstrings are weak in conjunction with an anterior tilt of the pelvis, then strengthen it by the following methods.

1. Lying prone with a pillow under the hips, tie exercise tubing around the ankle to be strengthened (if there is enough tubing both ankles can be done at the same time) and anchor the tubing to something a few inches off the ground towards the feet.

Start with the knee flexed about 10° and slowly bend it to about 90 degrees against the resistance. Make sure to stabilize the pelvis and low back by tightening the abdominals.

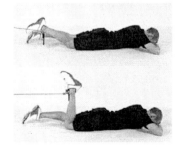

Fig. 13-49

Prone hamstring curls

3x 10-15 reps, 2-3x wk

2. This exercise can be done instead of or in conjunction with the previous exercise.

Lie supine with arms spread out on the floor for balance. Place both feet up on an exercise ball with the legs straight.

Tighten the stomach and lift the pelvis off the floor. Bend the knees and curl the ball towards the buttocks, then slowly straighten the legs to complete on rep. The pelvis should stay up off the floor and the spine properly aligned the entire time.

Ways to progress the exercise are (1) point the arms towards the ceiling (2) one leg at a time

Fig. 13-50 Hamstring curls w/feet on ball

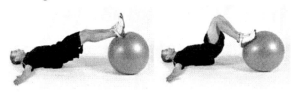

3x 10-15 reps

Piriformis

1. Sitting or lying prone with the knee flexed 90 degrees, tie tubing around the ankle to be strengthened or apply manual resistance from a partner. Externally rotate the leg against resistance.

Fig. 13-51 Hip external rotation against resistance

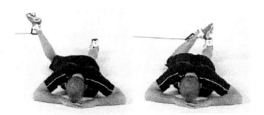

3x 10-15 reps, 2-3x wk

2. Start this exercise after completing 2-3 weeks of the previous exercise. Stand on one leg while twisting at the hips, rotating the ungrounded knee away the other knee, keeping the raised foot at the height of the opposite knee. Progress by adding cable resistance. See fig.'s 13-2 in the hip rotation posture section for photos.

3. Once the above exercise can be performed with ease, start "step up and overs". This exercise involves stepping over a knee-high object (broom handle set up on chairs, string tied at both ends, corner of bed, etc.) and touching the floor with the toes. The grounded hip is the focus as well as keeping the pelvis as level as possible and maintaining stability and balance throughout. The goals is to be able to step up and over an object about knee high without much change in lumbopelvic position.

See fig. 13-1 in the hip rotation posture section for photos.

PMAP for hip abduction

Stretch and or apply manual therapy to hip adductors, Q.L., TFL, piriformis, gluteus medius and minimus, and IT band where appropriate.

Activate and strengthen the superior fibers of the gluteus maximus as described on pg. 230.

For best results, correct any signs of upper or lower crossed syndrome, see box on pg.'s 200 and 201.

Start in the side-lying position, as in the test for gluteus medius strength. Place fingers on the lateral hip and lateral abdomen in order to monitor muscle contractions of the TFL, Q.L., and gluteus medius and minimus muscles.

The goal is to have the gluteal muscles fire before the other muscles, as well as be able to raise the leg at least 45° before strong Q.L. contractions take place to try to hike the hip.

Fig. 13-52 PMAP for hip abduction

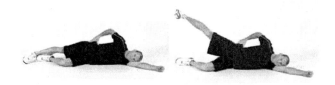

3x 10-15 reps

Gluteus medius

This exercise should not be started until PMAP for hip abduction is present. It is the exact same motion as the PMAP test, but now ankle weights and increased intensity can begin.

This is basic activation of the gluteus medius. Weightbearing exercises are the ultimate goal once simple strength has been established.

Lateral flexors

Utilize the same exercises that were performed for the weak Q.L. A modification of the first exercise can be made so that the side bending is pure rather than slightly backwards.

Functional Tests

Lower Abdominals

Any deficiencies in lower abdominal endurance can be trained as mentioned in the muscle testing section for this muscle by utilizing the appropriate number of reps.

Toe Raises

Strengthening the gastrocnemius is done exactly as the assessment test is performed for this muscle. Single or double leg raises are recommended, depending on the persons' ability.

Anterior Oblique Curl-ups

Use the same exercise as in the assessment. Strengthen as mentioned in the curl-up section of the muscle testing assessment, see pg.'s 177-179. More attention can be given to one side if appropriate.

Push-pull

Training for this type of stabilization strength is done exactly as in the assessments with the two or four sets of exercise bands. One side often needs more work in the single arm exercises. <u>Practice both squat and lunge positions.</u>

Curl-ups

Strengthen as mentioned in the curl-up section of the muscle testing assessment, see pg.'s 177-179.

Lunges

Strengthen by doing lunges.

Unstable surfaces can be added to the front foot to increase recruitment patterns.

Weight can be added to the hands or on top of the shoulders as in a straight bar.

Walking lunges have more shearing forces on the knee than stationary lunges, but also present a greater challenge for the neuromuscular system.

3x 10-15 reps, 1-3x wk (weight dependent)

Trunk Extension

Follow the exercises in the spine extension sections of the Stages III and IV.

Side plank

If the grade was less than 80% then start with the following exercises.

For each exercise, perform up to *10x 10 seconds on each side* with 3-5 seconds rest between each rep.

1. A modified version of the test position can be used for those who need it by bending the knees to 90 degrees and coming up on the bottom lower leg and knee instead of just the feet.

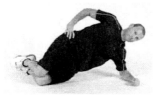

Fig. 13-53

Modified side plank

2. Use the same position as in the test (straight legs)
3. Using an exercise ball (the smaller the ball the more difficult the exercise), drape the bottom arm over the ball so that the bottom armpit is resting on the ball with that arm also hugging the ball, and the feet are in the same position as the assessment test. Place the top arm's hand on the ball to support the body.

Use the lateral flexors on the bottom side to bring the body up into a straight position like a board. When resting between reps the bottom knee should bend to relax and support the body, then straighten it once again after the 3-5 seconds of rest.

Push-ups

If the grade is less than 100%, then additional training is needed.

Compensations should be improved before attempting more push-ups. Here are some ideas for helping specific compensations.

• Head pushes forward – stretch the SCM, strengthen the deep neck flexors, and correct any faulty postures of the head or shoulders.
• Scapulas wing – strengthen the serratus anterior and trapezius muscles.
• Abdomen sags or buttock pushes up – strengthen abdominals, especially front planks and stretch the erector spinae if necessary.

Once the push-ups can be done without much compensation, start training with push-ups, men should start on their knees if necessary.

Squats

If either population tests below 100% then additional training is necessary. Take care of any compensations that are present before attempting more squats, or only perform the squats as far as the compensations will allow. This could mean only going down half way.

Training to improve quadriceps endurance is best done with but not limited to squats. Lunges, bridging exercises, and a number of other exercises described in Chapter 14 are also beneficial. See that section for details on frequency and intensity of training for the legs.

Proprioception

There is no one way that best trains the proprioception system; instead, it requires many different stimuli from many different positions and movements. This is why there are so many proprioception exercises in this manual and others.

Specific weaknesses can be observed in some of the exercises that can key in on other areas to strengthen or stretch, but in general, follow the routines in the proprioception section to improve overall proprioception. Close the eyes to make some of the exercises more difficult. And remember that most regular exercises can be turned into a proprioception exercise by adding unstable surfaces, standing on one leg, or closing the eyes (not always appropriate).

Cardio

Complex interval training or other types of cardiovascular training will not be mentioned in this manual because that is another book all in itself. Simple regimens will be explained throughout this manual.

Chapter 14   The Routines

The foundation of this exercise program is based on clinical evidence and proven therapeutic exercise techniques that have been developing for many years by the great minds in this field. The most recent of which are Richardson, Hodges, and Hides[138], whose research and motor control approach to treating low back disorders (LBD) lead to the foundation for Stages I-III of Exercise Progression. Stage IV is a more advanced exercise program that enables motivated individuals to progress to the highest levels of fitness.

The routines in this chapter are not limited to the low back, however; they can be used for 1) post-rehabilitating a low back injury or disorder, 2) progressing an imbalanced athlete or physically active person towards their goals, 3) progressing the general population towards a healthy level of overall fitness.

The main principle here is learning the proper motor control skills to safely stabilize and move the body through any action. This, of course, is desirable for all populations.

There are four stages to Exercise Progression that are each made up of different stages from the five components of strength, flexibility, proprioception, cardio, and DAM's. If the maximum time is taken for each stage, it is a *9-month program. The fist three stages focus on corrective exercising, education, and DAM's.*

Each component (strengthening, stretching, etc.) has its own duration and sequence that is progressed together with the other components. If one component is progressed too fast, then muscle imbalances will most likely be created instead of corrected.

The stage progression durations are gauged on the *least* amount of time required to learn and properly apply the exercises in that stage. If a person is not able to perform effectively in a stage, then they should not progress until ready, no matter how long it takes.

Stages I-IV are for the general population and emphasize overall health, fitness, flexibility, and strength. Those with activity-specific needs and the ability to take some time off from their activity should perform Stages I-III, followed by the activity-specific routines in this chapter.

If the person is an athlete or manual laborer who cannot stop or interrupt their activity, then they can alternate or combine the routines in Stages I-III with the appropriate activity-specific exercises in this chapter. However, this is not ideal and will take longer to learn and unlearn neuromuscular patterns, because the more advanced and compensation-prone activity-specific exercises would be performed before the body is ready.

Occasionally Stage I may be too simple and unnecessary for some, while Stage IV may be too difficult and unnecessary for others. Once finished with Stage III, general health and fitness can be maintained by rotating Stages I, II, and III; and, if appropriate, Stage IV should be rotated in every so often.

See the program design section at the end of this chapter for a variety of routines. Also see the additional chapters for each component's description and progression time table.

For those who do not enjoy exercise, and therefore will not continue practicing it, it is important to find a healthy alternative that promotes strength and movement, such as tai chi, yoga, qigong, pilates, etc.

Efficient movement is the goal here, not necessarily gym-like exercises, so any type of healthy movement is encouraged; although it is recommended to finish Stages I-III before attempting these healthy alternatives in order to build a solid neuromuscular foundation.

The previous chapters have described outlines of how to progress each component of Exercise Progression, and with some imagination it is possible to create a complete exercise program based on these outlines to suite one's own needs.

This chapter will, however, provide the reader with a general outline that combines all of the components into a progression suitable for just about anyone, including those with LBD and advanced athletes.

Exercise Progression

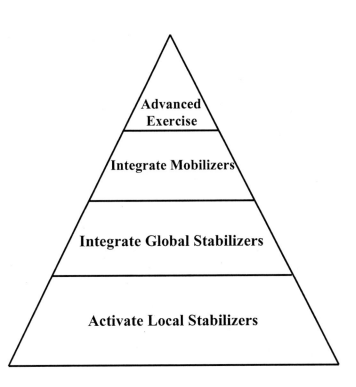

Stage I (1-4 wks)	**Activation of Local Stabilizers and DAM's**
	• Maintain neutral spine position while lying, sitting, and standing
	• Focus on activating transverse abdominis, multifidus, and gluteus maximus
	• Incorporate simple, isolated, and corrective stretching while maintaining a neutral spine position
	• Make any appropriate DAM's
Stage II (4-8 wks)	**Integration of Global Stabilizers**
	• Closed chain (weightbearing) strength exercises
	• Sagittal and frontal plane strength exercises only (no twisting)
	• Very slow/static/endurance training
	• Begin proprioceptive training, focus on maintaining a stable lumbar spine
Stage III (6-8 wks)	**Integration of Mobilizers**
	• Open and closed chain light weight strength exercises
	• Challenge lumbar spine with extremity movement and maintain proper spinal position and stability
	• Increase speed and gross movement
	• Integrate all planes of motion into strength training
	• Introduce segmental spinal movements
Stage IV (16 wks)	**Advanced Exercise**
	Part I Strength Training
	• Intense strength training
	• Dynamic flexibility training
	• Activity-specific training
	Part II Power Training
	• Activity-specific training
	• Explosive movements
	• Extreme CORE training

The Big Picture

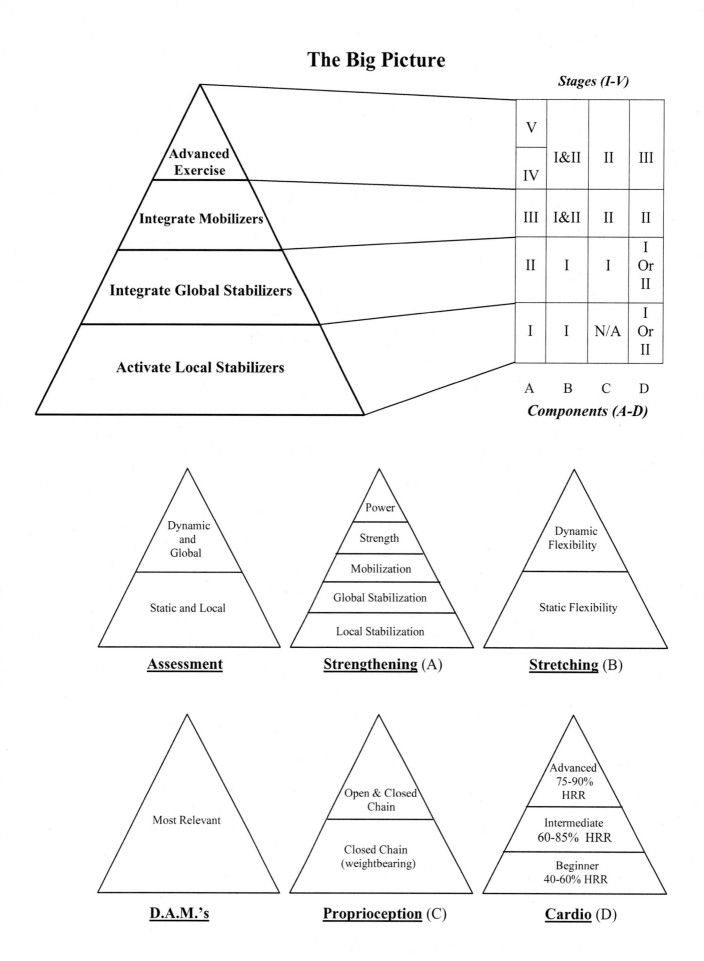

	A	B	C	D
V				
IV	I&II	II	III
III	I&II	II	II
II	I	I	I Or II
I	I	N/A	I Or II

Stages (I-V)

Components (A-D)

Assessment
- Dynamic and Global
- Static and Local

Strengthening (A)
- Power
- Strength
- Mobilization
- Global Stabilization
- Local Stabilization

Stretching (B)
- Dynamic Flexibility
- Static Flexibility

D.A.M.'s
- Most Relevant

Proprioception (C)
- Open & Closed Chain
- Closed Chain (weightbearing)

Cardio (D)
- Advanced 75-90% HRR
- Intermediate 60-85% HRR
- Beginner 40-60% HRR

238

General Routine Guidelines and Information

- The routines do not include every individual corrective action; instead they are a compilation of the most frequent corrections needed.
- It is possible to utilize the general routines here without an assessment and have a good chance of helping many people, but, of course, the assessments are recommended for those who have the skills to assess and create a more individualized program.
- If reps and sets are not listed for an option, then utilize those of the first option. For example, if exercise 3(b) is not followed by a # of recommended reps, then use those of 3(a).
- The first two stages do not include any arm movements against resistance (except an overhead shoulder press and rotator cuff exercise in Stage II) because initial spine stability and control is best trained for in the absence of open chain stresses. This can be a giant obstacle for those who are accustomed to regular weightlifting. It must be explained to this population that in order to reprogram the neuromuscular system, the impulses to the larger muscles must be greatly diminished while the smaller stabilizing muscles are reprogrammed; otherwise the larger muscles will continue to dominate all movement and create an unstable environment.
- Reprogramming the neuromuscular system can take up to three months (Stages I-II) for those with severe imbalances or injuries.
- Rotator cuff strength is essential to shoulder stabilization and will begin in Stage II even though it is not a true weightbearing exercise.
- Separate warm-up routines are not required until Stage IV due to the simple nature of the first three stages.
- The times listed after each workout category are estimates of the total time required for each category. This allows for precise exercise planning if time is restricted.
- If more than one multiple circuit is performed in a row, then different exercises can be used *or* the same circuit repeated if repetition is needed to properly learn certain movements and patterns.
- Many exercises have different variations listed: i.e., 1a, 1b, 1c, etc. These variations are, of course, optional and are provided for the many different types of goals and people encountered.

Activation of Local Stabilizers and DAM's

Description

For some people it is very difficult to trade their regular training routine for a corrective exercise program, even if it is only for a few weeks. This is when educating about the body seems to be the only hope to encourage change. Utilizing the corrective exercise/philosophy handout (see appendix) will reinforce the reasons for these exercises.

If any major imbalances or exercise-ready injuries are present, it is best to start with simple and isolated corrective exercises to ensure that dynamic functioning has a strong static foundation, then more complex corrective movements (Stages II and III) and intense weight training (Stage IV) can be incorporated without compromising musculoskeletal integrity. This corrective stage is done, ideally, with the exclusion of any additional exercise if major deficiencies exist, because this should be a time of rebuilding and refocusing the body towards balance, not high-intensity training or sports.

Unfortunately, the ideal cannot always be achieved (professional meets an athlete in mid-season), and corrective exercises must be performed in conjunction with a high-intensity program. The best way to combine the two is to make sure that the corrective exercises outnumber the other exercises by reps or total time. This will encourage proper muscle activation patterns (PMAP) and ensure a progression towards neuromuscular efficiency, but it will take more time and will not produce as efficient a neuromuscular system as a program that focuses solely on corrective exercising.

Ideally, the entire body is incorporated into a corrective exercise program no matter where the main problem is. For instance, the feet and lower body should be looked at for a chronic shoulder problem, because they can influence joint mechanics. But, again, situations occur where the optimal number of sessions is not available to properly progress or assess, and thus specific areas must be made a priority. This, of course, will limit long-term results, but is better than no corrective exercising at all and can be beneficial for the short term.

Guidelines

- If there is a *repetitive strain* soft tissue injury, then the acute stage of healing must be complete, along with exercise clearance and advice from a doctor, before starting this stage.
- If there is a *traumatic soft tissue injury*, the subacute stage of healing must be complete, along with exercise clearance and advice from a doctor, before starting this stage.
- Those with a LBD may take the full four weeks of this stage to progress, while the normal population takes much less; although, people with very poor posture and fitness can also take a long time in this stage.
- Following a proper assessment, simple and isolated stretches and activation exercises are given to eliminate neuromuscular compensations (synergistic dominance, reciprocal inhibition and facilitation, arthrokinetic inhibition, and referred pain inhibition), which will in turn improve ROM, posture, and functional deficiencies.
- Before starting an exercise program, mobilization techniques may need to be administered by a licensed professional in order to improve influential structural abnormalities.
- Manual therapy may also need to be implemented prior to or during an exercise program in order to improve major imbalances and release soft tissue adhesions and trigger points (TP's).
- Improving pain and dysfunction are the roots of all goals in this stage, even those who are pain free will have dysfunctions.
- Find the amount of exercise that promotes growth, not deterioration.
- A person who has to continue with an advanced activity or sport during this stage will require time spent on incorporating the local stabilizers into their daily movements. These programs should be done in conjunction with this stage's exercises.
- The only cardio performed in this stage should be walking, with a focus on integrating segmental stabilization (T.A. and multifidus), proper posture and breathing, foot stability, hip extension, torso rotation, etc. An athlete

in mid-season is an exception where more intense cardio should take place, as is someone with knee or hip problems, who cannot tolerate walking and requires cardio with less impact.

- Depending on the person, anywhere from one to ten different exercises may be appropriate.
- Utilize mostly isometric contractions in order to minimize global muscle recruitment.
- For a post-rehabilitation person, start the first week of exercises with only a few different movements each workout in order to monitor which ones aggravate symptoms. Remember, it can take up to several days to feel the full effects of a disc injury.
- Perform all exercises slowly.
- A temporary increase in pain is acceptable during active care rehabilitation for nonspecific back pain and sciatica.[77,78]
- Sometimes it is necessary to practice a DAM that is beyond a Stage I exercise level, for instance, how to squat and pick up a child, in order to allow an injury to heal faster.
- The muscle activation exercises listed in this stage are the minimum required. It is also common to need to train others in order to eliminate gross movement dysfunctions and prepare inhibited or dysfunctional antigravity muscles for the weightbearing exercises in Stage II. A detailed assessment will find the areas in need of activation.
- Emphasize proper nutrition and rest.
- Some people may need the same exercises for weeks at a time to properly learn them or heal, while others will learn fast and need a wide variety of exercises to stimulate growth and interest.
- Assess proper form on home exercises at least once a week.
- Explain that increased soreness is normal at the beginning and is often a sign of progress and muscle adaptation.
- Each person must meet all of the goals (at bottom of page) in order to move on to Stage II.

Priorities

1. Improve daily functioning, increase body awareness, and activate influential segmental muscles.
2. Educate about the individual's situation and their body in general, and utilize handouts.
3. Explain any dysfunctions found in the assessment, as well as the goals and strategies of the program.
4. Make any appropriate DAM's and incorporate them daily.
5. Apply manual therapy to key restricted joints or soft tissue adhesions and trigger points.
6. Stretch short or facilitated areas that contribute to faulty functioning and posture, as long as proper spinal stability can be maintained.
7. Balance tension in the most influential areas (cervical kyphosis and foot pronation greatly affect the low back) and correct major imbalances.

Variables

- Duration   1-4 weeks (depends on injury and ability)
- Frequency   Stretch (3-7x wk) Strength (3-7x wk) Cardio (3-7x wk)
- Intensity   40-60%

Choosing Exercises

- *Strengthening* – simple segmental stabilization and corrective activation exercises, Stage I
- *Stretching* – simple and isolated corrective stretches; ideally active stretches that activate inhibited muscles and incorporate the T.A. and multifidus into maintaining proper lumbopelvic alignment, Stage I
- *Proprioception* – first improve major imbalances; begin proprioception with Stage II
- *Cardio* – Stages I or II of cardio; brisk walking, unless an athlete is in mid-season or walking is not tolerated

- **DAM's** – whichever are necessary to start eliminating faulty recruitment patterns or prevent injury/re-injury

Goals

1. Maintain T.A. and multifidus activation in sitting and standing positions for 1 min. while breathing normally; multifidus activation should be symmetrical from left to right and L1-L5
2. PMAP for 1) hip abduction, 2) hip extension, 3) trunk flexion (supine)
3. At least 20 minutes of cardio at target heart rate (about 60% of maximum heart rate, unless contraindicated)
4. Efficiently perform any troublesome daily activities

Training Schedule

1. **Corrective Exercise**
2. **D.A.M.'s**
3. **Cardio**
4. **Cool-down Stretching**

M	T	W	Th	F	Sa	Su
1,3,4	2,3,4	1,3,4	2	1,3,4	1,4	3,4

1. Corrective Exercises (3-4x wk) <u>5-20 min</u> - In General, do the following;

a) Thoracic extensions (10x10 sec holds)

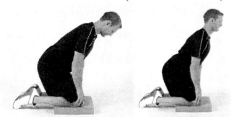

b) Wall stand (3-5 min)

- Pull in stomach
- Keep back flat
- Relax neck
- Don't tilt head backwards
- Feet 3inches from wall

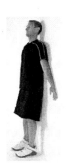

c) Free-Standing posture (Whenever you can)

- Use regular standing posture and imagine resisting the weight of gravity.
- Keep breathing relaxed.
- Incorporate into sitting postures

d) Breathing techniques   (3-5 min)

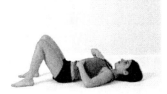

- Abdomen should rise first, followed by an expansion in the thoracic area and ribs

e) Pull in stomach and squeeze buttocks (3-5 min)

- Use regular standing posture.
- Keep breathing relaxed.

2. Daily Activity Modifications (D.A.M.'s)
↳ Whichever and whenever necessary

f) Multifidus & Transverse Abdominis Activation (10x10 sec holds)

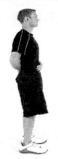

- Pull the lower abs inward toward the spine
- Focusing on the muscles directly lateral to the lower spine, contract them along w/the stomach, "pressurizing the CORE".

g) Leg lifts* (backwards) - (10x10 sec holds)

- Squeeze buttocks first
- Don't arch low back

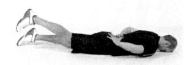

h) Leg lifts (sideways) - (10x10 sec holds)

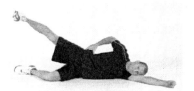

i) Forward bending w/stomach pulled in *
   10x (hold for 5 sec each)

- Practice sitting, standing and laying

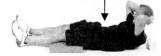

*Not always appropriate

j) Finding Neutral and Safety Zones

- Sitting, standing, functional positions and the like, tilt the pelvis upward, then downward, trying to find the most comfortable and strong feeling "center" position.

3. Cardio (3-7x wk) Brisk walking focusing on proper gait and postural patterns (<u>15-30 min</u>)

4. Cool-down, General, & Corrective Stretching (Major body parts as needed, include self-myofascial release wherever necessary) 3-7x wk/1-2x per day/1-4x 20-90 sec hold each stretch w/neutral spine (<u>10-60 min</u>)

Integration of Global Stabilizers

Description

Now that body awareness and PMAP of important segmental stabilizers have been established in Stage I, other imbalances and dysfunctions can be improved and the global stabilizers can be incorporated into weightbearing movements. The addition of proprioception training will prepare the body for gross functioning (Stage III). Correcting imbalances is still a goal here, but so is achieving strength and stability while moving in an upright and closed-chain manner. Stages II and III are an ideal foundation to fall back on when resting from more intense workouts.

Guidelines

- If there is a *repetitive strain* soft tissue injury, the acute stage of healing must be complete, Exercise Progression Stage I must be completed, and exercise clearance and advice from a doctor must be had before starting this stage.
- If there is a *traumatic soft tissue injury*, the subacute stage of healing must be finished, Exercise Progression Stage I must be completed, and exercise clearance and advice from a doctor must be had before starting this stage.
- There are two 2-4 week programs that follow the same principles and progress each strength and proprioception exercise to an unstable surface. Weeks # 1-4 = stable Weeks # 5-8 = unstable
- The specific corrective stretches and exercises from Stage I are continued and progressed.
- Increasing flexibility of the low back at this Stage is only a goal for those with muscular limitations, not low back injuries. Increased lumbar flexibility can cause more problems than not with many LBD.
- The minimum time (4 weeks) can be taken if the person is advanced and relatively balanced, but unless time is a factor, it is recommended to take the full eight weeks in order to establish a solid foundation.
- Just because somebody completed a certain exercise last week doesn't mean they're able to today. Injury flare-ups or fatigue days may require rest and simple movements only. Make sure that *health is the focus, not the exercises*.
- Exercise speed is still slow or isometric. Extremely slow motion reduces momentum and cheating.
- Utilize the sagittal or frontal planes for integrated uniplanar actions; rotation exercises start in Stage III.
- Assess proper form on home exercises at least once a week.
- Once ready, utilizing circuit training for the weightbearing exercises is optional but recommended.

Priorities

1. Continue with those from Stage I.
2. Challenge the body with proprioception-rich exercise in as many weightbearing ways (frontal or sagittal plane) as it can safely control and tolerate while maintaining the focus on: a) neuromuscular efficiency of core recruitment, b) corrective exercise, c) functional restoration.
3. Stabilize and strengthen the spine using high frequency and low intensity weightbearing exercises.
4. Strengthen the core while utilizing the least amount of movement and stress on the lumbar spine.
5. Continue static stretching and practicing DAM's.
6. Increase overall strength and cardiovascular endurance.
7. Ability to decelerate (eccentric) body weight in weightbearing positions; i.e., squats and lunges.
8. Build confidence in the body's ability to perform simple and complex tasks (fear can be a major contributor to chronic pain).
9. Sweat.

Variables

- Duration   4-8 weeks (depends on injury and ability)
- Frequency   Stretch (3-7x wk) Strength (3-7x wk) Proprio (5-7x wk) Cardio (3-7x wk)
- Intensity   50-75%

Choosing Exercises

The first 2-4 weeks of <u>strengthening and proprioception</u> are on stable surfaces; the second 2-4 weeks involves unstable surfaces.

- ***Strengthening*** – weightbearing closed-chain exercises that compress the spine and utilize vertical arm movements (i.e. squats or lunges w/a shoulder press) as well as continuing corrective activation exercises
- ***Stretching*** – simple and isolated corrective stretches; ideally active stretches that activate inhibited muscles
- ***Proprioception*** – weightbearing; one leg balancing and/or two legs on unstable surface, progress to eyes closed
- ***Cardio*** – Stages I or II of cardio; brisk walking or jogging unless specific exercises are appropriate
- ***DAM's*** – continue whichever are necessary

Goals

1. PMAP for sitting extension and flexion
2. Squats with arms up/very slow; 1) manual laborer/athlete =3-4 min (non-stop)
                        2) desk jockey (computer worker) = 2-2.5 min (non-stop)
3. Standing one-leg toe raises for 1x30 each side (15 slow, 15 fast)
4. Non-impact front lunges with arms up/very slow; 1x 10 quality reps on each side
5. Proprioception; one leg balance (stable surface) with eyes closed for 30 sec without assistance, each side
6. Non-impact side lunges with arms up/very slow; 1x10 good reps each side, pivoting side to side
7. Have the ability to properly perform all relevant stretches

➢ These exercises should be completed in succession with 15-30 sec rest between each

Weeks # 1-8

1. **Cardio** (3-7x wk) Use as a warm-up (<u>5-10 min</u>) or as a separate workout (<u>15-30 minutes</u>) brisk walking or jogging (ideally on trails or sensory-rich environments), focusing on proper gait patterns.

2. **Corrective Stretching** (Before exercise) *Actively* stretch any short/tight muscles that cause major imbalances or inhibitions, ideally as a group and then directly before a related exercise; such as stretching short psoas muscles *immediately* before lunges in order to facilitate the gluteus maximus (<u>4-10 min</u>).

3. **Proprioception** (5-7x wk) Weightbearing/closed chain only (<u>4-10 min</u>).

   A. 1 leg balancing, progress to eyes closed
   B. 2 leg balancing on unstable surface, progress to eyes closed
   C. 1 leg balancing on unstable surface, progress to eyes closed - *wks 5-8*

4. **Strengthening**

   Part I   Partial Weightbearing Exercises (5-7x wk) <u>3-5 min</u>

   A. Sitting on a ball, knees bent about 90° w/feet flat on floor; bounce (very small bounces) on ball while maintaining proper alignment, progress to arms overhead – 1 min
   B. Sitting on a chair, progress to unstable surface placed on chair; flex forward and extend backwards at the hips while maintaining neutral alignment – 1x 10 each direction
   C. Sitting on ball, come out sideways into a mini lunge. Maintain a neutral spine - 1x 10 each direction

   ➤ Part II can begin once each exercise in Part I can be performed in succession for the appropriate time. The Part I exercises can stop once they become easy.

   Part II   Weightbearing Exercises (3-5x wk) <u>15-25 min</u>

   • Squats - <u>2-3x 1-2 min</u>
   A. Supported, against wall (with or without ball behind low back), progress to arms up (begin unsupported once 1 min of supported squats is easy)
   B. Unsupported and stable, progress arms (begin unstable once 1 min of stable squats is easy)
   C. Unsupported and unstable, progress arms (alternate workouts between stable and unstable squats) - *wks 5-8*

   • Non-Impact Front Lunges - <u>2-3x 10 on each side</u>, start once unsupported squats can be performed for 1 min
   A. Supported (in doorway or holding onto an object)
   B. Unsupported and stable, progress to arms up
   C. Unsupported and unstable, progress to arms up - *wks 5-8*

     ➤ Squats and lunges can also be performed while holding a large ball or stick that is hit or pushed by the trainer and isometrically resisted by the individual.

   • Non-Impact Side Lunges - <u>2-3x 10 on each side</u>, start once front lunges can be performed for 1x 10
   A. Unsupported, pivoting side to side, progress arms upward and legs outward

   • Marching front Step-ups - <u>1-3x 1-2 min</u> – use a 4-8 inch box

     ➤ Perform squats plus either front *or* side lunges *or* front step-ups for each workout, not all in the same day.

   • Standing Toe Raises – <u>1-3x 20-30</u>, progress to one leg (15 slow 15 fast)
   • Rotator Cuff – <u>3x 1 min</u>, progress to unstable for *wks 5-8*

     ➤ All part II exercises are separated by <u>30-45 seconds rest</u>

5. **Cool-down, General, & Corrective Stretching** (major body parts as needed, include self-myofascial release wherever necessary) 3-7x wk/1-2x per day/1-4x 20-90 sec hold each stretch w/neutral spine (<u>10-60 min</u>)

6. **Daily Activity Modifications D.A.M.'s** (whichever and whenever necessary) <u>5-30 min</u>

Weeks # 1-8

Proprioception 4-10 min

A B C

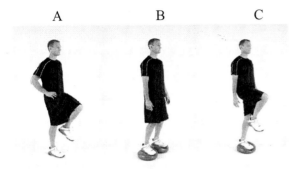

Strengthening Part I Partial Weightbearing
Exercises 3-5 min

A B

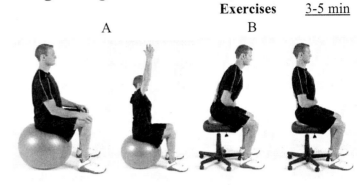

Strengthening Part I cont….

C

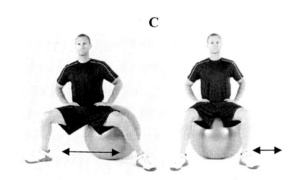

Part II Weightbearing Exercises 15-25 min

Squats 2-3x 1-2 min

A B

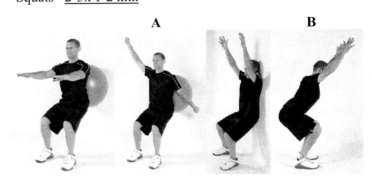

Strengthening Part II cont….

C

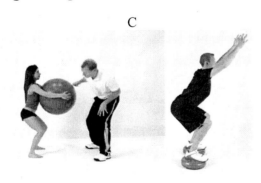

Non-Impact Front Lunges 2-3x 10 on each side

A B C

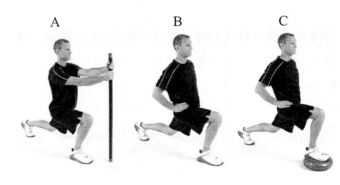

Non-Impact Side Lunges - 2-3x 10 on each side

A B

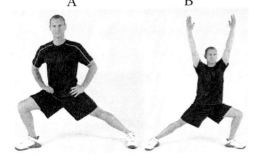

Marching front Step-ups
1-3x 1-2 min

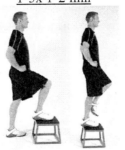

Calve Raises
1-3x 20-30

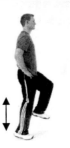

Rotator Cuff
3x 1 min

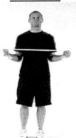

Integration of the Mobilizers
Parts I & II

Description

Gross movements in the form of weightbearing and non-weightbearing are introduced in this Stage in order to challenge the stabilization system to maintain proper alignment during extremity movements while the stabilization training continues to progress towards the needs of the individual. Corrective exercise is still appropriate. Part I (4 weeks) of this 8-12 week stage consists of functional circuits and non-dynamic stretching. The second 4-8 weeks introduces dynamic stretching and multiple circuits. Dynamic stretching does not begin until part II of this stage because the neuromuscular system has yet to learn the proper stabilization techniques for open-chain movements.

Guidelines

- If there is a *repetitive strain or traumatic soft tissue injury*, the subacute stage of healing must be complete, Exercise Progression Stages I and II must be completed, along with exercise clearance and advice from a doctor, before starting this stage.
- There are two Parts; Part I is 4 weeks and Part II is 4-8 weeks, depending on ability. There are also two categories of exercise: 1) CORE, 2) Total Body. Both are performed in the same workout.
- CORE program; Part I - simpler open chain exercises / Part II - more unstable and difficult exercises.
- Total Body program; Part II - progress exercises to highest level of difficulty but only moderate intensity; i.e., weight and velocity remain moderate; high intensity training begins in Stage IV.
- It is best to save rotation movements until complete stability is had in the simple motions.
- Each individual exercise in the "Total Body" category does not necessarily work the whole body. But, they should be organized so that the entire body is challenged evenly for each workout.
- Completing Stages I-II is recommended before starting this stage.
- Activity and sport-specific strength exercises (excluding power and plyometric exercises) begin here with little to no resistance in order to prepare for the more specific and intense power training in Stage IV.
- Only light to moderate weight is used along with multiple circuit training to enhance endurance; max strength is not a goal in this stage.
- Continue to increase the speed of movement but wait until Stage IV to begin explosive actions.
- Maintain important corrective isolated strength and flexibility exercises.

Priorities

1. Train the gross movers (mobilizers) to function on a stable spine and body by using moderate to no resistance and circuit training to enhance endurance.
2. Continue any necessary priorities from Stages I and II.
3. Achieve ability to control body weight in open and closed-chain multiplanar movements (push-ups, dips, squats, lunges, including rotation) with all types of muscle contractions (eccentric, isometric, and concentric).
4. Create an exercise program that resembles and improves daily life, not just gym strength.

Variables

- Duration
- Frequency
- Intensity

8-12 weeks
Stretch (3-7x wk) Strength (3-5x wk) Proprio (5-7x wk) Cardio (3-7x wk)
50-75%

Choosing Exercises

Part I

- *Strengthening*

  Functional Circuits: Progress through the 9 circuits
- *Stretching* - non-dynamic stretching with emphasis still on corrective isolation if necessary
- *Proprioception* – all types (open and closed chain)
- *Cardio* – Stage II (60-75%)
- *D.A.M.'s* – continue whichever are necessary

Goals

1. 10x (each side) one leg squat to toe touch
1. 1 minute of push-pull exercise w/10-20% body weight on the pulling portion
2. 10x (each side) stepping front lunges with a twist
3. 10x (each side) lower abdominals - 1 leg at a time, touching heal to floor while fully extending the leg
4. 1x 50 curl-ups (10strt/20 twist/20sidebnd)
5. 1x 25 (each side) quadruped superman

➤ These exercises should be completed in succession with 15-30 sec rest between each exercise and PMAP for all appropriate muscles.

Part II

- *Strengthening*

  Total body: open and closed-chain exercises, progress to unstable, 1 arm, and 1 leg where appropriate

  CORE: open-chain exercises on stable and unstable surfaces
- *Stretching* – non-dynamic and dynamic stretching
- *Proprioception* – all types (open and closed chain)
- *Cardio* – Stage II (60-75%)
- *D.A.M.'s* – continue whichever are necessary

Goals

1. 10x (each side) one leg squat to toe touch w/small weight in hand
2. 1 minute of push-pull exercise on unstable surface w/10-20% body wt. on the pulling portion
3. 1 x full ROM squat
4. 12 (total) side lunges with overhead press of 10-20lbs (F-Male) into 1 leg balance
5. Minimum of 10 proper push-ups w/elbows backwards (on knees for women)
6. 10x bent knee dead lift to overhead press and toe raise (10-20lbs/F-Male)
7. Lower abdominals – 1x starting w/legs straight and towards the ceiling (90º), lower legs to few inches off floor and hold for 2 seconds, lower and rest 1 second, then raise them back up to 90º, all the time maintaining the low back flat against the floor; *this is not a goal if LBP is still a factor*
8. 10x (each side) standing cable rotations w/15% body weight
9. 1x 25 (each side) opposite arm and leg reach on ball, unsupported

➤ These exercises should be completed in succession with 15-30 sec rest between each exercise and PMAP for all appropriate muscles.

1. **Cardio** (3-7x wk) Use as a warm-up (<u>5-10 min</u>) or as a separate workout (<u>15-45 minutes</u>) brisk walking or jogging (ideally on trails or sensory rich environments), focusing on proper gait patterns.

2. **Corrective Warm-up Stretching** (before exercise) *Actively* stretch any short/tight muscles that cause major imbalances or inhibitions, ideally as a group and then directly before a related exercise; such as stretching short pectorals *immediately* before thoracic extensions in order to facilitate the extensors (<u>4-10 min</u>).

3. **Proprioception** (5-7x wk) Weightbearing and non-weightbearing (<u>6-10 min).</u>

   A. Any proprioception exercises from Stage II
   B. Sitting on ball w/1 foot up, progress to 1 foot on a small ball
   C. Bridge w/shoulders on ball & feet flat on the floor w/knees bent 90°, progress to 1 leg up
   D. Foam roll w/1 foot up and both arms up
   E. Kneeling on ball w/both hands on stable surface
   F. Foam roll w/both feet on unstable surface

4. **Strengthening (Functional Circuit Training)** (2-3x wk) Light to moderate wt. – Start with Circuit # 1 and progress 1-8. Number nine is performed throughout.

5. **Cool-down, General, & Corrective Stretching** (major body parts as needed, include self-myofascial release wherever necessary) 3-7x wk/1-2x per day/1-4x 20-90 sec hold each stretch w/neutral spine (<u>10-60 min</u>)

1. Psoas	5. Torso Twist	9. Piriformis	13. Pectorals
2 Quadriceps	6. Hip Twist	10. Erector Spinae	14. SCM
3. TFL	7. Hamstrings	11. Q.L.	15. Upper Traps
4. Gastroc/Soleus	8. Hip Adductors	12. Latissimus Dorsi	16. Biceps/ Triceps

6. **Daily Activity Modifications DAM's** (whichever and whenever necessary) <u>5-30 min</u>

Training Schedule

1. Cardio	2. Corrective Exercises	3. Proprioception
4. Strengthening	5. Cool-down Stretching	6. D.A.M.'s

M	T	W	Th	F	Sa	Su
1-5	1-3, 6	1-5, 1 is optional	1-3, 6	1-5	1-3	2

Functional Circuits

- Take as little rest as possible between circuits and exercises
- Stretches are held for 20 seconds
- Exercises are 12-15 reps/side
- Utilize standing exercises as much as possible

- Circuit #'s 6 & 7 can incorporate the squat/lunge into the other exercises instead of by itself. Moving squats/lunges can also be used here.

- Start with # 1 and progress only if next circuit can be done without major compensations
- The #9 CORE circuit can be done anytime
- Repeat any circuit as many times as necessary

Circuit # 1 *(warm-up)*	**Circuit # 4** *(1 arm/2 leg/stable)*	**Circuit # 7** *(1 arm/2 leg/<u>un</u>stable or moving)*
1. Squats (25-50 reps) 2. Hip flexor stretch 3. Forward bend 4. Downward dog 5. Marching w/arms crossing knees (1 min) 6. One leg balance (30 sec per leg)	1. Push 2. Pull 3. Twist 4. Squat, lunge, or calve raises	1. Push 2. Pull 3. Twist 4. Squat, lunge, or calve raises
Circuit # 2 *(ten per leg each exercise)*	**Circuit # 5** *(2 arm/<u>1</u> leg/stable)*	**Circuit # 8** *(1 arm/2 leg/<u>un</u>stable or moving)*
1. Forward leg kick 2. Sideways leg kick 3. Backwards leg kick 4. Across leg kick	1. Push 2. Pull 3. Twist 4. Squat, lunge, or calve raises	1. Push w/a twist 2. Pull w/a twist 3. Twist 4. Squat, lunge, or calve raises w/a twist
Circuit # 3 *(2 arm/2 leg/stable)*	**Circuit # 6** *(2 arm/2 leg/<u>un</u>stable or moving)*	**Circuit # 9** *(CORE)* – 30-50 reps each side
1. Push (push-up/cable press/etc.) 2. Pull 3. Twist 4. Squat, lunge, or calve raises	1. Push 2. Pull 3. Twist 4. Squat, lunge, or calve raises	1. Lower Abs 2. Obliques 3. Lateral Abs 4. Back extension 5. Rotator cuff

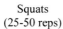
Circuit # 1 (warm-up)

| Squats (25-50 reps) | Hip flexor stretch (30-90 sec each) | Forward bend (30-90 sec) | Downward dog (30-90 sec) | Marching with rotation (45-90 sec) | One Leg Balance w/arm motion (30-60 sec per leg) |

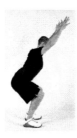 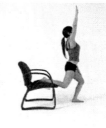 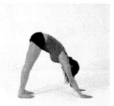 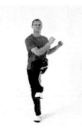 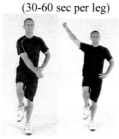

Circuit # 2 (10 per leg each exercise)

Double punches w/front kick (3 pics)   Side kick (1 pic)   Back kick (2 pics)

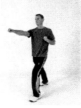 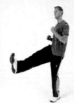

Front semi-circle kick

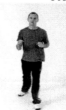 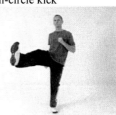

Circuit # 3 (2 arm/2 leg/stable) / 15-20 reps

Push   Pull   Twist   Lunge

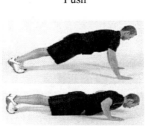 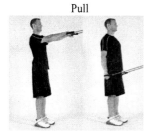 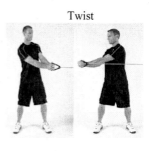 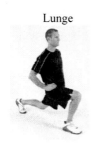

Circuit # 4 (1 arm/2 leg/stable) / 15-20 reps per side

Push   Pull   Twist   Squat

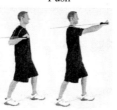 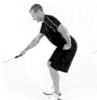 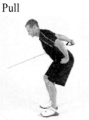 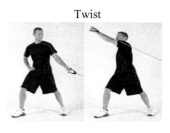 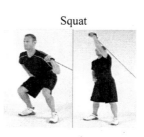

Circuit # 5 (2 arm/1 leg/stable) / 15-20 reps per side

Push Pull Twist One leg squat

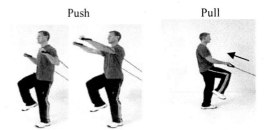
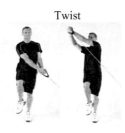
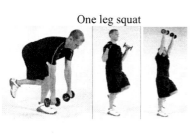

Circuit # 6 (2 arm/2 leg/<u>un</u>stable or moving) / 15-20 reps

Push Row Twist Squats on unstable surface

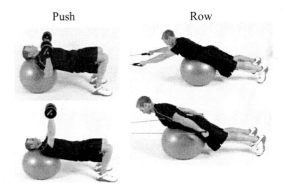
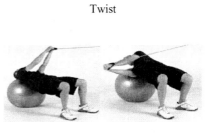
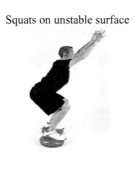

Circuit # 7 (1 arm/2 leg/<u>un</u>stable or moving) or (2 arm/1 leg/<u>un</u>stable or moving) / 15-20 reps per side

Push Row Twist Static Lunge on unstable surface with push-pull

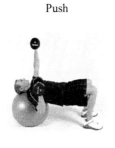
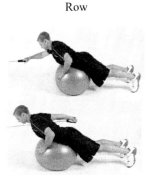
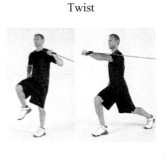
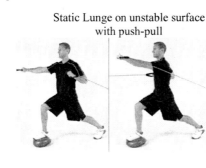

Circuit # 8 (1 arm/2 leg/<u>un</u>stable or moving) or (2 arm/1 leg/<u>un</u>stable or moving) / 15-20 reps per side

Push **w/a twist** Row **w/a twist** Twist Step-up into a twist and shoulder press

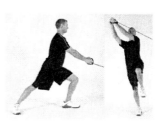

Circuit # 9 (CORE) – 30-50 reps or seconds each side

Circuit A

| Lower Abs (optional slant board) | Obliques (optional resistance) | Lateral Abs | Back Extension |

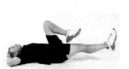
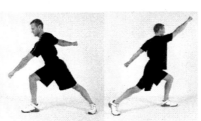
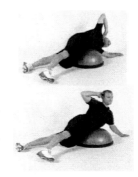
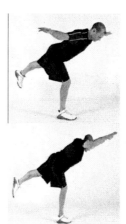

Rotator Cuff

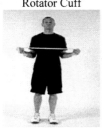

Circuit B

| Lower Abs | Obliques | Lateral Abs | Back Extension |

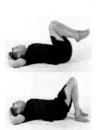
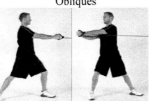
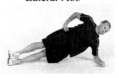
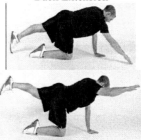

Circuit C

| Lower Abs | Obliques | Lateral Abs | Back Extension |

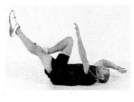
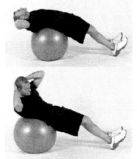
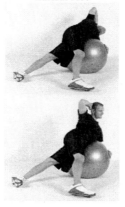
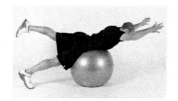

1. **Cardio** (3-7x wk) Use as a warm-up (5-10 min) or as a separate workout (15-45 minutes) brisk walking or jogging (ideally on trails or sensory rich environments), focusing on proper gait patterns.

2 **Corrective and Dynamic Warm-up Stretching -** *Actively* stretch any short/tight muscles that cause major imbalances or inhibitions, ideally as a group and then directly before a related exercise; such as stretching short erector spinae *immediately* before sit-ups in order to facilitate the abdominals (4-10 min).

3. **Proprioception** (5-7x wk) Weightbearing and non-weightbearing (6-10 min).

A. Any proprioception exercises from Stage II and weeks 1-4 of Stage III
B. Sitting on ball w/1 foot on small ball and light weight in 1 hand, passing or throwing to other hand
C. Bridge w/shoulders on ball, 1 leg up, and a light weight in 1 hand, passing to other hand
D. Foam roll w/1 foot up, both arms up, and added light weight to ipsilateral arm of the leg that is up
E. Kneeling on ball w/1 hand on stable surface and other performing a row w/light weight

4. **Strengthening - Multiple Circuit Training** (2-3x wk) Light to moderate wt. - perform 1 or 2 multiple circuits of 4 sequences with 4 exercises each (4 total body – rest 1 min - 4 total body – rest 1 min - 4 CORE – rest 1 min - 4 CORE – end – 16 exercises each multiple circuit); perform CORE circuits last (20min per multiple circuit)

5. **Cool-down, General, & Corrective Stretching** (major body parts as needed, include self-myofascial release wherever necessary) 3-7x wk/1-2x per day/1-4x 20-90 sec hold each stretch w/neutral spine (10-60 min)

1. Psoas	5. Torso Twist	9. Piriformis	13. Pectorals
2 Quadriceps	6. Hip Twist	10. Erector Spinae	14. SCM
3. TFL	7. Hamstrings	11. Q.L.	15. Upper Traps
4. Gastroc/Soleus	8. Hip Adductors	12. Latissimus Dorsi	16. Biceps/ Triceps

6. **Daily Activity Modifications DAM's** (whichever and whenever necessary) 5-30 min

7. **Dynamic Stretching Progression** (1-5x wk) 15-60 min – use as its own workout or with other workouts

Training Schedule

1. Cardio	2. Corrective Exercises	3. Proprioception
4. Strengthening	5. Cool-down Stretching	6. D.A.M.'s
7. Dynamic Stretching		

M	T	W	Th	F	Sa	Su
1-5	1-3, 6,7	1-5, 1 is optional	1-3, 6	1-5	1,7	2

Multiple Circuit # 1

Total Body Circuit	Total Body Circuit	CORE Circuit	CORE Circuit
1. Squat w/2 arm row	Lunges	Lower abs	Sport swing downward
2. Push-ups	Pull-ups or Rows	Curl-ups	Front Plank
3. Arm curls into shoulder press	Dips	1 or 2 leg push-ups	Hip-ups w/head on ball
4. Standing back dive	Lateral shoulder raises	Spine extension on ball w/ arms overhead	Standing superman w/ arms abducted

Total Body Circuit

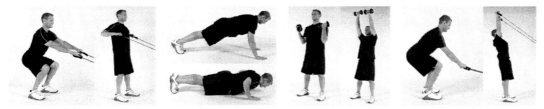

Total Body Circuit

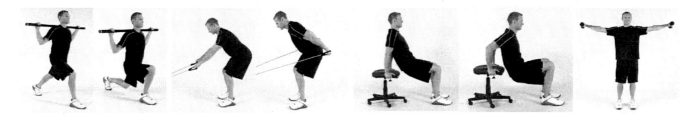

CORE Circuit

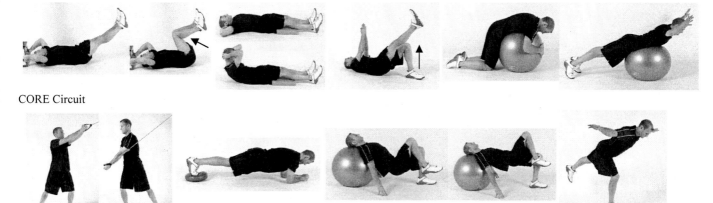

CORE Circuit

Sets = 1 per circuit   **Reps** = see individual exercises for details   **Multiple Circuits** = 1-2
Exercise Rest = 5-10 sec   **Individual Circuit Rest** = 30-60 sec   **Rest between Multiple Circuits** = 3-5 min
Note how each total body circuit includes exercises for legs, arms, chest, and back.

Multiple Circuit #2

Total Body Circuit	Total Body Circuit	CORE Circuit	CORE Circuit
1. Side lunges	1 leg squat to toe touch	Side planks	Sport swing upward
2. Push-ups w/a twist	1 arm row w/a twist	Torso rotations on ball	Side bends on ½ dome
3. Standing mid-back pulls (lower traps)	Bicep curls on 1 leg	Moving plank w/forearms on ball	Knee tucks w/feet on ball
4. Triceps pull-down	Push-pull	Quadruped superman	Prone hip extensions on ball

Total Body Circuit

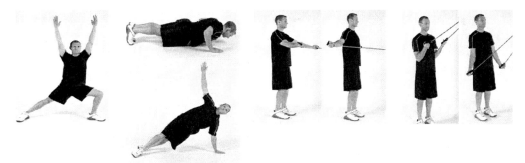

Total Body Circuit

CORE Circuit

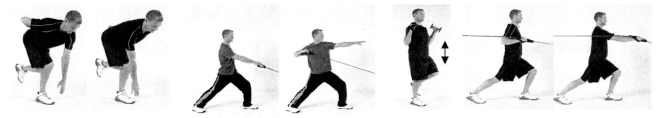

CORE Circuit

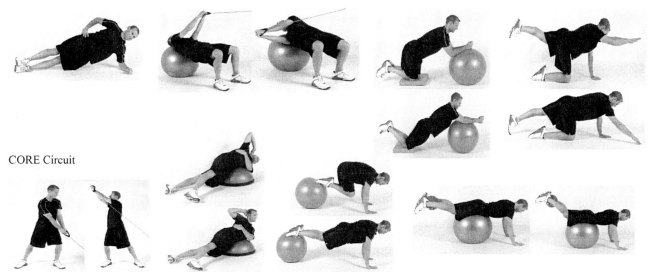

Sets = 1 per circuit   **Reps** = see individual exercises for details   **Multiple Circuits** = 1-2
Exercise Rest = 5-10 sec   **Individual Circuit Rest** = 30-60 sec   **Rest between Multiple Circuits** = 3-5 min
Note how each total body circuit includes exercises for legs, arms, chest, and back.

257

Multiple Circuit #3

Total Body Circuit	Total Body Circuit	CORE Circuit	CORE Circuit
1. Squat w/1 arm row	Stepping lunges	Reverse plank w/heels on ball	Lower abs
2. Push-ups w/hands on big ball	Push-pull	Curl-ups w/a twist	Knee tucks w/feet on ball (1 or 2 balls)
3. Standing toe raises	Standing back dive	Hip-ups w/head on ball	Side bends on ½ dome
4. Swimming on ball; straight 2 arm extension	Standing mid-back pulls (rhomboids)	Prone superman	Standing superman w/ arms abducted

Total Body Circuit

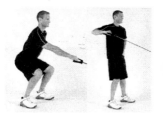 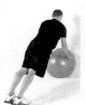 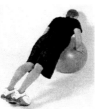 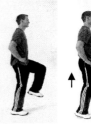 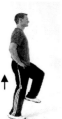 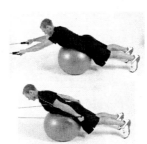

Total Body Circuit

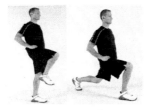 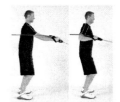 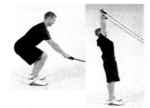 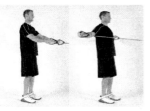

CORE Circuit

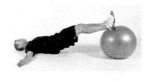 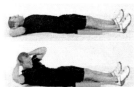 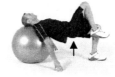 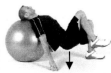 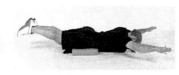

CORE Circuit

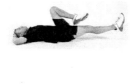 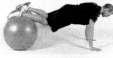 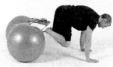 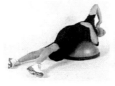 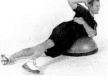 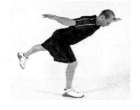

Sets = 1 per circuit **Reps** = see individual exercises for details **Multiple Circuits** = 1-2
Exercise Rest = 5-10 sec **Individual Circuit Rest** = 30-60 sec **Rest between Multiple Circuits** = 3-5 min
Note how each total body circuit includes exercises for legs, arms, chest, and back.

Multiple Circuit #4

Total Body Circuit	Total Body Circuit	CORE Circuit	CORE Circuit
1. 1 leg squat to toe touch	Bent leg dead lifts	Torso rotations on ball	Lower abs
2. Dumbbell press on ball	Pull-ups or Rows	1 or 2 leg push-ups	2 Ball balance
3. 1 arm rows w/a twist and 1 knee on bench	Incline push-ups w/feet on ball	1 arm sport swings	Dead bug (with or w/out ball)
4. Squats w/wt. held between legs	Standing mid-back pulls (middle traps)	Quadruped superman	Standing superman w/arms flexed

Total Body Circuit

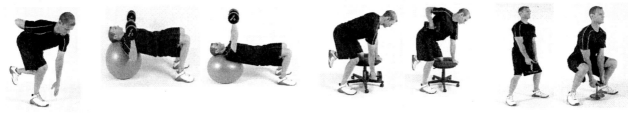

Total Body Circuit

CORE Circuit

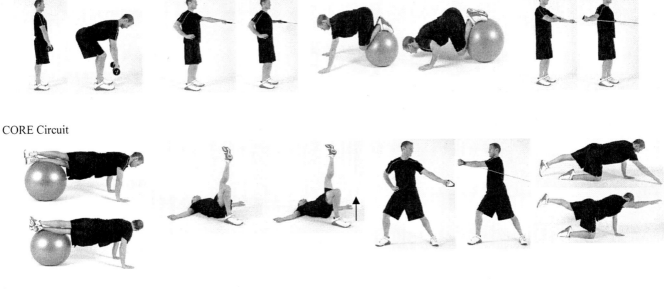

CORE Circuit

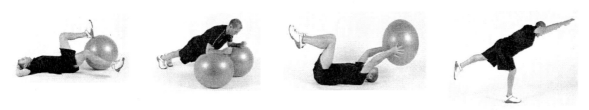

Sets = 1 per circuit   **Reps** = see individual exercises for details   **Multiple Circuits** = 1-2
Exercise Rest = 5-10 sec   **Individual Circuit Rest** = 30-60 sec   **Rest between Multiple Circuits** = 3-5 min
Note how each total body circuit includes exercises for legs, arms, chest, and back.

Multiple Circuit #5

Total Body Circuit	Total Body Circuit	CORE Circuit	CORE Circuit
1. Squat w/2 arm row	Side lunges into 1 leg balance	Lower abs	Side planks w/a twist
2. Push-ups w/a twist	1 arm row w/opposite leg extension	Sit-backs (slowly)	Hip-ups w/head on ball
3. Arm curls into shoulder press up onto box	Dips or triceps pushes	Dead bug w/arms holding big ball & moving	Front plank
4. Hamstring curls w/heels on ball	Standing mid-back pulls (lower traps)	Spine extension on ball w/1 arm dumbbell reach	Standing opposite arm/leg reach and tuck

Total Body Circuit

Total Body Circuit

CORE Circuit

CORE Circuit

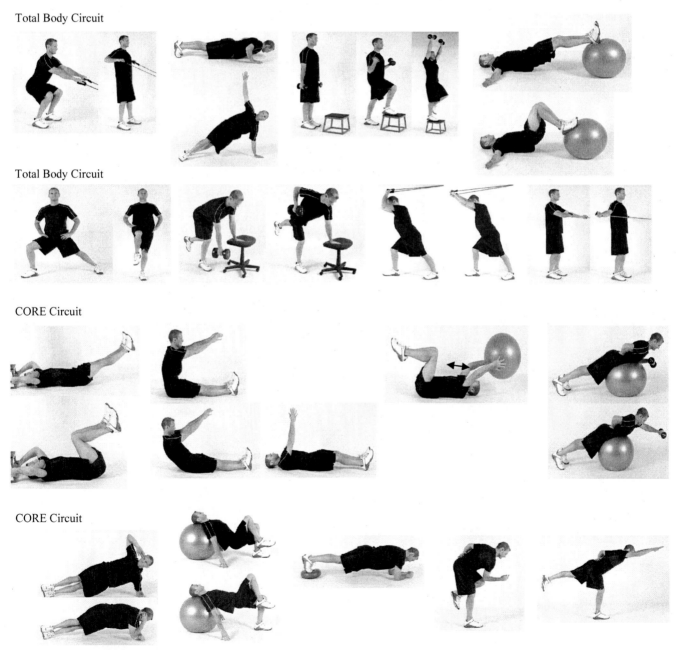

Sets = 1 per circuit   **Reps** = see individual exercises for details   **Multiple Circuits** = 1-2
Exercise Rest = 5-10 sec   **Individual Circuit Rest** = 30-60 sec   **Rest between Multiple Circuits** = 3-5 min
Note how each total body circuit includes exercises for legs, arms, chest, and back.

Multiple Circuit #6

Total Body Circuit	Total Body Circuit	CORE Circuit	CORE Circuit
1. Fast stationary lunges	Push-pull on unstable	Straight leg side crunches	Sport swing downward
2. Push-ups on 1 leg	Lateral shoulder raises	Squat into a sport swing upward	Side bends on big ball
3. 1 arm row w/a twist	1 arm triceps pull-across	Moving plank w/forearms on ball & knees unstable	Knee tucks w/a twist & feet on ball
4. Shoulder press on 1 leg	1 leg squat to toe touch and then shoulder press	"Tuck & opens"	Prone hip extensions on ball or table

Total Body Circuit

Total Body Circuit

CORE Circuit

CORE Circuit

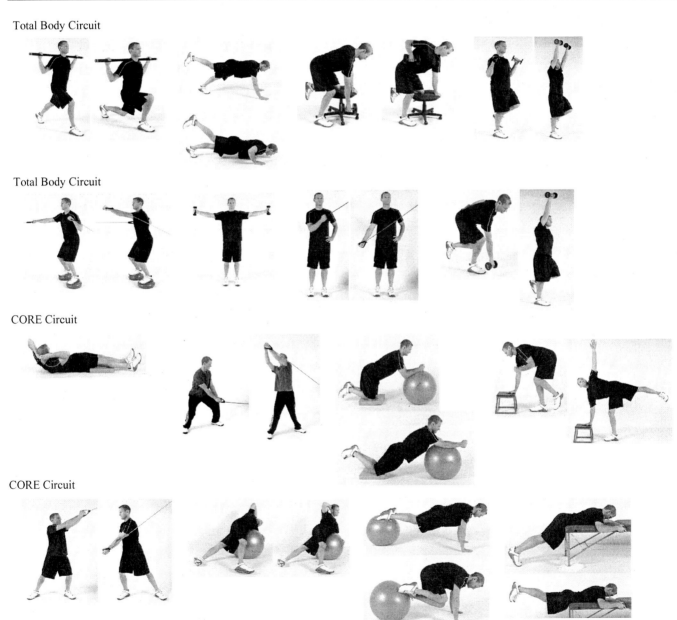

Sets = 1 per circuit   **Reps** = see individual exercises for details   **Multiple Circuits** = 1-2
Exercise Rest = 5-10 sec   **Individual Circuit Rest** = 30-60 sec   **Rest between Multiple Circuits** = 3-5 min
Note how each total body circuit includes exercises for legs, arms, chest, and back.

Multiple Circuit #7

Total Body Circuit	Total Body Circuit	CORE Circuit	CORE Circuit
1. Dumbbell press on ball	Side kick with arms pulling against resistance	Reverse plank w/1 or 2 heels on ball	Lower abs (optional slant board)
2. Swimming on ball; straight 2 arm extension	Super slow Push-ups w/ staggered hands	Curl-ups w/a twist on a ball	Pikes w/toes on ball
3. Standing toe raises (1 or 2 legs)	Bent leg dead lifts	Plank w/feet on ball and 1 hand on ground	Front plank w/forearms on 2 balls
4. Squats w/arms up on unstable surface	Lunge w/bicep curls	Superman on ball (all arms/legs up)	"Tuck & opens" (optional weights in hands)

Total Body Circuit

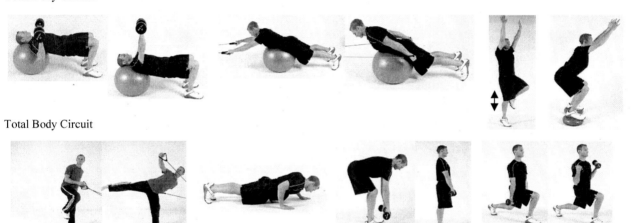

Total Body Circuit

CORE Circuit

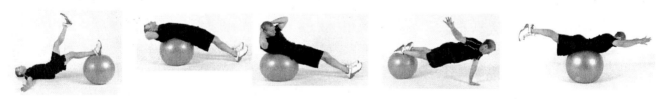

CORE Circuit

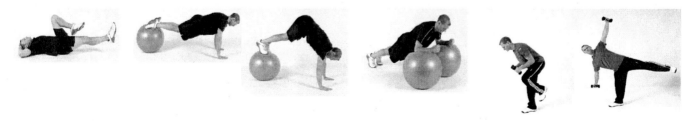

Sets = 1 per circuit   **Reps** = see individual exercises for details   **Multiple Circuits** = 1-2
Exercise Rest = 5-10 sec   **Individual Circuit Rest** = 30-60 sec   **Rest between Multiple Circuits** = 3-5 min
Note how each total body circuit includes exercises for legs, arms, chest, and back.

Multiple Circuit #8

Total Body Circuit	Total Body Circuit	CORE Circuit	CORE Circuit
1. Lunges w/a twist or chop	Squat w/1 arm row	Crunches on ball (optional weight in hands)	Ab pikes
2. 1 arm row w/knees on unstable surface	Push-ups into standing shoulder press	Side plank	Twisting planks w/feet grabbing ball
3. 1 arm chest press on ball	Standing backhand across and upward	Hip-ups w/arms up	Sport swings downward
4. Arm curls into shoulder press	1 arm sports swings	1 leg flying w/weights	Back extensions on ball (optional weight in hands)

Total Body Circuit

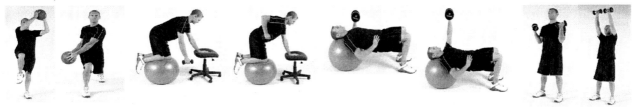

Total Body Circuit

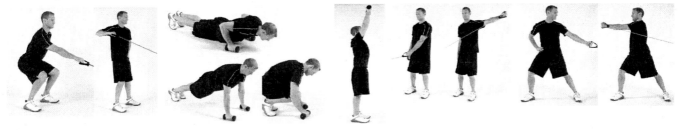

CORE Circuit

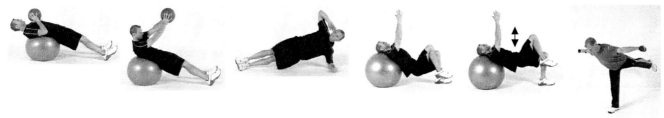

CORE Circuit

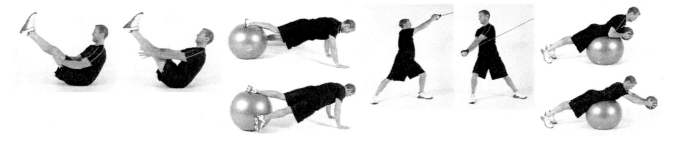

Sets = 1 per circuit   **Reps** = see individual exercises for details   **Multiple Circuits** = 1-2
Exercise Rest = 5-10 sec   **Individual Circuit Rest** = 30-60 sec   **Rest between Multiple Circuits** = 3-5 min
Note how each total body circuit includes exercises for legs, arms, chest, and back.

Advanced Exercise - Part I – Strength Training

Description

At this stage no major imbalances should exist, and the ability to dynamically control body weight should be possessed. Although this stage has similar exercises to Part II of Stage III, it is much more intense (↑ weight and velocity, more specific training goals, etc.) than the previous stages and is essential for those who wish to participate in challenging activities. Dynamic flexibility training is progressed along with advanced coordination, strength, cardiovascular, and activity-specific skills. Corrective exercising is only a concern in this stage for maintenance of prior corrections and can be done during the warm-up or warm-down routine or on an easy day.

Guidelines

- There should be no signs of injury during this stage.
- There is one 8-week program that can be completed in 4 weeks if: 1) extreme strength training is not a goal, 2) the person is ready for power training in Part II, or 3) the person wishes to return to Stage II or III exercises.
- The first 4 weeks of weight training focus on strength and control; the second 4 weeks focus on strength and speed of control; i.e., explosive contractions; this prepares the neuromuscular system for power.
- All major deficiencies and imbalances, D.A.M.'s, and pain should be resolved before starting Stage IV exercises.
- Completing Stages I-III is recommended before starting this stage.
- There are multiple aspects of strength training in this stage that should be uniquely combined for each individual. See the training schedules at the end of this chapter for ideas on how to mix up all the variables; i.e., upper and lower body, spinal extensions, abdominals, activity-specific exercise, and dynamic stretch routines.
- Increase the speed of movement; plyometrics (body weight only) are optional, but no transition contractions.
- High-intensity strength training is an option but is not for everyone; keep in mind that extreme strength is related to maximum power output.
- Intense low back and abdominal training are only for those who need to lift heavy or participate in sports, and they should periodically be alternated with less intense endurance exercises to allow for proper muscle development.
- Stretching can alternate between dynamic and corrective as needed.
- Do not perform high-intensity cardio on the same day as high-intensity strength training unless the workouts are separated by at least 6-8 hours and the person is extremely fit.
- Workouts should include intense and moderate levels of exertion throughout the week.
- Do the following exercises at the end of a workout in order to have proper stabilization strength throughout the entire workout: 1) Abdominals, 2) Back Extensors, 3) Rotator Cuff, 4) Forearms, 5) Neck
- Activity-specific populations should follow the special routines listed at the end of this chapter.

Priorities

1. Increase overall strength, flexibility, intensity, endurance, speed, coordination, and function to meet, not exceed, the needs of the individual. Some of the advanced exercises in this stage are too demanding for the general population and will cause unnecessary wear and tear on the body.
2. Achieve strength and stability during intense complex multiplanar movements with all types of muscle contractions (eccentric, isometric, and concentric).
3. Find a mixture of strength and activity-specific exercises that is unique for each individual's requirements.
4. Prepare the body for dynamic explosive movements against resistance (Part II) by utilizing simpler explosive movements in weeks 5-8 of this stage.

Variables

- Duration
- Frequency
- Intensity

4-8 weeks
Stretch (3-7x wk) Strength (3-5x wk) Cardio (3-7x wk)
60-100%

Choosing Exercises

- ***Strengthening*** – with the exception of: 1) complex explosive movements against resistance, 2) power/strength pairs, 3) CORE conditioning circuits, there is no limit to the type of exercise and training methods performed here. Utilize any training system (super sets, circuits, pyramids, etc.) and Stage IV strength exercises to gain the specific results desired
  * Because of all the different options here, no pictures are given, only word descriptions of exercises that have already been used in previous stages.
- ***Stretching*** – corrective and dynamic stretching. Learn to create a personalized dynamic stretch progression
- ***Proprioception*** – incorporate all types (open and closed chain) of proprioceptive exercises into the warm-up
- ***Cardio*** – primarily Stage III alternated with Stage II training days

Goals

- Goals are highly specific depending on each individual.

1. **Cardio -** use as a warm-up (5-10 min) or as a separate workout (30-90 min) 3-7x wk
2. **Warm-up**   1-2x 10 reps (5-10 seconds rest) 5-10 min
3. **Strengthening** – choose appropriate training system; i.e., split-routine, circuit training, etc., each will vary in total workout time; see following pages for examples of individual circuits and split-routines

   A. Upper Body (1-4x wk total)
   - (1) Chest
   - (2) Back
   - (3) Shoulders
   - (4) Triceps
   - (5) Biceps

   B. Lower Body (1-2x wk total)
   - (1) Squats
   - (2) Lunges or Step-ups onto box
   - (3) Toe raises
   - (4) Dead lifts
   - (5) Leg curls/extensions (optional)

   C. Spine Extensions (2-3x wk) unless circuit training, choose 3 different exercises from volume II from the back extension section of this stage.

   D. Abdominals (2-3x wk) unless circuit training, choose 4 different exercises from volume II from the back extension section of this stage.

4. **Dynamic Stretch Progression** (1-3x wk) 15-60 min – use as its own workout w/a cardio warm-up
5. **Cool-down, General, & Corrective Stretching** (major body parts as needed, include self-myofascial release wherever necessary) 3-7x wk/1-2x per day/1-4x 20-90 sec hold each stretch w/neutral spine (10-60 min)

Training Schedule

1. **Cardio**
2. **Warm-up**
3. **Strengthening (a-d)**
4. **Dynamic Stretch Routines**
5. **Cool-down/General Stretching**

Routines	M	T	W	Th	F	Sa	Su
Circuit	1-3 (a-d),6	1,6	2,3c,3d,5	1,5	1-3 (a-d),5	1,5	1,4
Cardio	1,4	1,5	1-3,5	5	1,4	1,5	1-3,5
Strength	1,2,3a,c,d,5	1,2,3c,d,5	2,3b,c,d,5	1,4	1,2,3a,c,d,5	1,4	5

➢ Strength (a-d); a = upper body   b = lower body   c = spine extensions   d = abdominals
➢ Depending on each person's goal, there are three main types of routines in Stage IV; the circuit routine utilizes circuits for endurance strength training, the cardio routine predominantly uses cardio training mixed with less focused strength training in order to maintain strength, and the strength routine focuses on maximum strength training and split-routines, see the end of this chapter for activity-specific routines.
➢ If health is the main goal, then each routine can be focused on for 1-2 weeks and then alternated, but if specific results are desired, then choose the appropriate routine and use it for at least 4 weeks.

Individual Circuits

Upper Body # 1	Upper Body # 2	Upper Body # 3	Upper Body # 4
1. Push-ups w/tubing	Push-pull on unstable	Push-ups w/hands on ball	Push-ups w/one hand on medicine ball
2. Regular lat pull*	Dips w/feet on ball	Sitting or standing row*	Bent over one arm row w/knee on bench
3. Standing mid-back pulls (lower traps)	Pull-ups	Lateral shoulder raises*	Swimming on ball; straight 2 arm flexion*
4. Arm curl into shoulder press*	Dumbbell press on ball*	Swimming on ball; straight 2 arm extension *	Standing mid-back pulls (rhomboids)

Lower Body #1	Lower Body # 2	Lower Body # 3	Lower Body # 4
1. Squats on discs holding weight or arms up	Step-ups onto box	Jumping lunges	Side lunges into 1 leg balance & overhead press
2. Bent leg dead lifts	Supine hamstring curls w/feet on ball	One leg push-up w/head on ball	One leg calf raise holding wt.
3. Standing toe raises	1 leg balance	Isometric squat as deep as functionally possible	1 leg squat to toe touch

Total Body #1	Total Body # 2	Total Body # 3	Total Body # 4
1. Chest	Biceps	Shoulders	Chest
2. Back	Triceps	Rotator cuff	Back
3. Legs	Legs	Legs	Shoulders
4. CORE	CORE	CORE	Legs

CORE #1	CORE # 2	CORE # 3	CORE # 4
1. Lower abs	Side planks w/a twist	Pikes w/toes on ball	Side bends on big ball
2. Curl-ups	Moving planks w/elbows on ball & knees unstable	Torso twists on ball against resistance	Plank w/feet on ball and 1 hand on ground
3. Front plank	Sport swing upward	Front plank w/forearms on 2 balls	½ Moon
4. Standing 2 arm 1 leg reach	Prone hip extensions on ball	Quadruped superman	Superman on ball (all arms/legs up)

Sets = 1 per circuit   **Reps** = goal dependent   **Circuits** = 3-4 (total, upper, or lower body) + 1-2 CORE circuits
Circuit Rest = 3-5 min (only perform 4 exercises at a time)

* These exercises can be done one arm at a time for one workout and two arms at a time for the next.

Split Routines

Chest	Back	Biceps	Triceps
1. Flat dumbbell press	Seated or standing rows	Dumbbell or barbell curls	Triceps pull-down
2. Incline press	Pull-ups or swimming pulls on ball	1 arm preacher curls	Dips
3. Fly's	Bent over one arm row w/knee on bench	Reverse close grip pull-ups	Bent-over overhead cable extensions
4. Push-ups w/hands on ball	Standing straight arm mid-back pulls	Mighty mouse curls	Kick-backs (1 knee on bench, standing bent over, or on ball)

Shoulders	Legs	Abdominals	Spine Extensions
Seated shoulder press	Squats	Lower abdominals	On floor
Lateral raises	Lunges	Lateral abdominals	On ball or apparatus
Front raises	Hamstring curls	Oblique abdominals	Standing
Reverse fly (rear delts)	Toe raises	Upper abdominals	

Sets = 3-5 per exercise   **Reps** = goal dependent   **Exercises** = 3-5 per body part   **Rest** = 1-5 min
Body Parts = 1-2 per workout + abdominals and spine extensions

Advanced Exercise - Part II - Power Training

Description

This stage may seem like it's only for extremists, but the power exercises are fundamental for any type of quick movement or slips and falls. The total body strengthening exercises that accompany the power training are designed to ensure that the strength gains from previous stages are maintained. The power exercises can be made easier for certain populations by performing them without weight or with very light weight and progressing from a moderate speed to as fast as controllable. If speed-strength (power) is the goal, then training must consist of lifting heavy loads (85-100%) and light loads (30%) as fast and controlled as possible in order to maximize results.[13,235-243] The rate at which one can produce strength (speed strength or power) is an essential neural adaptation for most individuals, along with the ability to properly utilize the CORE muscles at those speeds.

Guidelines

- This 8-week Stage is broken into two 4-week programs, each consisting of the same or similar total body strength and CORE exercises but different power training methods. See "Choosing Exercises" below and Chapter 6 for details.
- Completing at least 4 weeks of Stage IV, Part I is necessary before beginning this stage.
- It is useful to train the elderly in this Stage If they have gone through the previous three stages and are physically capable of performing Stage IV exercises. It can be very beneficial to take this population through activity-specific tasks that they need to perform at high speeds, such as starting an old lawnmower, handling grandchildren (medicine ball work), chopping wood, etc.
- This stage can last eight solid weeks or alternate with other stages every four weeks.
- Stretching can alternate between dynamic and corrective as needed.
- Do not perform high-intensity cardio on the same day as strength training unless the workouts are separated by at least 6-8 hours and the person is extremely fit.
- Cardio can alternate between intense and intermediate whenever necessary.
- Power exercise order: 1) Total body, 2) legs, 3) arms/CORE.
- Up to 30-45% of 1-rep max or 10% body weight is recommended for power exercises.[13]
- Max strength training in the power pairs exercises is only for those who need the combination of explosiveness and extreme strength.
- CORE conditioning circuits are only for those who participate in extremely intense activities.
- The exercise possibilities here are limited only by imagination and safety.
- Activity-specific populations should follow the special routines listed at the end of this chapter.
- Stage IV and V strength exercises are utilized.

Priorities

1. Develop power and CORE stamina by utilizing safe and functional exercises that prepare the body for high-speed movements and are unique to each individual's requirements.
2. Continue to increase dynamic flexibility and cardiovascular efficiency to meet the needs of the individual.
3. Maintain strength gains from Part I of Stage IV by continuing the same or similar exercises, as in the "Total Body Strengthening" section.

Variables

- Duration   4-8 weeks
- Frequency   Stretch (3-7x wk) Strength (3-5x wk) Cardio (3-7x wk)
- Intensity   75-100%

Choosing Exercises

Weeks 1-4

- *Strengthening*

  Strength/Power Pairs: strength exercise immediately followed by an explosive power exercise that is similar in biomechanics and explodes concentrically and eccentrically but utilizes a brief pause between the concentric and eccentric phase in order to eliminate the transition phase and build a foundation of stability for each contraction phase; try to imitate sport or significant activities

  Total body: exercises that retain the desired strength for each person

  CORE Conditioning: cardio that mimics related activities along with exercises that strengthen the trunk extensors, flexors, rotators, and side benders equally

- *Stretching* – utilize all types of stretching
- *Proprioception* – incorporate all types (open and closed-chain) of proprioceptive exercises into the warm-up
- *Cardio* – alternate Stages II and III

Goals

1. Quality and stability over quantity and speed
2. Develop the *speed, stability,* and *strength* components of power throughout the concentric and eccentric phases of the movement by utilizing a pause between each phase
3. Maintain previous total body strength gains

Weeks 5-8

- *Strengthening*

  Power Exercises: exercises that can be safely controlled through the transition phase of the exercise at high speeds and that mimic significant activities performed by the individual (squatting up and down as fast as controllably possible with no stopping, jumping is optional)

  Total Body: exercises that retain the desired strength for each person

  CORE Conditioning: cardio that mimics related activities along with exercises that strengthen the trunk extensors, flexors, rotators, and side benders equally

- *Stretching* – utilize all types of stretching
- *Proprioception* – incorporate all types (open and closed chain) of proprioceptive exercises into the warm-up
- *Cardio* – alternate Stages II and III

Goals

1. Quality and stability over quantity and speed
2. Develop the *speed* and *stamina* components of power throughout the transition phase of the movement
3. Maintain previous total body strength gains

1. **Cardio** <u>30-90 min</u> (3-7x wk)
2. **Warm-up** <u>5-10 min</u> (see weeks 5-8)
3. **Strength & Power Exercise Pairs**

- 1-2x wk
- 3-5 min rest
- 3-5 sets of 1-8 reps (max strength or strength) and 5-15 reps for each power exercise
- The strength exercise is immediately followed by the power exercise
- Each ballistic power exercise is performed with a brief moment of rest between the concentric and eccentric phase in order to set the foundation for transition stability strength (plyometrics)
- Choose exercises from the activity-specific section for those with specific needs
- Avoid all other major strengthening exercises on strength and power pair days

Group A	*Total Body*	Choose 2

Strength Exercise = a   Power = b - e

1a. Dumbbell or bench press
  b. Side lunge w/medicine ball push-throw
  c. Squat w/forwards jump and medicine ball push-throw straight forward
2a. Incline dumbbell or incline bench press
  b. Squat w/vertical jump & medicine ball push-throw upward (1 or 2 arm)
3a. Pull-ups , Lat pull down or Straight arm pull down
4a. Standing or Seated rows
  ➢ 3a & 4a have the same power exercise options (e-f)
  b. 1 arm row w/twist and one knee on a bench (lawn mower start)
  c. Overhead med ball throw forward at the floor
  d. Overhead backwards med ball throw; optional standing on unstable or jumping from stable
  e. Squat into 1 arm cable row w/a twist
  f. Standing on tip toes, squat down w/lat pull (reverse snatch)
5a. Standing chest uppercuts w/cables
  b. Overhead backwards medicine ball throw

Group B	*Lower Body*	Choose 1 Pair

Strength Exercise
  1. Squats (any type) 2. Lunges (any type)
  3. Leg press machine
Power Exercise
1. 2 leg box jumps, progress to 90° rotation in air
2. Squat jump w/180 degrees rotation in air, optional 360° & small weights or medicine ball in hands
3. Octagon jumps, progress to rotation in air
4. Jumping stationary lunges
5. 1leg step-ups onto box into a jump, arms overhead w/jumping leg landing on other side of box, optional small weights in hand
6. 1 leg jumps w/minimal knee bending; emphasize quickness in the lower leg, and progress to arms overhead holding a medicine ball
7. Jumping butt-kicks
8. Staggered jumps (focus on front leg)
9. Lunge jumps (focus on both legs)
10. Front kicks w/resistance on ankle

Group C	*Upper Body & CORE*	Choose 1

Strength Exercise = a   Power = b

1a. Dumbbell press alternating arms
  b. 1 arm cable rotations (alternate low, middle, and up high each set)
  c. Lunge into cable twist
  d. Squat into cable twist
2a. Dumbbell or bench press
  b. Standing medicine ball throw (1 or 2 leg)
  c. Standing medicine ball push-throw w/rotation
  d. Standing medicine ball overhead soccer throw or push forward
  e. Prone on ½ dome, ball, or back extension apparatus; extend spine and push ball forward
  f. Jumping push-ups (optional on knees)
  g. Jumping push-ups (on knees) w/hands on medicine ball
3a. Rows (any type), pull-ups, or pull-downs.
  b. Standing ball throw w/rotation at ground (1 or 2 legs)
  c. Kneeling medicine ball throw w/rotation at ground
  d. Overhead medicine ball throw at ground
4a. Any type of bicep exercise
  b. Overhead backwards med ball throw
  c. 1 arm cable rotations upward
5a. Any type of triceps exercise
  b. Overhead medicine ball (soccer throw) at wall
  c. Jumping push-ups w/hands close together

4. **Total Body Strengthening** (1-2x wk) 3-5 sets of 6-12 reps (45sec – 3 min rest) <u>40–100 min total</u>
   - (1) Squats or lunges (any type)
   - (2) Dead lifts or hamstring curls
   - (3) Push-ups or chest press (any type)
   - (4) Lat pull down or Pull-ups (any type - close/)
   - (5) Rows (any type)
   - (6) Shoulder press or lateral or front raise
   - (7) Rotator Cuff

   ➤ **7 Total Exercises**

5. **CORE Conditioning Circuits** (<u>35-50 min total</u>)
   - 1-2 x per wk
   - Rest 2-3 min between circuits and 5-10 sec between exercises
   - Choose 4 circuits and repeat only 1x each
   - Cardio and core exercises should be 75-90%
   - Plank and superman exercises that are timed are performed isometrically

Circuit #1	Circuit #2	Circuit # 3	Circuit # 4
3-5 min Cardio	3-5 min Cardio	3-5 min Cardio	3-5 min Cardio
Lower Abs 1 min	Standing superman w/arms abducted 6x 10 sec light wt.	Sport swings upward 1x 10 reps R/L	Plank w/feet on ball and 1 hand on ground 1 min R/L
Front plank w/forearms on 1 or 2 balls 1 min	Side plank 5x 10 sec R/L	Moving plank w/forearms on ball & knees unstable 1x 10-15 reps	Woodchops downward 1x 10-15 reps R/L
Supermans (any type) 6x 10 sec	Quadruped superman 1x 25 R/L	Standing superman 1x 15 R/L	½ Moon 1x 15 R/L

Circuit #5	Circuit #6	Circuit # 7	Circuit # 8
3-5 min Cardio	3-5 min Cardio	3-5 min Cardio	3-5 min Cardio
Curl-ups 1x 50	Side bends on ball 5x 10 sec R/L	Plank w/moving legs on 2 balls 1x 15 reps	Front plank w/feet on 1 or 2 balls 1 min
Reverse plank w/heels on ball 1 min	Pikes w/toes on ball 1x 15-25	1 arm sport swing straight 1x 10 reps R/L	Side bends on big ball 1x 10 reps R/L
Standing crunch & fly 30 sec R/L	Superman on ball (all arms/legs up) 1 min	Back Ext. on Ball w/wt. 1x 15 reps	Prone hip extensions on ball 1x10-15reps

6. **Dynamic Stretch Progression** (1-3x wk) <u>15-60 min</u> – use as its own workout w/a cardio warm-up
7. **Cool-down, General, & Corrective Stretching** (major body parts as needed, include self-myofascial release wherever necessary) 3-7x wk/1-2x per day/1-4x 20-90 sec hold each stretch (<u>10-60 min</u>)

Weeks 1-8

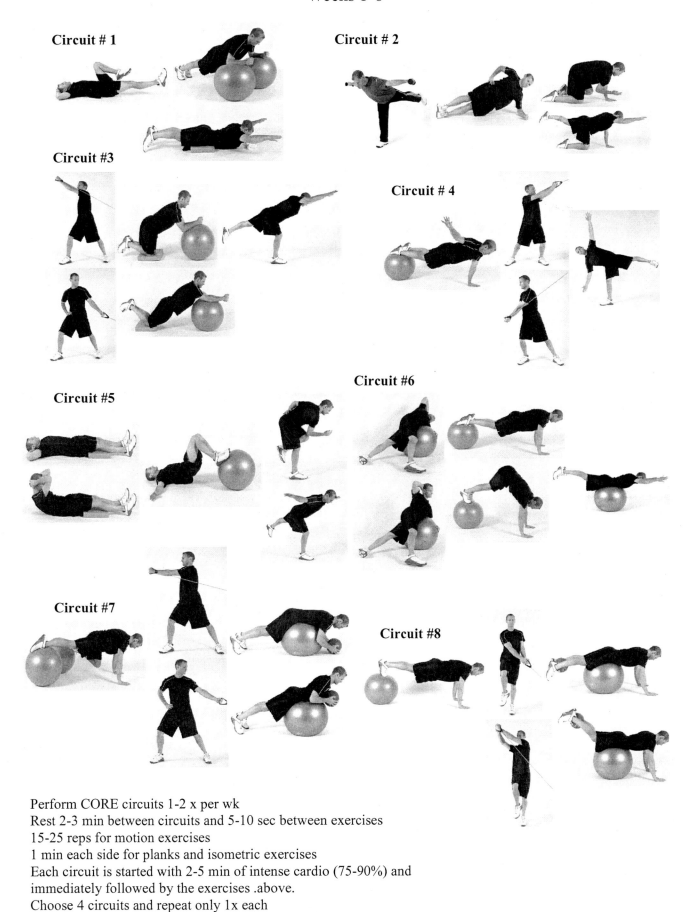

Circuit # 1

Circuit # 2

Circuit #3

Circuit # 4

Circuit #5

Circuit #6

Circuit #7

Circuit #8

Perform CORE circuits 1-2 x per wk

Rest 2-3 min between circuits and 5-10 sec between exercises

15-25 reps for motion exercises

1 min each side for planks and isometric exercises

Each circuit is started with 2-5 min of intense cardio (75-90%) and immediately followed by the exercises .above.

Choose 4 circuits and repeat only 1x each

Weeks 1-4

Group A - TOTAL BODY - Choose Two

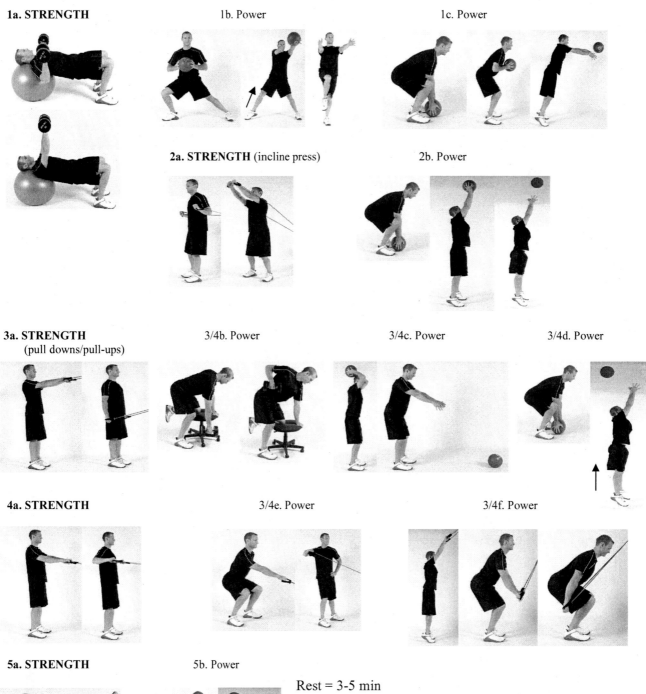

1a. STRENGTH

1b. Power

1c. Power

2a. STRENGTH (incline press)

2b. Power

3a. STRENGTH
(pull downs/pull-ups)

3/4b. Power

3/4c. Power

3/4d. Power

4a. STRENGTH

3/4e. Power

3/4f. Power

5a. STRENGTH

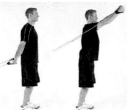

5b. Power

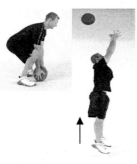

Rest = 3-5 min
Sets = 3-5 of 1-8 reps (max strength or strength) and
        5-15 reps for each power exercise
The strength exercise is immediately followed by the power exercise
Each ballistic power exercise is performed with a brief moment
    of rest between the concentric and eccentric phase in order to
    set the foundation for transition stability strength
    (plyometrics)

274

Group B - LOWER BODY - Choose one Pair

STRENGTH

1. Squats or Leg Press   2. Lunges

POWER

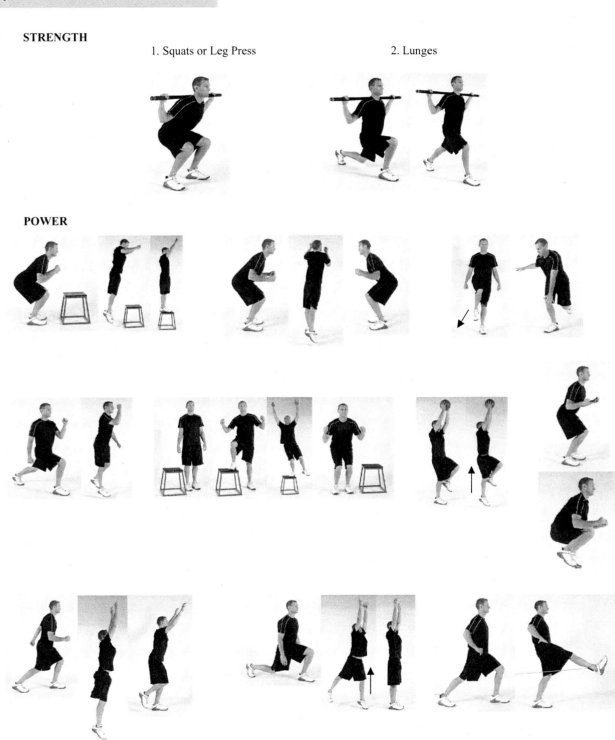

Rest = 3-5 min

Sets = 3-5 of 1-8 reps (max strength or strength) and
        5-15 reps for each power exercise

The strength exercise is immediately followed by the power exercise

Each ballistic power exercise is performed with a brief moment of rest between the concentric and eccentric phase in order to set the foundation for transition stability strength (plyometrics)

Weeks 1-4

Group C - UPPER BODY & CORE - Choose one Pair

1a. STRENGTH   1b. Power   1c. Power   1d. Power

2a. STRENGTH   2b. Power   2c. Power   2d. Power

                        2e. Power   2f. Power   2g. Power

3a. STRENGTH
(pull downs/pull-ups/rows)   3b. Power   3c. Power   3d. Power

4a. STRENGTH   4b. Power   4c. Power   **5a. STRENGTH**   5b. Power

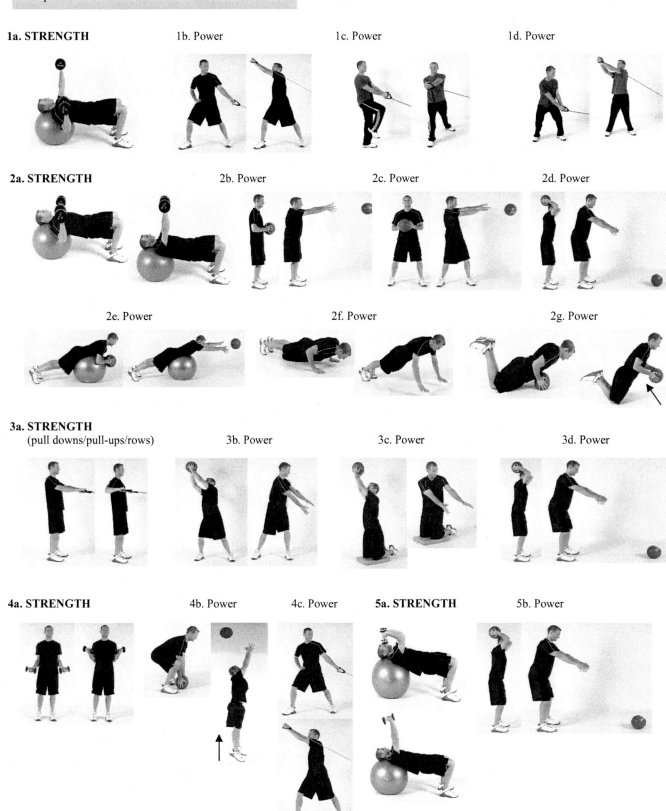

1. **Cardio** (3-7x wk) use as a warm-up (<u>5-10 min</u>) or as a separate workout (<u>30-90 min</u>) 3-7x wk
2. **Warm-up** 1-2 sets of 10-20 reps or 30-90 sec holds (5-10 sec rest) <u>5-10 min</u>

- (1) Squats (up to 50 reps) unstable surface is optional
- (2) Push-ups
- (3) Downward dog (calf stretch)
- (4) Static lunge with torso twists
- (5) Karate kicks w/punches
- (6) 1 leg flying hamstring stretch
- (7) Alternating lunge twists
- (8) One leg balance on ball
- (9) Marching w/torso twist
- (10) Any necessary dynamic stretches

3. **Power Exercises** (1-2x wk) 3-6 sets of 1-10 reps (3-5 min rest)
   OR power/stamina = 2-3 sets of 12-30 reps (2-3 min rest) <u>30 min-2 hr total</u>

- For each workout choose:
  - ➤ Choose exercises from the activity-specific section for those with specific needs
  - ➤ All concentric and eccentric contractions are explosive, focus on stabilizing through the transition phase as fast and controlled as possible (plyometrics)

Group A **Total Body** **Choose 2**	1. Squat into a vertical jump and ball push-throw upwards 2. Standing back dive against resistance 3. Squat w/forwards jump and medicine ball push-throw straight forward 4. Squat into a 1 or 2 arm medicine ball push upwards w/a jump 5. Side lunge w/medicine ball push-throw 6. Squat into 1 arm row (lawn mower start) 7. Standing on tip toes, squat down w/lat pull 8. Overhead backwards medicine ball throw, progress to standing on unstable surface, then jumping from stable ground
Group B **Lower Body** **Choose 1**	1. Squat jump w/180 degrees rotation in air, progress to 360 degrees and small weights or medicine ball in hands 2. Two leg box jumps, progress to 90 degrees rotation in air if appropriate 3. Octagon jumps, progress to rotation in air 4. Jumping stationary lunges w/weights in hands 5. 1 leg step-ups onto box into a jump w/arms overhead & jumping leg landing on other side of box, progress to small weights in hand 6. Front kicks w/resistance around ankle 7. 1 leg jumps w/minimal knee bending emphasizing quickness in the lower leg, progress to arms overhead holding a medicine ball 8. Staggered jumps (focus on front leg) 9. Lunge jumps (focus on both legs) 10. Jumping butt-kicks
Group C **Upper Body** **and** **CORE** **Choose 2**	1. One arm sport swing 2. Lunge into cable twist 3. Squat into cable twist 4. Standing medicine ball throw w/rotation at ground (wood chop) 5. Jumping push-ups (any type – big/small ball/staggered hands/etc.) 6. Standing medicine ball throw at wall directly behind (extreme twisting)

4. **Total Body Strengthening** (1-2x wk) 3-5 sets of 6-12 reps   (45sec – 3 min rest) 40–100 min total
   - (1) Squats or lunges (any type)
   - (2) Dead lifts or hamstring curls
   - (3) Push-ups or chest press (any type)
   - (4) Lat pull down or Chin-ups (any type)
   - (5) Rows (any type)
   - (6) Shoulder press or lateral raise
   - (7) Rotator Cuff

5. **CORE Conditioning Circuits** (35-50 min total)
   - Same as weeks 1-4

6. **Dynamic Stretch Progression** (1-3x wk) 15-60 min – use as its own workout w/a cardio warm-up

7. **Cool-down, General, & Corrective Stretching** (major body parts as needed, include self-myofascial release wherever necessary) 3-7x wk/1-2x per day/1-4x 20-90 sec hold each stretch (10-60 min)

Training Schedule

Weeks 1-8

1. **Cardio**   5. **CORE Conditioning circuits**
2. **Warm-up**   6. **Dynamic Stretch Routines**
3. **Power or Power Pairs**   7. **Cool-down/General Stretching**
4. **Total Body**

Routines	M	T	W	Th	F	Sa	Su
General (A)	1-3,7	1,6	2,4,7	2,5,7	1-3,7	1,7	6
General (B)	2,3,5,7	1,6	2,4,7	1,7	2,3,5,7	1,7	1,6
General (C)	1-3,7	2,4,7	1,2,5,7	2,6	1-3,7	2,5,7	1,6

- Routine (A) is the easiest listed here while (B) is more difficult because it involves CORE conditioning twice a week and in the same workout as the power exercises.
- Routine (C) is challenging in a different way; it involves strength training 5x per week, although only one component per workout.
- If it is not possible to exercise the number of times per week as listed above, then a double workout day can be used to combine a cardio day with a weight training day; power exercises and total body exercises should not be combined on the same day, and each double workout day should consist of 6-8 hours of rest between workouts and increased nutritional intake and rest.

Group A - TOTAL BODY - Choose Two

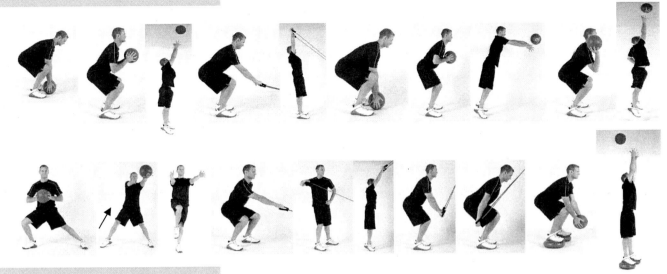

Group B - LOWER BODY - Choose One

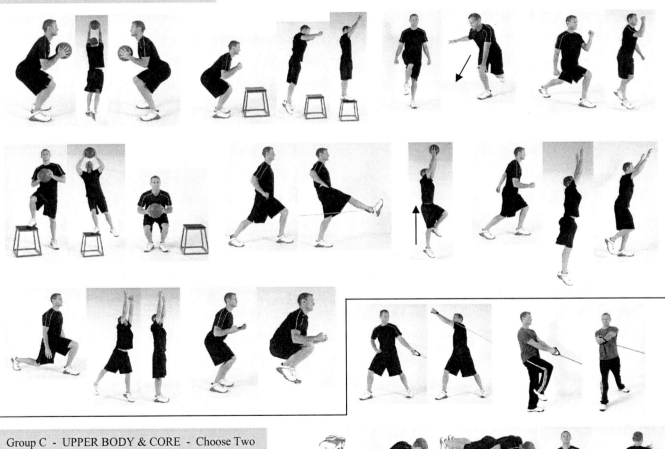

Group C - UPPER BODY & CORE - Choose Two

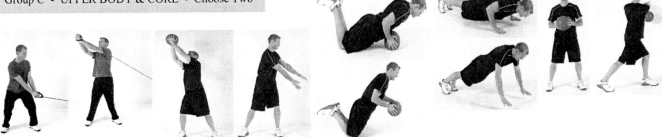

Program Design for General Maintenance

Once all of the stages have been completed, by a non-activity-specific individual, it is time to decide on how to maintain results without losing strength or overtraining. There are numerous ways to combine the different components and stages in order to achieve health and fitness goals.

The following routine has been developed for those who wish to exercise for the benefits of general health and fitness and who have completed all four stages of Exercise Progression.

Focus	M	T	W	Th	F	Sa	Su
Everything	Cardio (III) Proprio (II) Strength (II) Stretch (I)	Cardio (II) Stretch (II)	Proprio (II) Strength (III) Stretch (I)	Cardio (III) Stretch (II)	Cardio (II) Strength* (IV or V) Stretch (I) *alternate by week	Cardio (III) Stretch (I)	Stretch (II)
Cardio & Stretching	Cardio (III) Proprio (II) Stretch (II)	Cardio (II) Stretch (I)	Cardio (III) Proprio (II) Stretch (II)	Rest	Cardio (III) Proprio (II) Stretch (I)	Cardio (II) Stretch (I)	Stretch (II)
Cardio & Strength	Cardio (II) Strength(II)	Cardio (III) Stretch (I)	Cardio (II) Strength(IV)	Stretch (II)	Cardio (III) Strength(II)	Cardio (II) Stretch (I)	Stretch (I)

(#) = Stage #
- The components are in the order that they should be completed in for each workout from top to bottom.
- Each week can be performed for up to a month or rotated every week with a different routine, or
- One whole stage can be focused on for 1-4 weeks and then alternated with another stage for 1-4 weeks, or
- Proprioception, stretching, and cardio can be the focus one week while the following week is strengthening, stretching, and cardio.
- Unless highly conditioned, do not combine high intensity cardio, stretching, or strengthening on the same day.
- Alternating between easy, moderate, and intense exercise allows the body to recuperate while maintaining results.

Description

Activity-specific training should begin once Stage III has finished and replaces Stage IV by way of the training schedule on pg. 281, which combines activity-specific workouts with regular Stage IV workouts. The activities listed in this chapter are mostly sports but can also include construction and warehouse workers.

　　For those who compete and need to have peak performances at specific times, it is best to learn how their body responds to different quantities, types, and intensities of exercise. The interactions between the different components will vary depending on the person and what sport or activity is performed. For example, some sports compete a few times a week, while others only have big competitions once a month.

　　There are many methods that claim to produce peak results at a given time, but everyone is unique and therefore requires individualized progressions and programs for peak performance.

　　For instance, some people respond well to resting (less quantity and more quality), while others lose their edge and become slightly deconditioned if they alter their training the same amount as the other group.

　　The appropriate program can only be fine tuned through trial and error, not adhering to guidelines in this or any other manual; however, the guidelines here and elsewhere are the foundation to base individualized programs on.

Guidelines

- Activity-specific training includes various mixtures of the following components:
    1. Activity-specific workout = 1-3x wk
    2. Core conditioning circuits = 1-2x wk
    3. Total body strengthening = 1-2x wk
    4. Split-routine* = 3-5x wk
    5. Circuit training* = 2-3x wk
    6. Cardio = 3-6x (includes "activity-specific" activity if aerobic)
    7. Stretching = 5-7x wk
    8. Activity-specific drills (fundamentals; i.e., passing and dribbling for soccer or basketball) 1-3x wk
    9. Overall strengthening workouts = 3-5x wk (includes #'s 1-5)
    * The split-routine and circuit training programs are separate systems with different goals that should be rotated every 1-4 weeks, not within the same week.
- All beginners or post-rehabilitating individuals with activity-specific goals should start with Stage I and finish Stage III, then begin the activity-specific training.
- The activity-specific portion of each workout should involve power exercises and can also include power-pair training for those who are ready for Part II of Stage IV.
- The training schedules for this phase of training (pg. 283) can be used instead of or alternated with the schedules in Stage IV (pg. 278). In other words, this is an additional or replacement stage for athletes and those in need of a more activity-specific workout.
- Although only a few activities are described here, almost any sport or activity can be trained for by following the "Training Schedule" on pg. 283 and replacing the "Activity Specific Workout" with a circuit training workout each time it comes up in the routine, or with another appropriate activity-specific workout not listed in this manual.
- Weight training for most activities (excluding football and other max-strength activities) should involve 2-3 sets of each exercise (total body or split routine) with 12/10/8 reps, increasing the weight each set, and occasionally super-setting opposing muscle groups.
- The drills portion of each workout is only briefly described for each activity because a coach is best suited to teach "in action" training.

Priorities

- Same as Stage IV.

Variables

- Duration
- Frequency
- Intensity

Varies depending on season and activity
Stretch (3-7x wk) Strength (3-5x wk) Cardio (3-7x wk)
75-100%

Choosing Exercises

- Same as Stage IV, with the addition of activity-specific exercises and drills.
- The following box gives general guidelines for most activities.

Off/Early-Season	Mid-Season	Last Month of Season (taper)
• Most intense strength and weight training • Building endurance for activity • Strength = 2-5 x per wk • CORE = 3 x per wk	• More moderate than intense weight training w/the focus on maintaining strength and increasing endurance or power if appropriate • Strength = 1-3 x per wk • CORE = 3 x per wk	• Least frequent weight training w/the focus on race type reps (quality over quantity) • Strength = 1x per wk • CORE = 2-3 x per wk

Goals

- Goals are highly specific depending on each individual and their activity.

Training Schedule

1. Cardio
2. Warm-up
3. Power Exercises
4. Total Body
5. CORE Conditioning circuits
6. Dynamic Stretch Routines
7. Cool-down/General Stretching
8. Activity-specific workout
9. Activity-specific drills (fundamentals)
10. Split-Routine for strength training
11. Circuit Training

Routines	M	T	W	Th	F	Sa	Su
Activity-specific Strength & Endurance Training (A)	1,2,4,7	2,5,9,7	1-3,7	1,6,9	1,2,8,7	2,5,9,7	6
Activity-specific Strength Training (B^1)	1,2,10,7	2,9,10,7	1,6	2,10,7	2,9,10,7	1,7	1,6
Activity-specific Strength Training (B^2)	1,2,5,9,7	2,8,7	1,6	2,5,9,7	1,2,8,7	1,6	2,7
Activity-specific Endurance Circuit Training (C)	1,2,11,7	1,2,9,6	2,11*,7 * = optional	1,2,5	1,2,11,7	1,2,9,6	2,7

- (B^1) focuses on strength and (B^2) focuses on skills; both are needed for complete training.
- Activity-specific routines (B^1) and (B^2) should be alternated every 1-2 weeks for combined strength and activity-specific training results; use (B^1) & (B^2) workouts as a single routine when combining with (A) & (C).
- Only use the (B^1) routine in the off-season or early portion of a season; unless the activity is year-round.
- Activity-specific routines (C) and (B^1) and (A) should be alternated every 1-4 weeks for combined strength and activity-specific training results.
- Use the activity-specific workout and drills portion from the previous pages to fit into their corresponding places in the training schedule above. The rest of the components are just as they were in Stage IV.

- PHILOSOPHY

- CREATING BALANCE

- HEALTH vs. FITNESS

- STRETCHING

- WORKOUT ROUTINE

- PROPRIOCEPTION

- HEALING TIMES

- DYNAMIC STRETCH ROUTINE

- COOL-DOWN STRETCHING

- LOW BACK STRETCHES

- WARM-UP ROUTINE

- CHAIR JOCKEY WORKOUT

- PAIN & DYSFUNCTION CYCLE

Facts

- If a muscle is in a shortened position (bad posture or repetitive use) for a prolonged time, it will become tight and it's antagonist weak. This is the basis for muscle imbalances throughout the body.

- Pain can be referred from tension areas to other "non-related" areas (headaches).

- Generally, pain causes inhibition in stabilizer muscles and hyperactivity in the mobilizers.

- It can take up to ten years to feel the affects of bad posture.

- Bad posture affects digestion and many other internal functions

The Six Components

- Assessment
- Strength
- Stretching
- Proprioception (coordination)
- Daily Activity Modifications (D.A.M.'s)
- Cardio

The Program

Exercise can be just another form of movement that adds to the repetitive strain we place on the body every day. OR, it can be a regenerating activity that enhances the form and function of the body.

Exercise Progression trains the body to function how it was designed to; efficiently and pain free.

Unless specific exercises are performed and individual imbalances corrected, the body will succumb to the daily tortures of sitting, slouching, and improper movement patterns that slowly lead to the irreversible consequences of arthritis, altered spine curvatures, joint abnormalities, poor neuromuscular function, aches and pains, etc.

The corrective exercises used in Exercise Progression are unique and not common to gyms or most other types of exercise arenas, including physical therapy.

They are unique and they are only given after a detailed assessment, i.e. no general protocols.

Everyone gets exactly what their body needs to find balance and function efficiently.

Depending on the person, these corrective exercises (Stages I and II) will take anywhere from four to sixteen weeks to greatly improve the overall function and balance of the body.

Once function and form have reached a peak, advanced exercise and training are recommended to further improve the body so that it is ready for all the demands life puts on it.

Details

Simply put, the body's soft tissue system (muscles, tendons, ligaments, and fascia) is connected from head to toe, deep to superficial, and cannot be dysfunctional in one area without creating a chain reaction of compensations throughout the rest of the body.

There are two main types of muscles in the body; stabilizers and mobilizers. Stabilizers are used in posture and are what keep the body in proper alignment for everything from sports to digestion and breathing. Mobilizers are the larger muscles that move the body about.

The way the body works is that during *poor* posture and prolonged sitting, the stabilizers "go to sleep" and the mobilizers become overactive. This dynamic eventually settles in and infects all movements of the body, even standing, which means that many bones and joints will be out of place and unstable, ALL THE TIME.

Once these patterns are engrained, it does not take long for aches and pains to arrive "suddenly" for no apparent reason. Thankfully, these aches and pains are often predictable and fixable.

Routinely stretching the overactive areas and activating the "sleeping" muscles will restore posture and function to optimal levels.

Changing Posture

The key to changing posture is "yagottawannadoit." Random attempts to change do not even make a dent in the armor of habitually formed poor posture and faulty movements that we acquire through the fatigue of daily rituals.

A postural breakthrough requires constant efforts in the direction of positive reinforcement of a specific position or movement that improves the way the body lives by placing it in its most efficient space for functioning.

This can be learned by (1) recognizing the maladaptive patterns, (2) practicing new and improved patterns, and (3) constantly being aware of the attitudes and habits that bring the body back to the maladaptive patterns.

These inefficient patterns are a result of our lifestyle and cannot be changed without altering some thoughts and habits of our everyday routines.

This means that we must be dissatisfied with our current state and direction of health and commit to a change for the better; otherwise our old habits will eventually take over and bring the body back to it's "comfort zone."

Posture is an attitude, and therefore cannot be changed without a new thought process. It is well known that people with multiple personalities have different postures and even medical conditions that go with each personality. This shows that we become what we think and believe.

You can shape yourself, or you can be shaped by bad habits.

Corrective Exercise

Corrective exercise is essential for establishing a strong functional foundation at all levels, no matter how novice or elite a person's capabilities are. Anyone in pain or with less than optimal functioning, should start with corrective exercises.

Many aches and pains are caused by simple muscle recruitment problems. Bad posture and lack of stimulation to the stabilizing muscles cause the more superficial and larger "mover" muscles to take over.

These larger muscles unfortunately are not designed to hold postures and stabilize joints very well. Because of this, they tire quickly, therefore creating that nagging ache, and they move the body around (sports, daily activities, etc.) without maintaining stability throughout the body.

Depending on the person, it can take anywhere from 10-20 weeks to become functionally efficient at whatever movements they need to do. Once the body is more balanced, it will function with less wear and tear, and lead to fewer injuries, aches, and pains. At that point, more advanced exercising can begin.

The corrective exercises challenge the body enough to grow muscle (in new places) but also allow it to recover from repetitive training and bounce back stronger than before.

No matter the person, it is always necessary to cycle through corrective exercising. For example, athletes should focus heavily on corrective exercise in the off season and only when necessary during the season.

Health vs. Fitness

The following definitions are as described by the Merriam-Webster's Collegiate Dictionary, 1995.

- Health - "the condition of being sound in body, mind, and spirit; *esp* : freedom from physical disease or pain"
- Fit - "sound physically and mentally: Healthy"
- Fitness - "the quality or state of being fit" and "the capacity of an organism to survive and transmit its genotype to reproductive offspring as compared to competing organisms"

It is easy to see why fitness becomes associated with health but often times does not truly promote it. The above definition of "fit" leaves out the spiritual dimension but is still considered "healthy", while the fitness definitions are based on the degree in which one is fit and competing with others.

These definitions, which are probably the most accepted in society, show that health is three dimensional but fitness is only two dimensional, and if someone has a high level of fitness then they must be fit and therefore healthy. This type of "fitness health" is driven by the mind, and without getting too philosophical, is lacking a spiritual component which keeps the body in line with true health as opposed to "fitness health." The main difference is not spiritual awareness, which is a bonus, but rather enjoying the pursuit of health instead of pursuing results from fitness. It is easy to get caught up in trying to fight or delay death with exercise and diet instead of simply enjoying the process of living healthfully.

In order to be healthy one must have balance between the physical, mental, and spiritual aspects of their life. In regards to the physical dimension of health, it must have a balance between 1) nutrition 2) movement 3) rest. If any one is lacking or excessive, health is unattainable. For most of us the goal should be health instead of fitness training whenever possible, but it may be necessary for athletes and those who are physically active to find a balance between extreme training and health training, and therefore both types (fitness and health) of programs should be learned and then alternated properly.

Health is always in flux and requires constant adjustments through nutrition, movement, intensity, and thought process. There is a point where the amount of exercise or activity is detrimental to health, see graph below.

Health vs. Fitness

Graph notes:

1. Optimum health requires much less exercise than optimum fitness.
2. Too much exercise can be just as detrimental as little or no exercise.

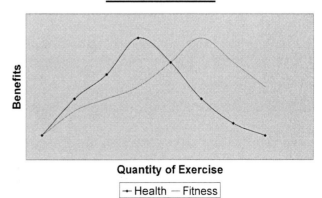

Quantity of Exercise

← Health — Fitness

HEALTH vs. FITNESS

Exercise Goals

- **Health** - To stress the body in a way that encourages *all* of its systems to function most efficiently.
- **Fitness** - To stress the body in a way that achieves specific external results (esthetics, speed, strength, endurance, etc.).

These two goals can have very different impacts on the body, but ideally they complement one another. When exercising for health there is no such thing as a bad workout unless an injury or overtraining results. Understanding this perspective makes it easier to avoid the disappointment of failing to achieve, or overexertion to gain specific results (weight, time, repetitions, etc.).

When exercising for fitness the body's internal functions are often sacrificed to reach external goals. Exercising at too high of intensity and/or for too long a time can drain the entire body of its vitality, which can be replenished if treated appropriately, but will eventually have long term negative effects on overall health if this type of training is habitual. Unfortunately those who train at this level either do it on a consistent basis, which doesn't allow enough time for re-vitalization and speeds up wear and tear, or do it infrequently which often results in injuries. These people can look healthy on the outside, but to an experienced observer their body's systems are noticeably inefficient.

A few things are needed if health is a goal.

1. Patience
2. Knowledge of appropriate exertion levels (mostly intuitive)
3. Understanding that health relies on fitness more than fitness relies on health.
4. Realizing that *health is a state of being* and *fitness is being in a physical state.*

In order to obtain health the ego must be left out of goal setting. The ego wants to protect and maintain the self-image it has created throughout a lifetime. Examples of some ego images and goals are:

- Looking good (compared to others of course)
- Being good at something (compared to others of course)
- Achieving a physical goal, even at the expensive of health.

These goals are accepted and encouraged by most of society because of one main idea; succeeding or winning for whatever it takes. This may be necessary to seriously compete in athletics or extreme activities, but it must be realized that these two examples do not promote health and should not be participated in unless the relationship between health and fitness is understood and accepted.

A wise person will have the ability to achieve both health and fitness goals at the same time. Some example goals are;

- Lower resting heart rate, blood pressure, body fat (if obese), and have more daily energy.
- Train for an event i.e. marathon, race, sport, etc, to the best of my capabilities while listening to my body for signs of overtraining and not be disappointed if I can't compete because the goal was to train to the best of my capabilities, not achieve results.

With all of this being said, it is possible to be *relatively* healthy if extreme training (most athletes) is properly utilized. The point to be made here is that extreme training is not necessary to become healthy and it is associated with less than optimal health, which could still be considered healthy, just not as healthy as possible.

The choice is simple; live for the mind (external results), or live for the body (internal results).

The physical aspect

Thinking about it energetically, the brain sends impulses to the muscle telling it to move, receptors in the muscle are constantly sending impulses back to the brain informing it about the muscle's position, speed of movement, length, and tension.[18,19] Receptors in the muscle also send signals back to the spinal cord that shoot right back to the muscle, totally bypassing the brain, these are reflex arcs, the simplest being the *stretch reflex*.[18,19]

The stretch reflex *increases* tension in the muscle being lengthened, and has a static and dynamic component[16,27] so as long as the muscle is moving it will have some tension in it that interferes with its passive stretch potential. This tension will increase proportionally with the speed of the stretch.[16,27] Therefore, *a slow stretch should be applied to inhibit tension in the muscle* (autogenic inhibition) and facilitate its elongation.[17] Also holding the stretch for at least twenty seconds will stimulate the golgi tendon reflex and inhibit the muscle spindle's stretch reflex, which will create an adaptation in the muscle spindles and allow the muscle to stretch further without initiating the stretch reflex.[27]

These reflexes help the body function on a daily basis (maintaining posture and muscle tone)[18,19] but can limit stretching if they are not understood. If the reflexes are not taken advantage of, then stretching is just like any other movement, it will move the muscle without any affect on its long term length.

Experience leads the author to believe that the reflex arcs are hypersensitive when the mind is busy, therefore allowing a smaller stimulus to activate the reflex and decrease the muscle's stretch potential. In order to best override the stretch reflex the mind must be relaxed. When the mind is focused on body awareness the muscles can relax along with the reflex arcs, allowing for a maximal stretch. Injuries and sharp pains are exceptions, even if they can be tuned out, they shouldn't.

While relaxation is often a goal of stretching, the rest of the body should not be limp during the stretch. For instance, while stretching the low back it is often beneficial to activate the abdominal muscles in order to stabilize the intervertebral segments against excessive motion.

The mental aspect

Stretching is best done with a quiet mind and some knowledge of how the muscles respond to lengthening. The mind and body are always communicating, and when the mind is busy their connection is weakened. What one did and what one has to do are thoughts that often cause a level of anxiety undetectable to a busy brain but are enough to interfere with the reflex arcs. Stretching can act as a time out from the daily routine and unite the physical with the mental. Instead of the muscles reacting to the brain (stress), the brain should *interact with* the muscles when stretching. For instance, during a stretch if it becomes uncomfortable, one can back off, breath through it, or hold it anyway while gritting the teeth and hardly breathing (yes, you). This last technique usually adds more stress than it takes away. Instead, interact with the muscle by breathing smoothly and clearing the mind, this takes practice. Then it is possible to feel the muscle and each tightness surrounding it. Without reacting to the tightness the breath can be used to sooth the muscles and establish a new and improved length that wasn't possible with the old reflex arc, not to mention increase circulation and body awareness.

This doesn't have to be an enlightening experience, rather a timeout from the outside world and a union with the inside. This moment should be enjoyed; it's a great thing to be able to improve health just by breathing and paying attention to the body. *Without this "timeout" stretching is just another movement that can add stress to the body.*

This is of course an ideal way to stretch that is not always possible, but time should be taken to have ideal sessions whenever possible.

❖ In general, if stretching is not the minds focus and enjoyable, then it will not fully benefit the body.

Stretching

Types of Flexibility

Non-dynamic

Passive, self-myofascial release, active, isometric, and active assisted stretching techniques are all non-dynamic. This type of flexibility is less complex and usually achieved in one movement plane, sometimes two, and is best used to correct posture imbalances and elongate muscles because of its relatively simple methods. It does not transfer very well into dynamic or multi-planar flexibility because it lacks the neuromuscular coordination. Non-dynamic flexibility is the foundation of stretching and should be the first goal of any novice or injured person.

Dynamic

Dynamic techniques, like Yoga movements, are the only way to achieve dynamic flexibility. This type of flexibility is controlled by the neuromuscular system and allows the muscles to elongate while controlling the body's speed, direction, balance, and coordination. Therefore, coordination is required to avoid injury. All three planes of movement should be challenged in a way that prepares the body for real life situations, such as reaching behind the wash machine to pick up fallen clothing. Dynamic flexibility cannot be totally converted into non-dynamic flexibility because the maximum length allowed by the muscle is rarely reached in a dynamic stretch.

➢ Both types are needed for overall flexibility.

Example: An athlete has a daily routine of non-dynamic stretching for the entire body and can pass every basic ROM test there is, but he/she does not do any dynamic stretching. If they are blessed with great coordination and flexibility it is possible to escape wear and tear or clumsy injuries. But, if they are like most people, they will need to practice dynamic flexibility, otherwise a situation will eventually occur that puts the body into a position it has neither the strength, flexibility, or coordination to control, all of which could have been trained through dynamic stretching.

How far is enough to get a good stretch?

The goal isn't to go as far as one can, rather as far as one should. The end-feel of a stretch is the best guide to how far and even if stretching should be done. If the end-feel is a structural blockage or sharp pain, then stretching can do more harm than good. But if the end-feel is a leathery restriction, like muscle, then stretching should help the limitation.

Stretch the muscle to the barrier (*first point* of moderate tension), hold until the muscle "let's go" or about 20-30 seconds is reached, then, relax it or gently stretch it to the next point of noticeable tension. More is not always better when it comes to twisting, bending, pulling, pushing, and everything else that is possible to do to the body. It can be a fine line between injury and improvement depending on the condition of the surrounding tissues and the stretching techniques used. Stretching to the limit will often create instability in the involved joint(s) due to surpassing the ability of the antagonistic muscle to stabilize the joint(s). A great way to prevent overstretching is to stretch slowly and smoothly, get the muscles warm, and *make sure the surrounding muscles (especially the antagonist) can support the joint in that position.*

Breathing

If breathing isn't relaxed and synchronized with the stretch, then results will be poor. The exhalation helps relax the muscle and is most beneficial during the elongation phase. While holding a stretch for the appropriate time the inhalation should be similar to the exhalation in force and duration (3-5 seconds in, 3-5 seconds out, with a pause in between). This isn't always possible at the beginning of a difficult stretch, but by the last few seconds a rhythm should be achieved, otherwise the muscles won't completely relax and **accept** the new length. At first it will seem impossible to relax in some of the new positions, but by focusing on proper breathing it is possible to reach the muscle's greatest stretch potential.

Growth Stimulating Variables

- Intensity
- Velocity
- Volume (repetitions, sets)
- Rest
- Plane of Motion
- ROM
- Exercise Selection
- Exercise Order
- Frequency
- Balance and Coordination

All of these variables should be mixed up about once a month for strength training to keep the body challenged and prevent overtraining or boredom.

Plane of Motion

There are three different planes of motion; all three are utilized in functional movements. If one plane is underdeveloped, that direction of movement will most likely lead to wear and tear or injury. A comprehensive exercise program needs to include and systematically progress each plane of motion.

The three planes of motion:

1. *Sagittal* – forward/backward
2. *Frontal* – side to side
3. *Transverse* – rotation

Adaptation to Specific Variables

Adaptation	# of exs's	Sets	Reps	Load % of 1 rep max	Rest	Tempo	X/wk (total)
Max Strength	3-6	4-6	1-5	85-100%	3-5 min	3-1-1	3-5
Strength	3-4	3-4	6-8	75-85%	45 sec- 5 min	3-1-1	3-5
Hypertrophy	3-6	3	9-12	70-85%	45-90 sec	4-2-2	3-5
Endurance	2-4	1-3	12-25	50-80%	1-3 min	3-2-1	3-4
Stabilization	3-5	1-3	12-25	40-70%	0-1.5 min	Slow	3-5

* Number of times per wk varies depending on how many muscles are strengthened each workout.

Stretching Guidelines

STATIC	DYNAMIC
• Hold each stretch for at least 20 seconds. • Do not use before a strength workout or sport. • This is the easiest type of stretching to learn and results in the least amount of injuries. • Always make sure you are warm before stretching. • Without relaxed breathing the body's reflex system will not accept the new length of the muscle and your efforts will be wasted. • Static stretches are ideal for improving posture and aches and pains. • One example of a static stretch is laying on your back and pulling one leg up into the air and holding it for 20-30 seconds (hamstring stretch).	• Each stretch is held for only 6-8 seconds while other muscles coordinate to hold the body in various positions, i.e. yoga-type poses. • Dynamic stretching is ideal for warm-up or as its own workout because it challenges the body to maintain good alignment while utilizing important stabilizing muscles. • Always make sure you are warm before stretching. • Dynamic stretching is more advanced than static stretching and is associated with more injuries. • This type of stretching is essential for anyone who wishes to be able to play sports or have functional flexibility.

Workout Routine

Guidelines

- Always warm-up at least 5-10 minutes prior to weightlifting or stretching in order to increase the body's temperature and coordinate the neuromuscular system. Proper warm-ups include; jumping rope, dribbling a basketball, jogging, cardio, performing easy exercises in all three planes of motion which prepare the body for the upcoming workout, etc.).
- Stretching should be done 1) before a workout (if something feels extremely tight) by using short, dynamic movement stretches instead of 20-30 second holds (holding a stretch for 20-30 seconds is great for a cool down but tends to weaken that muscle for the following hour or so), 2) as its own workout, i.e. yoga, or 3) after a workout by using long, static holds, i.e. 20-30 seconds in one position.
- Always do abs/low back and rotator cuff exercises at the end of a workout, otherwise they will fatigue in the middle of the workout and loose their ability to stabilize the body during the main exercises.
- If you feel too tired to workout, then you probably are. Focus on stretching and recovery that day.
- Get plenty of water and rest before, during, and after a workout. The workout is only 1/3 of physical fitness; the body also needs rest and proper nutrition.
- For strengthening, components "a-e" can be done 1-2x wk while "f" can be done 3-4x wk (see below).
- Strengthening can be done by using numerous techniques. Basic weight training and circuit training are described here because they are the easiest and most beneficial for the average person.
- For general results, alternate between circuits and basic weight training every 1-4 weeks.
- The following exercise components are the basics for a healthy fitness routine.

Exercise Components

1. **Cardio/Sports** (3-6x wk)
2. **Stretching** (5-7x wk)
3. **Balance/Coordination** (2-3x wk)
4. **Strengthening** (2-5x wk total)
   - a) chest (push)
   - b) back (pull)
   - c) arms (curl/extend)
   - d) shoulders (raise)
   - e) legs
   - f) abs/low back

Sample Workout Schedule

	M	T	W	Th	F	Sa	Su
A	1-3,4(a,b,f)	1 & 2	3, 4(e,f)	1 & 2	1-3,4(c,d,f)	2 & rest	1-3
B	Circuit	1-3	1 & Circuit* * optional	1-3	Circuit	rest	1-2

Training Techniques for Strengthening

Basic Weight Training (A)

Goal = Strength or Toning

- 45 sec-3 min rest (↑ intensity = ↑ rest)
- 2-3 different exercises per muscle group
- 3-4 sets of each exercise
- 6-12 sets total for each muscle group
- 6-15 reps, except abs/low back, which can often be done to failure.

Circuit Training (B)

Goal = Endurance and Toning

- 2-4 circuits each workout
- 2-4 different exercise per circuit
- 5-10 sec rest between exercises
- 2-3 min rest between circuits
- 12-20 reps each exercise
- Utilize entire body within each circuit
  ### OR
- Focus on one or two parts each circuit and rotate body parts each circuit.

Proprioception is often referred to as a sixth sense that creates our physical awareness by constantly communicating the body's position to the brain via receptors located throughout the body, even in fascia[30,31,32] and spinal ligaments.[29] It allows the body to regain balance during a slip or to touch the nose while the eyes are shut.

It is mostly an unconscious system that functions along with the vestibular system (inner ear) to provide the sensory input needed to respond to our physical environment. Whether the body responds appropriately or not depends on the condition of these two systems along with the conditioning of the neuromuscular system.

The proprioceptive system has the ability to cause specific muscles to contract or relax through unconscious reflexes[18,19] and is the same system responsible for the stretch reflex. For example, when stretching the hamstrings too far or too fast, muscle spindles will cause a reflex contraction of the hamstrings to control and resist the movement.

Significance of Proprioception

If one was to lose most or all of their proprioception they would not be able to reach for a drink while talking to someone and still maintain eye contact with that person. They would have to constantly watch their hand (because the proprioceptive system isn't telling the brain where it is) and consciously move it towards the cup through the feedback of the eyes. Then do the same thing on the way up to the mouth.

This is basic proprioception that most people have and don't need to train for but it shows the main principle of proprioception that is strived for, and that is being able to perform efficiently during complex movements without having to think about it.

For example, specific repetitive training can improve proprioceptive ability and teach the neuromuscular system how to properly jump, throw, and land while only having to think about who to throw it to, not how to do it. Or it can train the system to instantly and unconsciously react to slips and falls.

With the exception of sleeping, the body is constantly utilizing proprioceptors for simple, complex, unconscious, and conscious movements. It is for this reason that Exercise Progression spends a lot of time developing this sixth sense in order to develop a more efficient neurological system to control the muscles.

Many people do not have the ability to properly access their neurological system and recruit the specific muscles needed in order to strength train efficiently because they have been inactive for a prolonged time or have numerous compensations throughout the body.

This is where posture balancing exercises followed by proprioception training will 'wake up' the neurolomuscular system and encourage better strength straining results.

The soles of the feet are the foundation for proprioception while standing, so there must be an emphasis on proper foot positioning. It is commonly called "small (or short) foot" and is helpful for increasing afferent input (neurological input to the brain), mostly from the sole.[4,41]

The short foot position is accomplished by bringing the ball of the foot towards the heel, without curling the toes, which will raise the arch a little bit and place the entire body in a position that is well suited for coordination and balance.

Of course overall posture must be aligned in order for the body to be properly placed over the feet. This takes practice and often requires repeating many times while sitting before it can be done standing.

Summary

Every movement or exercise involves the proprioceptive system, so a key to improved performance and function is to *properly* stimulate the system to obtain a specific coordination.

The saying "If you don't use it you lose it" definitely applies to proprioception. As we grow older or more sedentary our proprioceptive team "sits on the bench" more than it "plays" and thus becomes deconditioned and slow to react. This can be improved with specific training no matter how long it has been inactive or how old the person or injury is.

Proprioceptive training is a necessity if the maximum benefits of exercising or rehabilitation are desired because it allows the muscles to fire on all cylinders. Proprioceptive training is also great for warming up the neuromuscular system prior to exercise.

If someone has abnormally poor proprioception and coordination it is useful to their diet; B12 deficiencies are associated with a poor sense of balance and joint position awareness, clumsiness, and decreased reflexes to name a few of the many side affects.[128]

Strain - Also called a pull, partial tear, complete tear, or rupture of the ***MUSCLE* or *TENDON*.**

Grade 1 Strain (mild)	Grade 2 Strain (moderate)	Grade 3 Strain (severe)
• Slightly overstretched with no tearing of the muscle or tendon • No loss of function • Painful • 2-10 days healing time	• Tearing of the muscle or tendon at its attachment to the bone • Some loss of function • Painful • 10 days-6 weeks healing time • Surgery is sometimes needed	• Rupture and separation of the muscle or tendon from the bone • Near to total loss of function • Less pain than a grade 1 or 2 strain • 6-12 weeks healing time • Surgery is required

Sprain - A severe overstretching of a ***LIGAMENT.*** Pain, swelling, or bruising are common symptoms.

Grade 1 Sprain (mild)	Grade 2 Sprain (moderate)	Grade 3 Sprain (severe)
• Some tearing of the ligament, 0-20% • No loss of function • 2-6 weeks healing time	• Partial tear of the ligament, 20-75% • Some loss of function • 6-10 weeks healing time • Surgery is sometimes needed	• Complete tear of the ligament or complete separation from the bone, 75-100% • Total loss of function • 10-16 weeks healing time • Surgery is required • Severe sprains can pull loose a fragment of bone causing a sprain/fracture

Healing Time Table

Tissue	Injury	Healing Time
Muscle	Grade 1 strain	2-10 days
	Grade 2 strain	10 days – 6 weeks
	Grade 3 strain	6-12 weeks
Ligament	Grade 1 sprain	2-6 weeks
	Grade 2 sprain	6-10 weeks
	Grade 3 sprain	10-16 weeks
Tendon	Sprains	See muscle strains
	Acute tendonitis	2-6 weeks
	Chronic tendonitis	6-12 weeks
	Tennis elbow (chronic)	3-6 months
Bursae	Acute/mild bursitis	1-2 weeks
	Chronic bursitis	6-8 months
Nerve	Inflammation/trauma	3 months – 1 year
Vertebral disc	Herniation	3-12 months

The Healing Process

Whether the body is ailing from muscle, ligament, bone, or any other pathology, *the key to healing is creating an environment in that area that is most conducive to receiving nutrient-rich blood flow and energy.* This is done by;

1. Avoiding aggravating factors, i.e. picking at the scab (running on an inflamed knee, doing anything that causes pain in the injured area, etc.).
2. Finding habits that relieve symptoms. For example, spinal extension positions are usually very helpful for those with lumbar disc herniations or bulges.
3. Good nutrition, such as; fresh fruits and vegetables that aren't cooked to death, less dairy and red meat (these can cause inflammation and stagnation in the blood), less fried and microwaved foods (destroys nutrients), more water, etc.
4. Stretching and or strengthening any areas that will improve blood flow and balance tension surrounding the area.
5. Spending a couple of minutes each day focusing on the problem area by sending it positive energy and asking yourself what you can learn from it.

While all five of the above factors are essential, there is one that is often overlooked. Number five is one that most people don't think about and yet it is one that they tend to do the opposite of.

Think about how an injury or pain will or should prevent a person from doing something they normally do on a regular basis, i.e. sports, physical activities, job, or even sleeping. This limitation is usually not enjoyable for the person so they tend to resent the injury or pain; not to mention any fear and anxiety associated with it due to the unknown healing time and the "when will I be normal again" thoughts.

Many people will go so far as to despise an injury because it keeps them from doing something they love. When the brain despises a part of the body, what type of energy do you think it sends to it? Yeah, it's not very healing to say the least.

Resentment and anxiety are obviously not ideal in creating a healing environment, so the next step is to try to learn something from the injury so that the brain will see it as beneficial. That's what pain is anyway. It is a signal from the body to the brain telling it that something is wrong, and it's likely that the physical pain is related to a lesson in life, such as slowing down or being open to different ways.

It is important to be aware of the ego and its desire to attain certain "superficial" goals that may get in the way of healing or becoming healthy in general. For example, it is common for injured people to try to achieve their fitness goals despite the signals

from their body telling them to slow down and take some time off.

Once the injury or pain is seen as an "incite to better health", powerful life lessons can be learned in the way of; 1) learning to slow down in general, this often allows doors of opportunity to open that would not have opened otherwise, 2) learning to be more empathetic to others, 3) learning to focus on health instead of external goals, 4) realizing that without suffering one cannot appreciate what they have or learn to act in spite of fear and pain, etc.

This is all fine and dandy, but one more difficult change needs to be made, and that's finding a new activity or habit to replace the old non-supportive one(s) until the injury is healed.

It is very conducive to health to enjoy more than one activity so that these activities can be cycled routinely in order to break up the repetitive wear and tear on specific body parts from each activity. For instance, it's usually great for a tennis player with a bad knee to take up certain cardio machines or swimming. This is however impossible if that person is focused on tennis instead of their health. The reality is this;

Focus on health, and you will receive it. Focus on unhealthy things, and you will eventually receive signals (usually pain) from your body telling you that you need to focus on your HEALTH!

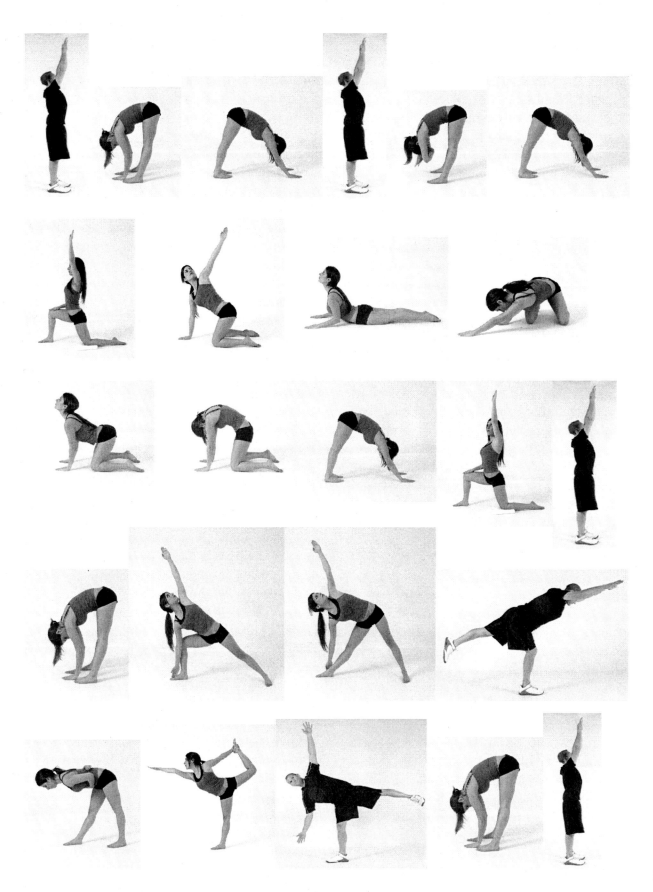

296

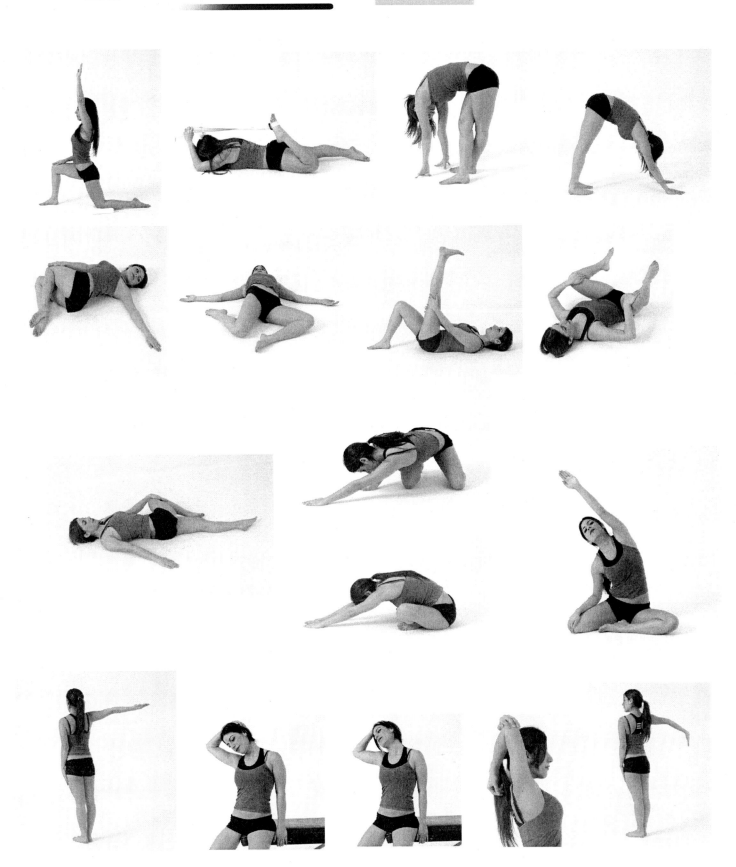

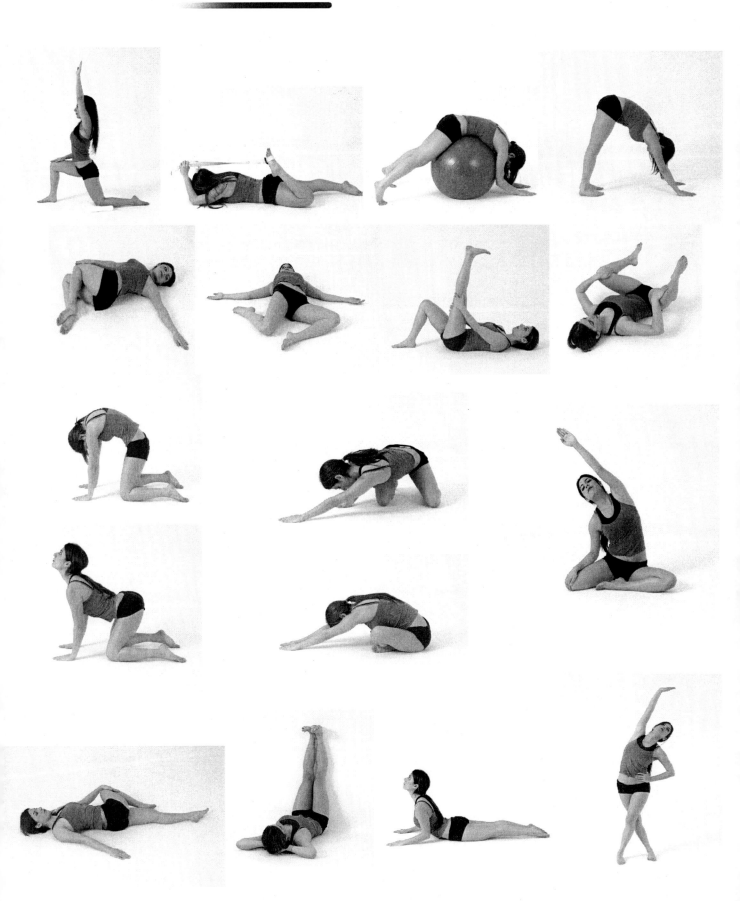

1. Squats
(30-50 reps)

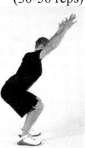

2. Push-ups (hold for 10 seconds 10x)

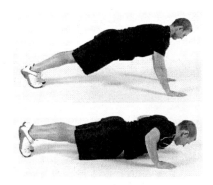

3. Downward Dog
(hold for 30-90 seconds)

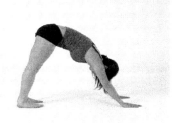

4. Static lunge
(10-20 twists/side)

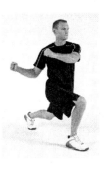

5. Karate Kicks w/punches
(10-20 kicks per side)

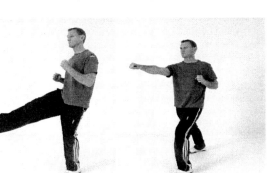

6. 1 leg flying hamstring
stretch
(30 seconds each side)

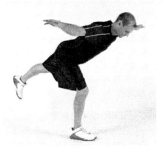

7. Alternating lunge twists
(10-20 reps)

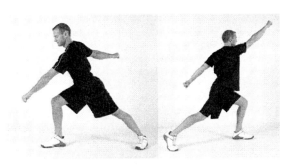

8. One leg balance on ball
(one minute each leg)

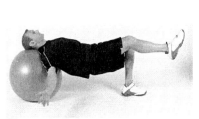

9. Marching w/torso twist
(60-90 seconds)

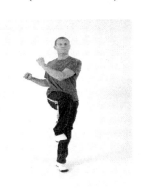

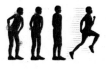

The Chair Jockey Workout

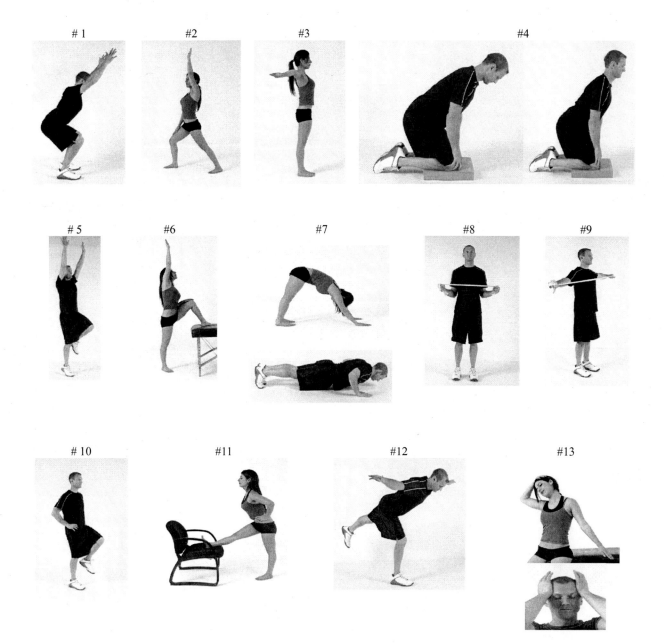

1   #2   #3   #4

5   #6   #7   #8   #9

10   #11   #12   #13

Meet the Chair Jockey

A chair jockey is someone who spends too much time sitting on a daily basis. Prolonged sitting causes "deloading" of the tissues, which occurs from lack of gravity stress on the body and results in a weakening of the stabilizing muscles. This deloading reduces the body's ability to resist gravity during sports or simply standing, and works on the following principles;

Sitting = non-weight bearing = poor muscle recruitment & posture = ↓ energy/productivity = ↑ injuries

Standing = weight bearing = ↑ leg and spine strength = ↑ energy & mental capacity = ↓ pain & injuries

The Chair Jockey Workout is designed to be simple and time efficient. It can be used throughout the day in the office or at home to keep the body's stabilizing muscles strong and activated. This routine improves posture and reduces stress at the precise areas needed to reverse the harmful effects of sitting and repetitive movements, which add up at the end of the day and week and cause dull aches or even pain in the low back, neck, and shoulders. It is the best answer to a busy schedule of sitting and a life full of aches and pains.

It should take no more than 6 or 7 minutes each time and should be done in the order shown. They can be repeated throughout the day to break up the constant strain of non-gravity induced poor posture. These exercises are also ideal for traveling because they can be done in a hotel room without any equipment, although exercise tubing is good to have.

Exercise Descriptions

- Hold all stretches for 20-30 seconds with *relaxed* breathing

1. *Squat*
   - These can be done with the arms pointing upward or straight in front of the chest.
   - Suck in the stomach, squat down, and stick the hips backwards as if sitting into a chair.
   - Don't let the knees go past the toes.
   - Move slowly and pause at the bottom, stretching the arms away from the body.
   - Keep the shoulders relaxed and the head in-line with the spine (pointing downward)
   - Repeat as many as time or effort permits.

2. *Front thigh stretch*
   - This stretch can also be done with the back knee on the ground.
   - Suck in the stomach and squeeze the buttocks on the side of the leg in back.
   - Reach upward, don't arch the low back, and slightly twist the torso away from the front leg.

3. *Chest stretch*
   - Stand tall, stomach sucked in slightly, and relax the rest of the body.
   - Squeeze the shoulder blades together and hold 5-10 seconds, continue breathing. Repeat 5-10 times.

4. *Upper spine extension*
   - Kneeling on a pad, suck in the stomach and brace the upper body with hands on knees.
   - Slouch forward to assume the rest position.
   - Keeping the lower back stationary and stable, use the vertical muscles along the spine to push the chest outward (extending the mid/upper back).
   - Keep the head in line with the spine.
   - Hold for 10 seconds and repeat 5-10 times.

5. *Toe raises*
   - Using 1 or 2 legs, (reaching upward is optional), raise yourself up onto the ball of your foot and repeat up and down *slowly* 15-30 times.
   - Keep the stomach sucked in and stay on the inside of the ball of the foot.

6. *Front thigh stretch*
   - See # 2, but use a chair.

7. *Push-up/Calve stretch*
   - Starting in the calve stretch, try to push the heels into the floor and the chest towards the thighs.
   - Keep the stomach sucked in with relaxed breathing.
   - Transition into a push-up position (on knees or straight legs), and move up and down as slow as possible in order to work the back also.
   - Do as many as time or effort permits.

8. *Rotator cuff strengthening*
   - Tubing is optional, but optimal.
   - Keeping the elbows at your side, start with the hands in front of the belly button and rotate the arms so that the fists go away from the body.
   - Hold at the end point for a few seconds and repeat slowly 15-30 times.

9. *Shoulder blade squeezes*
   - Tubing is optional, but optimal.
   - Palms can face up or down.
   - Keeping the stomach sucked in with upright, yet relaxed posture, start with the arms in front of the chest and squeeze the shoulder blades together and bring the arms backwards, posture should not change.
   - Hold at the end point for a few seconds and repeat 10-15 times slowly.

10. *One leg balance*
    - Keeping the hips level, stand on 1 leg for 30-60 seconds, progressing to eyes closed.
    - Focus on good body and foot posture.

11. *Leg stretch*
    - This can be done facing (not shown) and or twisting away from the chair.
    - Place the foot up on a chair, keep the spine upright and slightly lean towards the foot.
    - Stretch the foot up and down to add a stretch to the calves.
    - Keep the stomach sucked in and don't slouch the low back.

12. *Spine/Back exercise*
    - Keeping the stomach sucked in without slouching the low back, squeeze both glutes and raise one leg.
    - Hold the arms outward by squeezing the shoulder blades together.
    - Keep the head in line with spine.
    - Push the raised leg and arms out and away from the body. Hold for 15-30 seconds each side.

13. *Neck stretching and facial relaxation*
    - Sitting, gently tug on the back of the head in all directions searching for tight spots in the neck muscles.
    - Hold each tight spot for 20-30 seconds and focus on breathing.
    - The other hand can be used to massage the area being stretched.
    - After the neck is stretched, massage the temples while making every possible facial expression in order to energize and relax tension in the head.
    - Lastly, focus the eyes on something distant to relax them.

Tips for Sitting

1. ALWAYS use a lumbar support for the low back.
2. Shift position constantly to distribute stress to various areas.
3. When picking something off the floor or bending down, place one hand on a knee and slightly lift up the buttocks while maintain an arched low back.
4. Don't twist. Always face whatever task is at hand by turning the body as a unit.
5. Don't read papers that are flat on the desk. Prop them up so the head isn't flexed all the way forward and down.
6. Have the keyboard and mouse at the same level as the elbows when they are naturally hanging at your side. Also keep them at a forearms distance away from your body so that no reaching occurs.
7. Use arm rests to take pressure off the low back.
8. Keep the monitor about 18 inches from your eyes and make sure lighting is sufficient so that they are more relaxed.
9. If you are on the phone a lot, support your "phone arm" with an elbow on the desk and switch sides often.
10. Posture is an attitude that creates a physical state. Be aware of deadlines and stress weighing down the body into poor posture. Use relaxed breathing and thoughts of what you are grateful for to improve posture and reduce stress.
11. Take frequent breaks to introduce movement to the body and keep its systems working efficiently, i.e. The Chair Jockey Workout.
12. Drink plenty of water.
13. Do the following exercises at the end of the day to reverse some of the damages caused by sitting.

Leg Elevation on Wall

Laying on a flat surface, scoot the buttocks as close as possible to a wall and prop the legs up. Lay in this position for 5-10 minutes to facilitate circulation of stagnant blood.

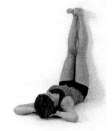

Standing Wall Posture Exercise

Standing with feet 3 inches from wall, keep the entire spine, back, and neck touching the wall by using the lower abdominals to "tuck in your tail". Hold for 3 minutes in a natural manner.

Pain & Dysfunctional Cycle

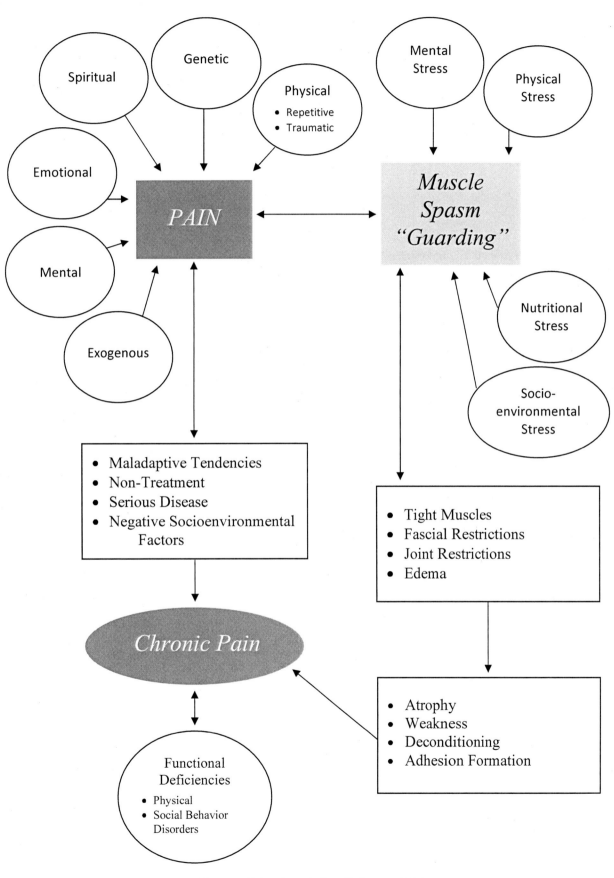

A combination of ideas from Calliet, Chaitow, and Liebenson.

EXERCISE PROGRESSION WORKOUT SHEET
STAGE I

Name _____

Date _____   History _____

Corrective Exercises																							
Thoracic extensions (a)																							
Wall stand (b)																							
Posture practice (c)																							
Breathing (d)																							
Stomach & butt squeeze (e)																							
Stomach & back tighten (f)																							
Leg lifts backwards (g)																							
Leg lifts sideways (h)																							
Forward bending (i)																							
Neutral & safety zones (j)																							
Cardio																							
Stretching																							
DAM's/Other																							
Date																							

EXERCISE PROGRESSION WORKOUT SHEET
STAGE II Weeks 1-8

Name _____

Date _____ History

Cardio	
Stretching	
Proprioception (a,b or c)	
Strengthening	
Part I	A.
	B.
	C.
Part II	
Squats (a,b or c)	
Front Lunges (a,b or c)	
Side Lunges	
Marching Front Step-ups	
Toe Raises	
Rotator Cuff	
Stretching	
DAM's/Other	
DATE	

EXERCISE PROGRESSION WORKOUT SHEET
STAGE III   Part I

Name _____

Date   History

Cardio		
Stretching		
Proprioception (a-f)		
Strengthening Functional Circuits (1-9)		
Stretching		
DAM's/Other		

Date _____

EXERCISE PROGRESSION WORKOUT SHEET

STAGE III   Part II

Name

Date   History

Cardio																							
Stretching																							
Proprioception (a-e)																							
Strengthening																							
1st Multiple Circuit																							
2nd Multiple Circuit																							
Stretching																							
DAM's																							
Dynamic Stretching																							
Date																							

EXERCISE PROGRESSION WORKOUT SHEET

STAGE III   Part II (DEMO)

Name _____

Date _____ History _____

	70%	65%		75%	70%	65%	
Cardio	run/30min	bike/45min		swim/30min	run/30min	Hiking	
Warm-up Stretching	5 min		5 min		5 min		
Proprioception Strengthening	B - 2 min C - 2 min	C - 2 min D - 2 min	B - 2 min D - 2 min		B - 2 min C - 2 min		
1st Multiple Circuit	1 15x45lb/20 15x10lb/15x10 10/max max/15/5lb 2min/50 reps 2 min/2 min 5x10sec/10 5x10sec/25 3 15x55/15x25 30rep/50rep max/ max 10x50lb/15x10				2 10/max 15x10lb/12x25 1min/12x12lb 12x20lb/10x10 5x10sec/15rep 15rep/10rep 10x20lb/15rep 25rep/15rep 4 12rep/12x10lb 10rep/12x25lb 12x45lb/max 12x20lb/15x10		
2nd Multiple Circuit	1min/50reps 2min/2min 2min/20reps 2min/12reps				50rep/12x30lb 10rep/25rep 2 min/ 2 min 15x15lb/12rep		
Stretching	#'s 1-16 20 min	#'s 1-16 30 min	#'s 1-16 30 min		#'s 1-16 20 min	#'s 1-16 30 min	
DAM'S							
Golf pick-up		3x10					
Box pick-up off floor		1x10					
Dynamic Stretching				30 min			1 hr
Date	mon 3-23-06	tue 3/24	wed 3/25	th 3/26	f 3/27	sat 3/28	sun 3/29

WORKOUT SHEET
STAGE IV - Part I · Weeks 1-8

Name_____   Date_____   History_____

Cardio							
Warm-up							
Proprioception							
Strengthening Upper/Lower Body							
Date							

WORKOUT SHEET

STAGE IV - Part I - Weeks 1-8

Strengthening Spine Extensions						
Back ext. on ball or apparatus						
Same as above, but 1arm w/wt.						
Standing bent over rows						
Standing bent over w/arms adb.						
Standing superman - opp reach						
Standing superman - 2 arm						
1/2 Moon						
Prone on ball hip/leg extension						
Hugging table into 2 leg ext						
Standing back dive						
Prone superman on floor						
Quadruped superman						
On ball; 2 arm/1 leg reach						
On ball; 2 arm/2 leg reach						
Prone on ball w/med ball push						
Abdominals						
Lower abdominals						
Straight leg sit-ups w/sit-back						
Straight leg curl-ups						
Crunches on ball						
Woodchops (from up high)						
Sport swing (from middle)						
Sport swing (from down low)						
Supine torso twists on ball						
1 leg torso rotation w/cable						
Side plank						
Side plank w/a twist						
Side plank up on 1 straight arm						
Front plank						
Front moving plank - stable						
Front moving plank - unstable						
Front unstable plank - lower						
Front unstable plank -upper						
Feet on ball & 1 hand on floor						
Reverse plank w/heels on ball						
Standing side bends w/wt						
Side bends - ball or slant board						
Knee tucks w/feet on ball						
Pikes w/toes on ball						
2 ball balance w/1 arm free						
Dynamic Stretching						
General Stretching						
Date						

WORKOUT SHEET

STAGE IV - Part II - Weeks 1-4

Name

	Date	History

Cardio												
Warm-up												
Strength/Power Pairs												
Total Body												
Total Body												
Lower Body												
Upper/CORE												
Total Body Strengthening												
Squats or Lunges												
Dead Lifts or Hamstring curls												
Push-ups or Chest Press												
Lat-Pull or Pull-ups												
Rows												
Shoulder press or Lateral or Front raises												
Rotator Cuff												
CORE Conditioning												
Dynamic Stretching												
Stretching												
Date												

WORKOUT SHEET
STAGE IV - Part II - Weeks 5-8

Name

Date

History

Cardio															
Warm-up															
Power															
Total Body															
Total Body															
Lower Body															
Upper/CORE															
Upper/CORE															
Total Body Strengthening															
Squats or Lunges															
Dead Lifts or Hamstring curls															
Push-ups or Chest Press															
Lat-Pull or Pull-ups															
Rows															
Shoulder press or Lateral or Front raises															
Rotator Cuff															
CORE Conditioning															
Dynamic Stretching															
Stretching															
Date															

References

1. Petty N, Moore A. Neuromusculoskeletal Examination and Assessment. Churchill Livingstone, Edinburgh. 1998
2. Umphred, D.A. Neurological Rehabilitation, ed. 3. Mosby-Year Book, Inc. 1995
3. Magee, David, J. Orthopedic Physical Assessment 3rd Edition/W.B. Saunders Company. 1997
4. Chaitow L, DeLaney JW. Clinical Applications of Neuromuscular Techniques, Vol. II – The lower body. Churchill Livingstone, 2002.
5. Jones M. Medical Exercise Specialist (MES) workshop/manual. American Academy of Health, Fitness and Rehab Professionals (AAHFRP). 2004
6. Kisner, C, and Colby, L.A. Therapeutic Exercise: Foundations and Techniques, ed. 3. F.A. Davis Company, Philadelphia. 1996
7. Simons, G, David, Simons S, Lois, and Travell G, Janet. Myofascial Pain and Dysfunction: The Trigger Point Manual. *The upper half of the body.* ed. 2. vol. 1. Williams and Wilkins, Baltimore. 1999
8. Simons, G, David and Travell G, Janet. Myofascial Pain and Dysfunction: The Trigger Point Manual. *The lower extremities,* ed. 2. vol. 2. Williams and Wilkins, Baltimore. 1992
9. Tor-bjorn M. Hanson and Pat Laufenberg. The Four Seasons: Unlocking the Secrets to Human Potential/One source Potentials, Inc. Tor-bjorn M. Hanson. 1989
10. Kottke FV. The rationale for prolonged stretching for correction of shortening of connective tissue, *Arch. Phys. Med. Rehabil.* 47:345. 1966
11. Chaitow L, DeLaney JW. Clinical Applications of Neuromuscular Techniques, Vol. I – The upper body. Churchill Livingstone, 2002
12. Chaitow, Leon. Soft-Tissue Manipulation: A Practitioner's Guide to the Diagnosis and Treatment of Soft-Tissue Dysfunction and Reflex Activity/Thorsons Publishing Group, Wellingborough, Northhamptonshire – Rochester, Vermont. 1987
13. Clark MA, Lucett S, Corn R, Cappuccio R, Humphrey R, Kraus SJ, Titchenal A, and Robbins P. NASM course manual; Optimum performance training for the health and fitness professional, ed. 2. National Academy of Sports Medicine, 2004
14. Lewit K. Manipulative Therapy in Rehabilitation of the Motor System. London, Butterworth 1985
15. Lewit K. Postisometric relaxation in combination with other methods. Manuelle Medezin 2:101. 1986
16. Alter MJ. Science of Flexibility, ed. 2. Human Kinetics. 1996
17. Basmajian JV. Therapeutic Exercise ed. 3. Williams and Wilkins, Baltimore. 1978
18. Sherwood, Lauralee. Human Physiology: From Cells to Systems, ed. 2. West Publishing Company, Minneapolis/St. Paul. 1993
19. Marieb, Elaine. Human Anatomy and Physiology, ed. 3. The Benjamin/Cummings Publishing Company, Inc., California. 1995
20. Schilling B.K and M.H. Stone. Stretching: Acute Effects on Strength and Power Performance. Strength and Conditioning Journal: 22(1): 44-47. 2000
21. Kokkonen, J. and A.G. Nelson. Acute stretching exercises inhibit maximal force performance. *Med. Sci. Sport Exerc.* 28(5):S1130. 1996
22. Nelson, A.G., J.D. Allen, A. Cornwell, and J. Kokkenen. Inhibition of maximal torque production by acute stretching is joint-angle specific. 26th Annual Meeting of the Southeastern Chapter of the ACSM, Destin, FL, January. 1998
23. Fowles, J.R., and D.G. Sale. Time course of strength deficit after maximal passive stretch in humans. *Med. Sci. Sports Exerc.* 29(5):S155. 1997
24. Halbertsma, J.P.K., A.I. van Bolhuis, and L.N.H. Goeken. Sport stretching: Effect on passive muscle stiffness of short hamstrings. *Arch. Phys. Med. Rehabil.* 77(7): 688-692. 1996
25. Wiemann, K., and K. Hahn. Influences of strength, stretching, and circulatory exercises on flexibility parameters of human hamstrings. *Int. J. Sports Med.* 18:340-346. 1996
26. Clark, MA. Integrated Neuromuscular Stabilization Training (Power). National Academy of Sports Medicine (Publishers). Thousand Oaks, CA. 2000
27. Clark, MA. Integrated Flexibility Training. National Academy of Sports Medicine (Publishers). Thousand Oaks, CA. 2000

28. Grays Anatomy, 38th edn. New York: Churchill Livingstone. 1995
29. Solomonow, M., Zhou, B., Harris, M., Lu, Y., and Barrata, R.V. The ligamento-muscular stabilizing system of the spine. *Spine*, 23:2552-2562. 2000
30. Bonica, J. The management of pain, ed. 2. Lea and Febiger, Philadelphia. 1990
31. Earl, E. The dual sensory role of the muscle spindles. Physical Therapy Journal 45:4. 1965
32. Wilson, V. Inhibition in the CNS. Scientific American 5:102-106. 1966
33. American College of Sports Medicine. ACSM's Guidelines for Exercise Testing and Prescription. ed. 7. Lippincott Williams and Wilkins. 2005
34. Smith, ML, Mitchell, JH. Cardiorespiratory adaptations to exercise training. In: Durstine JL, ed. *Resource Manual for Guidelines for Exercise Testing and Prescription.* ed. 2. Baltimore: Williams and Wilkins. 1993
35. Copeman, W.S.C., and Ackerman, W.L. Fibrositis of the Back. *Quarterly Journal of Medicine.* 13:37-51. 1944
36. Bond, D.W. *The Problem with the Back Mouse.* In: Massage and Bodywork. December/January, 76-79. 2004
37. McGill SM. Low Back Disorders: Evidence-based prevention and rehabilitation. Human Kinetics. 2002
38. Vleeming A, Snijders C, Stoeckart R, Mens J. The role of the sacroiliac joints in coupling between spine, pelvis, legs and arms. In: Vleeming A, Mooney V, Dorman T, Snijders C, Stoeckart R (eds) Movement, stability and low back pain. Churchill Livingstone, Edinburgh. 1997
39. Cailliet, R. Low Back Pain Syndrome ed. 5. F.A. Davis.1995
40. Plaugher G. and Lopes M. Textbook of Clinical Chiropractic: *A Specific Biomechanical Approach.* Williams and Wilkins, Baltimore, Maryland. 1993
41. Liebenson C. Rehabilitation of the Spine: A practitioner's manual. Lippincott Williams and Wilkins. 1996
42. Lewit K. *Role of Manipulation in Spinal Rehabilitation.* In: Liebenson C. Rehabilitation of the Spine: A practitioner's manual. Lippincott Williams and Wilkins. 1996
43. Janda V. *Evaluation of Muscular Imbalance.* In: Liebenson C. Rehabilitation of the Spine: A practitioner's manual. Lippincott Williams and Wilkins. 1996
44. Fairbank JCT, Park WM, McCall IW, et al.: Apophyseal injection of local anesthetic as a diagnostic aid in primary low-back pain syndromes. *Spine* 6:598-605. 1981
45. Panjabi M M. The stabilizing system of the spine. Part I. Function, dysfunction, adaptation, and enhancement. *Journal of spine disorders* 5:383-389. 1992
46. Cholewicki J. Mechanical stability of the in vivo lumbar spine. PhD Dissertation. University of Waterloo, Ontario, Canada. 1993
47. Liebenson C. Journal of Bodywork and Movement Therapies. 1(2), 87-90 January. 1997
48. Janda V. Muscles, central nervous motor regulation and back problems. In Korr IM. (ed): Neurobiologic Mechanisms in Manipulative Therapy. New York, Plenum. 1978
49. Kendall FP, McCreary EK. Muscles: Testing and Function. ed. 3. Williams and Wilkins. 1983
50. Chek P. Scientific back training. *Correspondence Course.* Encinitas CA: C.H.E.K. Institute. 2000
51. Spitzer WO, LeBlanc FE, Dupuis M: Quebec Task Force on Spinal Disorders: Scientific approach to the assessment and management of activity-related spinal disorders: A monograph for clinicians. Spine 12(Suppl 7):S1 1987
52. Liebenson C, Oslance J. *Outcomes Assessment in the Small Private Practice.* In: Liebenson C. Rehabilitation of the Spine: A practitioner's manual. Lippincott Williams and Wilkins. 1996
53. Hislop HJ, Montgomery J: Daniels and Worthingham's Muscle Testing: Techniques of Manual Examination, ed. 6. W.B. Saunders Company, Philadelphia, Pennsylvania. 1995
54. Gray, H. Gray's Anatomy: The Classic Collector's Edition. *Anatomy, Descriptive and Surgical.* Bounty Books, New York. 1977
55. Vasilyeva L. and Lewit K. *Diagnosis of Muscular Dysfunction by Inspection.* In: Liebenson C. Rehabilitation of the Spine: A practitioner's manual. Lippincott Williams and Wilkins. 1996
56. Lowman CL. The sitting position in relation to pelvic stress. *Phsyiother Rev* 21:30-33. 1941
57. Greenman P. Principles of Manual Medicine. ed. 2. Williams and Wilkins, Baltimore. 1996
58. Plaugher G. and Lopes M. *Scoliosis.* In: Plaugher G. and Lopes M. Textbook of Clinical Chiropractic: A Specific Biomechanical Approach. Williams and Wilkins, Baltimore, Maryland. 1993
59. Norris C. The muscle debate. Journal of Bodywork and Movement Therapies 4(4):232-235. 2000
60. Jull G, Janda V. Muscles and motor control in low back pain: assessment and management. In: Twomey LT,

Taylor JR. (eds): Physical therapy of the low back, Clinics in Physical Therapy. Churchill Livingstone, New York. 1987

61. Janda V. Muscle Function Testing. London, Butterworth. 1983

62. Field D. Anatomy. *Palpation and surface markings.* ed. 2. Butterworth-Heinemann, Oxford. 1997

63. Myers T. Anatomy Trains: *Myofascial Meridians for Manual and Movement Therapists.* Churchill Lingingstone. 2001

64. Vleeming A, Mooney V, Dorman T, Snijders C, Stoeckart R (eds) Movement, stability and low back pain: the essential role of the pelvis. Churchill Livingstone, New York. 1997

65. Gluck N, Liebenson C. Paradoxal muscle function. Journal of Bodywork and Movement Therapies 1(4): 219-222

66. Guides to the Evaluation of Permanent Impairment. ed. 3. Chicago, American Medical Association. 1988

67. Liebenson C. Manual resistance techniques in mobilization. In: Chaitow L (ed) Muscle energy techniques. Churchill Livingstone, Edinburgh. 2001

68. LaBan MM, Raptou AD, Johnson EW. Electromyographic study of function of iliopsoas muscle. *Arch Phys Med Rehabil* 46:676-679. 1965

69. Nachemson A, Elfstron G. Intravital Dynamic Pressure Measurements in Lumbar Discs. Stockholm, Almqvista Wiksell. 1970

70. Vera-Garcia FJ, Grenier SG, McGill SM. Abdominal muscle response during curl-ups on both stable and labile surfaces. *Phys Ther* 80(6):564-9. 2000

71. Axler CT, McGill SM. Low back loads over a variety of abdominal exercises: searching for the safest abdominal challenge. *Medicine and Science in Sports and Exercise* 29(6): 804-811. 1997

72. Juker D, McGill SM, Kropf P, Steffen T. Quantitative intramuscular myoelectric activity of lumbar portions of psoas and the abdominal wall during a wide variety of tasks. *Medicine and Science in Sports and Exercise* 30(2): 301-310. 1998

73. Liebenson C, Chapman S. Lumbar Spine: Making a Rehabilitation Prescription, Program 1. *Rehabilitation of the Spine/Video series* Williams and Wilkins. 1998

74. Byl NN, Sinnot PL. Variations in balance and body sway. *Spine* 16:325-330. 1991

75. Slausberg C. Educational Handout sheet. 2002

76. Merriam-Webster's collegiate dictionary. ed. 11. Merriam-Webster, Incorporated, Springfield, Massachusetts, U.S.A. 2004

77. Bigos S, Bowyer O, Braen G, et al: Acute Low Back Problems in Adults. Clinical Practice Guideline. Rockville, MD, U.S. Department of Health and Human Services, Public Health Service, Agency for Health Care Policy and Research. 1994.

78. Clinical Standards Advisory Group: Back Pain. London, HMSO. 1994

79. Jacob G, McKenzie R. Spinal Therapeutics Based on Responses to Loading. In: Liebenson C. Rehabilitation of the Spine: A practitioner's manual. Lippincott Williams and Wilkins. 1996

80. Adams M, Bogduk N, Burton K, Dolan P. The Biomechanics of Back Pain. Churchill Livingstone, Edinburgh. 2002

81. White A, Gordon S. Synopsis: Workshop on idiopathic low back Pain. *Spine,* 7:141-149. 1982

82. Bogduk N, Twomey L. Clinical anatomy of the lumbar spine. ed. 2. Churchill Livingstone, New York. 1991

83. Adams M, Hutton W. The relevance of torsion to the mechanical derangement of the lumbar spine. *Spine,* 6: 241-248. 1981

84. Kirkaldy-Willis W, Bernard, Jr. T. Managing Low Back Pain. ed. 4. Churchill Livingstone, San Francisco. 1999

85. Adams M, Dolan P, Hutton W. Diurnal variations in the stresses on the lumbar spine. *Spine* 12 (2): 130-37. 1987

86. Buckwalter, J. Spine update: Ageing and degeneration of the human intervertebral disc. *Spine,* 20: 1307-1314. 1995

87. Marchand F, Ahmed AM. Investigation of the laminate structure of lumbar disc annulus fibrosis. *Spine,* 15:402-410. 1990

88. Solomonow M, Zhou B, Harris M, Lu Y, and Baratta R. The ligamento-muscular stabilizing system of the spine. *Spine,* 23:2552-2562. 2000

89. Kapandji I.A. The Physiology of the Joints, Vol. III. The Trunk & The Vertebral Column. Churchill

Livingstone. 1974

90. McGill S, Brown S. Creep response of the lumbar spine to prolonged lumbar flexion. *Clinical Biomechanics,* 7:43. 1992

91. Farfan H. Mechanical disorders of the low back. Philadelphia: Lea and Febiger, 1973.

92. Panjabi M, Krag M, Chung T. Effects of disc injury on mechanical behavior of the human spine. *Spine,* 9:707-713. 1984

93. McCall I, Park W, Obrien J. Induced pain referral from posterior lumbar elements in normal subjects. *Spine,* 4:441. 1979.

94. Cripton P, Berlemen U, Visarino H, Begeman P, Nolte L, and Prasad P. Response of the lumbar spine due to shear loading. In: *Injury prevention through biomechanics* (pg.111). Detroit: Wayne State University. 1995

95. Yingling V, McGill S. Mechanical properties and failure mechanics of the spine under posterior shear load: Observations from a porcine model. *Journal of Spinal Disorders,* 12 (6):501-508. 1999

96. Yingling V, McGill S. Anterior shear of spinal motion segments: Kinematics, kinetics and resulting injuries observed in porcine spine model. *Spine,* 24 (18):1882-1889. 1999

97. Biering-Sorensen F. Physical measurements as risk indications for low back trouble over a one-year period. *Spine* 9:106-119. 1984

98. Luoto S, Heliovaara M, Hurri H, Alaranta H. Static back endurance and the risk of low back pain. Clinical Biomechanics 10:323-324. 1995

99. Okada M. An electromyographic estimation of the relative muscular load in different human postures. *J Human Ergol* 1:75-93. 1972

100. Nemeth G. On hip and lumbar biomechanics. A study of joint load and muscular activity. *Scand J Rehabil Med* 10 (Suppl):1-35. 1984

101. Chaitow L (ed) Muscle energy techniques. Churchill Livingstone, Edinburgh. 2001

102. Clark M. A scientific approach to understanding kinetic chain dysfunction. National Academy of Sports Medicine (Publishers). Thousand Oaks, CA. 2000

103. Dorland's Illustrated Medical Dictionary. ed 25. WB Saunders, Philadelphia. 1974

104. Battie M, Bigos S, Fisher L, Spengler D, Hansson T, Nachemson A, and Wortley M. The role of spinal flexibility in back pain complaints within industry: A prospective study. *Spine,* 15:768-773. 1990

105. Biering-Sorenson F. Physical measurements as risk indications for low-back trouble over a one-year period. *Spine,* 9 106-119. 1984

106. Gracovetsky S. The spinal engine. Wien: Springer-Verlag. 1988

107. Adams M, McNally D, Chinn H, and Dolan P. Posture and the compressive strength of the lumbar spine. *Clinical Biomechanics,* 9: 5-14. 1994

108. Gunning J, , Callaghan J, and McGill S. The role of prior loading history and spinal posture on the compressive tolerance and type of failure in the spine using a porcine trauma model. *Clinical Biomechanics,* 16 (6): 471-480. 2001

109. Gracovetsky S. Function of the Spine. J Biomed Eng 8:220. 1986

110. McGill S, Kippers V. Transfer of loads between lumbar tissues during the flexion relaxation phenomenon. *Spine,* 19(19):2190. 1994

111. Nachemson A, Morris J.M. In vivo measurements of intradiscal pressure. *Journal of Bone and Joint Surgery,* 46A:1077. 1964

112. Nachemson A, Andersson G.B.J. and Schultz A.B. Valsalva manoeuvre biomechanics: Effects on lumbar trunk loads of elevated intra-abdominal pressure. *Spine,* 11 (5):476. 1986

113. Krag M, Byrne K, Gilbertson L, and Haugh L. Failure of intraabdominal pressurization to reduce erector spinae loads during lifting tasks (pg. 87). In: *Proceedings of the North American Congress on Biomechanics.* Montreal, August 25-27. 1986

114. Heinking K, Jones III J, Kappler R. Pelvis and sacrum. In: Ward R (ed) American Osteopathic Association: foundations for osteopathic medicine. Williams and Wilkins, Baltimore. 1997.

115. Janda V. Muscle strength in relation to muscle length, pain and muscle imbalance. In: Harms-Rindahl K (ed): Muscle Strength. New York, Churchill Livingstone. 1993.

116. Eisler P. *Die Muskein des Stammes.* Gustav Fischer, Jena, 1912 (p. 653-656). In: Simons, G, David and Travell G, Janet. Myofascial Pain and Dysfunction: The Trigger Point Manual ed. 2 vol. 2. Williams and Wilkins. 1999

117. McKenzie RA. The Lumbar Spine: *Mechanical Diagnosis an d Therapy.* Spinal Publications, Ltd., New Zealand. 1981

118. Shea M. Myofascial Release: *a manual for the spine and extremities.* Shea Educational Group, Juno Beach, Florida. 1993

119. Barnes M. The basic science of myofascial release. *Journal of Bodywork and Movement Therapies.* 1(4):231-238. 1997

120. Lowen A. Bioenergetics. *The revolutionary therapy that uses the language of the body to heal the problems of the mind.* Penguin Books, New York. 1976

121. Basmajian JV. Muscles Alive. Williams and Wilkins, Baltimore. 1974

122. Nachemson A. Electromyographic studies on the vertebral portion of the psoas muscle. *Acta Orthop Scand* 37:177-190. 1966

123. Jones L. Spontaneous release by positioning. The DO 4:109-116. 1964

124. Goodheart G. Applied kinesiology. Workshop procedure manual, 21st edn. Privately published, Detroit. 1984

125. Walther D. Applied kinesiology synopsis. Systems DC, Pueblo, Colorado. 1988.

126. Jones L. Strain and counterstrain. Academy of Applied Osteopathy, Colorado Springs. 1981

127. Roskopf G. MAT, Muscle Activation Techniques; "The Science behind MAT. Online. Available: www.muscleactivation.com. 2006

128. Cousins, G. Conscious Eating. North Atlantic Books, Berkeley, California. 2000

129. Dolan P, Earley M, Adams M A. Bending and compressive stresses acting on the lumbar spine during lifting activities. J. Biomech 27:1237-1248. 1994

130. Mannion AF, Adams MA, Dolan P. Sudden and unexpected loading generates high forces on the lumbar spine. Spine 25:842-852. 2000

131. Dolan P, Adams MA. Recent advances in lumbar spine mechanics and their significance for modeling. Clin Biomech 16 (Suppl. 1):S8-S16, 2001

132. Krag MH, Cohen M C, Haugh L D et al. Body height change during upright and recumbent posture. Spine 15: 202-207.1990

133. Adams MA, Dolan P. Time-dependent changes in the lumbar spine's resistance to bending. Clin Biomech 11: 194-200. 1996

134. Dolan P, Adams M A. Influence of lumbar and hip mobility on the bending stresses acting on the lumbar spine. Clin Biomech 8: 185-192. 1993.

135. Adams M A, McNally D S, Chinn H et all. Posture and the compressive strength of the lumbar spine. Clin Biomech 9:5-14. 1994

136. Granata K P, Marras W S. The influence of trunk muscle coactivity on dynamic spinal loads. Spine 20:913-919. 1995

137. Bogduk N. Clinical Anatomy of the Lumbar Spine and Sacrum, ed. 3. 1997.

138. Richardson C A, Hodges P, Hides J. Therapeutic exercise for lumbopelvic stabilization. *A motor control approach for the treatment and prevention of low back pain.* ed 2. Churchill Livingstone, New York. 2004

139. Comeford M, Mottram S. Functional stability re-training. Manual Therapy 6(1)3-14. 2001

140. Comeford M, Mottram S. Movement and stability of dysfunction-contemporary developments. Manual Therapy 6(1)15-26. 2001

141. McGill S, Juker D, Kropf P. Quantitative intramuscular myoelectric activity of quadratus lumborum during a wide variety of tasks. Clinical Biomechanics 11:170-172. 1996

142. Basmajian JV, DeLuca CJ. Muscles Alive. ed.5. Williams and Wilkins, Baltimore. 1985

143. Letts RM, Quanbury AO. Paraspinal muscle activity . *Phys Sportsmed* 6(9): 80-90. 1978

144. Bogduk N, Macintosh J E, Pearcy M J. A universal model of the lumbar back muscles in the upright position. Spine 17: 897-913. 1992

145. Calliet R. Soft tissue pain and disability. ed. 3. F.A. Davis Company. 1996

146. Hides J, Stokes M, Saide M, Jull G, Cooper D. Evidence of lumbar multifidus muscle wasting ipsilateral to symptoms in patients with acute/subacute low back pain. Spine 19:165-172. 1994

147. Hides J, Richardson C A, Jull G. Multifidus muscle recovery is not automatic following resolution of acute first episode low back pain. Spine 21:2763-2769. 1996

148. Macintosh J, Valencia F, Bogduk N, Munro R. The morphology of the human lumbar multifidus. Clinical Biomechanics 1:196-204. 1986

149. Johnson J. The Multifidus: *Back Pain Solution.* New Harbinger Publications, INC, California. 2002

150. Hodges P, Richardson C A. Relationship between limb movement speed and associated contraction of the trunk muscles. Ergonomics 40: 1220-1230. 1997

151. Moseley G, Hodges P, Gandevia S. Deep and superficial fibers of lumbar multifidus are differentially active during voluntary arm movements. Spine 27:E29-E36. 2002

152. Aurin A, Latash M. Directional specificity of postural muscles in feed-forward postural reactions during fast voluntary arm movements. Experimental Brain Research 103:323-332. 1995

153. Hodges P, Cresswell A G, Thorstensson A. Preparatory trunk motion accompanies rapid upper limb movement. Experimental Brain Research 124:69-79. 1999

154. Rantanen J, Rissanen A, Kalimo H. Lumbar muscle fiber size and type distribution in normal subjects. *European Spine Journal* 3:333-335. 1994

155. Weber B R, Grob D, Dvorak J, Muntener M. Posterior surgical approach to the lumbar spine and its effect on the multifidus muscle. *Spine* 22:1765-1772. 1997

156. Coste J, Delecoeuillerie G, Cohen de Lara A, LePark J M, Paolaggi J B. Clinical course and prognostic factors in acute low back pain: An inception cohort study in primary care practice. *British Medical Journal.* 308:577-588. 1994

157. Gilbert J R, Taylor D W, Hildebrand A, Evans C. Clinical trial of common treatments for low back pain in family practice. *British Medical Journal.* 291:791-794. 1985

158. Danneels L A, van der Straeten G G, Cambier D C, Witvrouw E E, Cuyper H J. CT imaging of trunk muscles in chronic low back pain patients and healthy control subjects. *European Spine Journal.* 9:266-272. 2000

159. Donisch E W, Basmajian J V. Electromyography of deep back muscles in man. *Am J Anat.* 133:25-36. 1972

160. Nitz A J, Peck D. Comparison of muscle spindle concentrations in large and small human epaxial muscles acting in parallel combinations. *American Surgeon.* 52:273-277. 1986

161. Rolf I. The body is a plastic medium. Boulder, CO: Rolf Institute. 1959

162. Currier D, Nelson R, eds. Dynamics of human biologic tissues. Philadelphia: FA Davis. 1992

163. Varela F, Frenk S. The organ of form. Journal of Social Biological Structure. 10:73-83. 1987

164. Tesh K M, Dunn J, Evans J H. The abdominal muscles and vertebral stability. *Spine,* 12 (5):501. 1987

165. Macintosh J E, Bogduk N, Gracovetsky S. The biomechanics of the thoracolumbar fascia. *Clinical Biomechanics,* 2:78. 1987

166. McGill S M, Norman R W. The potential of lumbodorsal fascia forces to generate back extension moments during squat lifts. *Journal of Biomechanical Engineering,* 10:312. 1988

167. Bogduk N, Macintosh J E. The applied anatomy of the thoracolumbar fascia. *Spine,* 9:164. 1984

168. Yahia L H, Newman N, Rivard C H. Neurohistology of the lumbar spine. Acta Orthopedica Scandinavica, 59:508-512. 1988

169. Lockhart R D, Hamilton G F, Fyfe F W. Anatomy of the Human Body. J.B. Lippincott Company. Philadelphia. 1972

170. Pate D. Radiographic terms for disc herniations. *Dynamic Chiropractic.* Nov 15, vol 17, issue 24. 1999

171. Roy S H, DeLuca C J, Snyder-Mackler L, Emley M S, Crenshaw R L, Lyons J P. Fatigue, recovery and low back pain in varsity rowers. Medicine and Science in Sports and Exercise. 22:463-469. 1990

172. Hodges P, Gandevia S C. Changes in intra-abdominal pressure during postural and respiratory activation of the human diaphragm. *Journal of Applied Physiology.* 89:967-976. 2000

173. Hodges P. Changes in motor planning of feedforward postural response of the trunk muscles in low back pain.Experimental Brain Research. 141:261-266. 2001

174. Hodges P, Richardson C A A. Inefficient muscular stabilisation of the lumbar spine associated with low back pain: a motor control evaluation of transversus abdominis. *Spine* 21:2640-2650. 1996

175. Hodges P, Moseley G L, Gabrielsson A H, Gandevia S C. Acute experimental pain changes postural recruitment of the trunk muscles in pain-free humans. Experimental Brain Research, in press. 2003

176. Hodges P, Richardson C A A. Feedforward contractionof transverse abdominis is not influenced by the direction of arm movement. Experimental Brain Research. 114:62-370. 1997

177. Hodges P, Richardson C A A. Contraction of the abdominal muscles associated with movement of the lower limb. *Physical Therapy.* 77:132-144. 1997

178. Hodges P, Butler J E, McKenzie D, Gandevia S C. Contraction of the human diaphragm during postural adjustments. *Journal of Physiology.* 505: 239-548. 1997

179. Gahery Y, Massion J. Co-ordination between posture and movement. Trends in Neuroscience. 4:199-202. 1981

180. Gurfinkel V S. The mechanisms of postural regulation in man. Soviet Scientific Reviews. Section F. Physiology and General Biology. 7:59-89. 1994

181. Hodges P, Gandevia S C. Activation of the human diaphragm during a repetitive postural task. *Journal of Physiology*. 522:165-175. 2000

182. Hodges P, Heijnen I, Gandevia S C, Reduced postural activity of the diaphragm in humans when respiratory demand is increased. *Journal of Physiology*. 537:999-1008. 2001

183. Sapsford R R, Hodges P, Richardson C A A, Cooper D H, Markwell S J, Jull G A. Co-activation of the abdominal and pelvic floor muscles during voluntary exercises. Neuromuscular and Urodynamics. 20:31-42. 2001

184. Hodges P. Sapsford R R, Pengel H M. Feedforward activity of the pelvic floor muscles proceeds rapid upper limb movements. In: Proceedings of the VIIth International Physiology Congress, Sydney, Australia. 2002

185. Cresswell A G, Oddsson L, Thorstensson A. Compensatory responses to sudden perturbations of the trunk during standing. In: Horak W M, Horak F. (eds) Posture and gait: control mechanisms. University of Oregon Books, Portland, OR, pp 380-383. 1992

186. Hodges P. Is there a role for transverses abdominis in lumbo-pelvic stability? Manual Therapy 4: 74-86. 1999

187. Morris J M, Benner F, Lucas D B. An electromyographic study of the intrinsic muscles of the back in man. *Journal of Anatomy*. 96:509-520. 1962

188. Hodges P, Cresswell A G, Daggfeld K, Thorstensson A. In vivo measurement of the effect of intra-abdominal pressure on the human spine. *Journal of Biomechanics*. 34:347-353. 2001

189. Hodges P, Eriksson A E M, Shirley D, Gandevia S C. Intra-abdominal pressure can directly increase stiffness of the lumbar spine. *Journal of Biomechanics*, in press. 2003

190. Shirley D, Hodges P, Eriksson A E M, Gandevia S C. Spinal stiffness changes throughout the respiratory cycle. *Journal of Applied Physiology*, in press. 2003

191. Sihvonen T, Partanen J, Hanninen O, Soimakallio S. Electric behaviour of low back muscles during lumbar pelvic rhythm in low back pain patients and healthy controls. Archives of Physical Medicine and Rehabilitation. 72:1080-1087. 1991

192. Johansson H, Sjölonder P, Sojka P. A sensory role for the cruciate ligaments. Clinical Orthopaedics and Related Research 268:161-178. 1991

193. Massion J. Postural control systems in developmental perspective. Neuroscience and Biobehavioural Reviews. 22:465-472. 1998

194. Panjabi M M. The stabilizing system of the spine. Part II. Neutral zone and stability hypothesis. *Journal of spine disorders* 5:390-397. 1992

195. Santaguida P L, McGill S M. The psoas major muscle: a three dimensional geometric study. *Journal of Biomechanics*. 28:339-345. 1995

196. Stokes I A, Henry S M, Single R M. Surface EMG electrodes do not accurately record from lumbar multifidus muscles. *Clinical Biomechanics*. 18:9-13. 2003

197. Yoshihara K, Shirai Y, Nakayama Y, Uesaka S. Histochemical changes in the multifidus muscle in patients with lumbar intervertebral disc herniation. *Spine*. 26:622-626. 2001

198. Zhao W, Kawaguchi Y, Matsui H, Kanamori M, Kimura T. Histochemistry and morphology of the multifidus muscle in lumbar disc herniation: Comparitive study between diseased and normal sides. *Spine*. 25: 2191-2199. 2000

199. Lehman G, McGill S M. Quantification of the differences in EMG magnitude between upper and lower rectus abdominis during selected trunk exercises. *Physical Therapy*. 81: 1096-1101. 2001

200. Gustein R R. The role of abdominal fibrositis in functional digestion. *Miss Val Med J*. 66: 114-124. 1944

201. Melnick J. Trigger areas and refractory pain in duodenal ulcer. *NY State J Med* 57:1073-1076. 1957

202. Travell J. Symposium on mechanism and management of pain syndromes. *Proc Rudolf Virchow Med S oc*. 16:126-136. 1957

203. Németh G. On hip and lumbar biomechanics. A study of joint load and muscular activity. *Scand J Reh abil Med* (Supp. 1) 10:1-35. 1984

204. Myers T. The deep six. Part I. In: Massage and Bodywork. June/July. 94-100. 2003

205. Myers T. The deep six. Part II. In: Massage and Bodywork. August/September. 94-108. 2003

206. Kapandji I.A. The Physiology of the Joints, Vol. II. The lower limb, ed. 5. Churchill Livingstone, Edinburgh. 1987

207. Mann RA, Moran GT, Dougherty SE. Comparative electromyoghraphy of the lower extremity in jogging, running, and sprinting. *Am J Sports Med.* 14:501-510. 1986

208. Sutherland DH, Cooper L, Daniel D. The role of the ankle plantar flexors in normal walking. *J Bone Joint Surg [Am].* 62:354-363. 1980

209. Sutherland DH. An electromyoghraphic study of the planter flexors of the ankle in normal walking on the level. *J Bone Joint Surg [Am].* 48:66-71. 1966

210. Cordo PJ, Nashner LM. Properties of postural adjustments associated with rapid arm movements. *J Neurophysiol* 47:287-382. 1982

211. Thie J. Touch for Health: A practical guide to natural health with acupressure touch and massage. DeVorss and Company ed. 3. 1998

212. Chek P. Scientific core conditioning; *Correspondence Course.* Encinitas CA: C.H.E.K. Institute. 1998

213. Kirkaldy-Willis W. Pathology and pathogenesis of low back pain, Ch. 5. In: Kirkaldy-Willis W, Bernard, Jr. T. Managing Low Back Pain. ed. 4. Churchill Livingstone, San Francisco. 1999

214. Nachemson A. The load on lumbar discs in different positions of the body. *Clinical Orthopedics and Related Research,* 45:107. 1966

215. Kelsey J.L. An epidemiological study of the relationship between occupations and acute herniated lumbar intervertebral discs. *International Journal of Epidemiology,* 4:197-205. 1975

216. Holmes AD, Hukins DWL, Freemont AJ. End-plate displacement during compression of lumbar vertebra-disc-vertebra segments and the mechanisms of failure. *Spine,* 18:1280135. 1993

217. Videman T, Nurminen M, Troup JDG. Lumbar spinal pathology in cadaveric material in relation to history of back pain, occupation and physical loading. *Spine,* 15 (8):728. 1990

218. Pope MH. Risk indicators in low back pain. *Annals of Medicine,* 21:387-392. 1989

219. U.S. Department of Labor. Back injuries associated with lifting. (Bulletin 2144). Washington, DC: Government Printing Office. 1985

220. Andersson GB. Epidemiologic aspects of low back pain in industry. *Spine,* 6:53-60, 1981

221. Marras WS, Lavender SA, Leurgens SE, Fathallah FA, Ferguson SA, Allread WG, Rajulu SL. Biomechanical risk factors for occupationally related low back disorders. *Ergonomics,* 38:377-410, 1995

222. Punnett L, Fine LJ, Keyerserling WM, Herrin GD, Chaffin DA. Back disorders and non-neutral trunk postures of automobile assembly workers. *Scandinavian Journal of Rheumatology,* 33:442-448. 1991

223. Snook SH. Low back in industry. In: White AA, Gordon SL. (Eds.), *Symposium on idiopathic low back pain.* St. Louis: Mosby. 1982

224. Gordon SJ, et al. Mechanism of disc rupture-A preliminary report. *Spine,* 16:450. 1991

225. Adams MA, Hutton WC. Gradual disc prolapse. *Spine,* 10:524. 1985

226. Adams MA, Mannion AF, Dolan P. Personal risk factors for first-time low back pain. *Spine* 24:2497-2505, 1999

227. Mannion AF, Dolan P, Adams MA. Psychological questionnaires: do 'abnormal' scores precede or follow first-time low back pain? *Spine* 21:2603-2611. 1996

228. Nachemson A, Vingard E. Influences of individual factors and smoking on neck and low back pain. In: Nachemson A, Jonsson E, (eds). Neck and back pain: the scientific evidence of causes, diagnosis and treatment. Lippincot, Williams and Wilkins, Philadelphia, 79-96. 2000

229. Papageorgiou AC, Croft PR, Thomas E et al. Influence of previous pain experience on the episode incidence of low back pain: results from the South Manchester Back Pain Study. *Pain* 66:181-185, 1996

230. ReigoT. The nature of back pain in general population: a longitudinal study. PhD thesis, Linkoping University. 2001

231. Waddell G, Burton AK. Occupational health guidelines for the management of low back pain at work-evidence review. Faculty of Occupational Medicine, London, 2000

232. Croft PR, Macfarlane GJ, Papageorgiou AC et al. Outcome of low back pain in general practice: a prospective study. BMJ 316:1356-1359. 1998

233. Burton AK, Tillotson KM, Main CJ et al. Four-year follow up of patients with low back pain – outcomes and predictors. *Spine* (submitted) 2001

234. Cox JM. Low back pain: Mechanism, diagnosis, and treatment. ed. 5. Williams and Wilkins, Baltimore, 1990

235. Stone MH, Plisk SS, Stone ME, Schilling BK, O'Bryant HS, Pierce KC. Athletic performance development: Volume load-1 set vs. multiple sets, training velocity and training variation. *NCSA J* 20(6):22-31. 1998

236. Kaneko M, Fuchimoto T, Toji H, Suei K. Training effect of different loads on the force-velocity relationship and mechanical power output in human muscle. *Scand J Sports Sci* 5(2):50-5. 1983

237. Sale DG. Neural adaptation in strength and power training. In: *Human Muscle Power.* Jones NL, McCartney N, McComas AJ (eds). Champaign, IL: Human Kinetics. 1986

238. Chu DA. Explosive power and strength. Champaign, IL: Human Kinetics. 1996

239. Ebben WP, Watts PB. A review of combined weight training and plyometric training models: complex training. *Strength and Cond* 20(5):18-27. 1998

240. Stone MH. Considerations in gaining a strength power training effect. *NSCA J* 4(1):22-4, 54, 1982

241. Schmidtbleicher D. Training for power events. In: *Strength and power in sports.* Chem PV (ed). Boston: Blackwell Scientific. 1992

242. Ebben WP, Blackard DO. Complex training with combined explosive weight and plyometric exercises. *Olymp Coach* 7(4):11-2, 1997

243. Ebben WP, Blackard DO. Paired for strength: a look at combined weight training with plyometric exercises with a focus on vertical jump improvement. *Train Cond* 8(3):55-63, 1998

244. Hakkinen K, Komi PV. Electromypgraphic changes during strength training and detraining. *Med Sci Sports Exerc* 15(6):455-460. 1983

245. Hakkinen K, Allen M, Komi PV. Changes in isometric force and relaxation time, electromyographic and muscle fiber characteristics of human skeletal muscle during strength training and detraining. *Acta Physiol Scand* 125:573-585. 1985

246. Hakkinen K, Komi PV. Training-induced changes in neuromuscular performance under voluntary and reflex conditions. *Euro J Exerc Physiol* 55: 147-155. 1986.

247. Enoka RM. Muscle strength and its development: new perspectives. *Sports Med* 6: 146-168. 1988.

248. Rutherford OM, Jones DA. The role of learning and coordination in strength training. *Euro J Appl Physiol* 55: 100-105. 1986.

249. Narici MV, Kayser B. Hypertonic response of human skeletal muscle to strength training in hypoxia and normoxia. *Eur J Appl Physiol* 70:213-219. 1995

250. Narici MV, Roi GS, Landoni L, Minetti AE, Cerretelli P. Changes in force, cross-sectional area and neural activation during strength training and detraining of the human quadriceps. *Euro J Appl Physiol* 59:310-319. 1989

251. Komi PV, Vitasalo JT, Rauramaa R, Vihko V. Effect of isometric strength training on mechanical, electrical, and metabolic aspects of muscle function. *Euro J Appl Physiol* 40: 45-55. 1978.

252. Moritani T, deVries HA. Neural factors versus hypertrophy in the time course of muscle strength gain. *Amer J Phys Med* 58(3) 115-129. 1979

253. Staron RS, Karapondo DL, Kraemer WJ et al. Skeletal muscle adaptations during early phase of heavy resistance training in men and women. *J Appl Physiol* 76:1247-1255. 1994

254. Mayhew TP, Rothstein JM, Finucane SD, Lamb RL. Muscular adaptation to concentric and eccentric exercise at equal power levels. *Med Sci Sports Exerc* 27:868-873. 1995

255. Sale, DG. Neural adaptation to resistance training. *Med Sci Sports Exerc* 20(5):S1 35-45. 1988

256. Milner-Brwon HS, Stein RB, Yemm R. Changes in firing rate of human motor units during linearly changing voluntary contractions. *J Physiol* 230:371-390. 1973

257. Bernardi M, Solomonow M, Nguyen G. Motor unit recruitment strategies change with skill acquisition. *Euro J Appl Physiol* 74:52-59. 1996

258. Haig A, et all. Prospective evidence for change in parasinal muscle activity after herniated nucleus pulpous. *Spine* 18: 926-930. 1993.

259. Tran N. Scoliosis. Online. Available: www.spinalmedicine.com/articles/scoliosis.html. 1997

260. Dalton E. Straight Talk; *Symptomatic Scoliosis.* In: Massage and Bodywork. April/May, 62-70. 2006

261. Richardson C A, Snijders C J, Hides J A, Damen L, Pas M S, Storm J. The relation between the transverses abdominis muscles, sacroiliac joint mechanics, and low back pain. Spine 27:399-405. 2002

262. Richardson C A, Jull G A, Richardson B A. A dysfunction of the deep abdominal muscles exists in low back pain patients. In: Proceedings of the World Confederation of Physical Therapists, Washington, DC, pg 932. 1995

263. Hides J, Jull G A, Richardson C A. A clinical palpation test to check the activation of the deep stabilizing muscles of the spine. International Sports Medicine Journal 1:(4). 2000

264. Green RJ, Webb JN, Maxwell MH. The nature of virus-like particles in the paraxial muscles of idiopathic scoliosis. J. Pathol. 1979, Sep;129(1):9-12

265. Webb JN, Gillespie WJ. Virus-like particles in paraspinal muscles in scoliosis. Br Med J. 1976 Oct 16;2(6041):912-913

266. Stirling AL, et al., Association between sciatica and Propionibacterium acnes. Lancet 2001:V357.

267. Baechle TR and Earle RW. (2000) Essentials of Strength Training and Conditioning: 2nd Edition. Champaign, IL: Human Kinetics

268. Bompa TO. 1999 Periodization Training for Sports. Champaign,IL: Human Kinetics

269. Fleck SJ and Kraemer WJ. (2004) Designing Resistance Training Programs, 3rd Edition. Champaign,IL: Human Kinetics

270. Knuttgen HG and Kraemer WJ. terminology and measurement in exercise performance. J Appl Sport Sci Res. 1987 1:1-10

271. Newton RU, Murphy AJ, Humphries BJ, Wilson GJ, Kraemer WJ, Hakkinen K. Influence of load and stretch shortening cycle on the kinematics, kinetics and muscle activation that occurs during explosive upper-body movements. Eur J Appl Physiol Occup Physiol. 1997;75(4):333-42

272. Garhammer J. A review of power output studies of Olympic and powerlifting: Methedology, performance prediction and evaluation tests. J Strength Cond Res. 1993 7(2):76-89

273. Adams K, O'Shea JP, O'Shea KL and Climstein M. The effect of six weeks of squat, plyometric and squat-plyometric training on power production. J Appl Sport Sci Res. 1992 6:36-41

274. Clutch D, Wilson C, McGown C and Bryce GR. The effect of depth jumps and weight training on leg strength and vertical jump. Res Quarterly. 54:5-10

275. Wilson GJ, Newton RU, Murphy AJ, Humphries BJ. The optimal training load for the development of dynamic athletic performance. Med Sci Sports Exerc. 1993 Nov;25(11):1279-86

276. Behm DG, Sale DG. Velocity specificity of resistance training. Sports Med. 1993 Jun;15(6):374-88

277. Bosco C and Komi PV. (1980) Influence of countermovement amplitude in potentiation of muscualr performance. Biomenchanics VII proceeding (pp129-135). Baltimore:University Park Press

278. Schmidtbleicher D. Training for power events. In Komi PV (ed) Strength and Power in Sport (pp381-395). Oxford, UK: Blackwell Scientific

279. Evans, RC. Illustrated Essentials in Orthopedic Physical Assessment. St. Louis, Missouri: Mosby, 1994.

280. Hoppenfeld, S. Physical Examination of the Spine and Extremities. San Mateo, CA: Appleton & Lange, 1976.

281. Cipriano, J. Photographic Manual of Regional Orthopaedic and Neurological Tests. 2nd edition. Atlanta Georgia: Williams and Wilkins, 1991

282. Liebenson, C. Vleeming's active SLR test as a screen for lumbopelvic dysfunction. *Dynamic Chiropractic*, Feb. 24, 2003. www.chiroweb.com/archives/21/05/13.html.

Glossary/Index

A

Acute pain, 78
Agonist, 4, 13, 27, 34, 48, 49, 185
Annulus, 86-88, 94
Antagonist, 2-4, 7, 8, 27, 34-37, 39-41, 46, 48, 57, 59, 75, 140, 225, 285, 290
Arthrokinetic inhibition, 3, 4, 13, 75, 240
Assessment
        asymptomatic, 21, 24
        breathing, 176
        charts, 194-196
        functional strength, 28-29, 187-193
        muscle testing, 27-28, 176-187
        palpation, 27, 174-176
        posture, 26-27, 149, 153-164
        red flags, 26, 149
        ROM, 27, 164-174
        symptomatic, 21
Asymptomatic, 3, 20-22, 24, 73, 128, 147, 153, 207, 213

B

Bed rest, 93
Big picture, 238
Biomechanics of lifting, 83-85
Breathing, 36, 38

C

Central nervous system (CNS), 5,6,10, 11, 13-15, 20, 99, 104
Chronic pain, 1, 21, 22, 73, 99, 157, 244, 303,
Closed chain – *Exercises performed where the hand or foot is fixed and does not move. The hand/foot remains in constant contact with the surface, usually the ground or the base of a machine. These exercises are typically weight bearing exercises.*

Concentric, 36, 53
Contralateral – opposite side
CORE, 13-15, 56, 80
Corrective exercise, 2-3, 22
Curl-ups, 105, 108, 177, 178, 202, 227, 228, 230, 234 - *There are two main phases of a sit-up. The first is the curling of the trunk, which should mostly involve the abdominals, and is called the 'curl-up.' The second phase is flexion at the hip, which can occur only from activation of the hip flexor muscles, and is called the 'sit-up.' Completing the second phase creates more*

intradiscal pressure and compression forces than simply doing the trunk curl.

D

D.A.M.'s - Daily Activity Modifications, 68
Deconditioning, 93, 303
Deloading, 10, 78, 301
Diaphragm, 11, 13, 15, 79, 84, 90, 97, 101-103, 107, 112, 113, 176
Disc/Herniations, 7, 16, 40, 75, 78, 82, 84-90, 92-94, 101, 107, 116, 123, 124, 126, 127, 147-149, 151, 197-200, 227, 241, 294, 295

E

Eccentric, 36, 53
End plate (vertebrae), 86, 87, 94
Energy sling of the back, 116, 120, 145
Erector spinae (E.S.), 4, 8, 9, 11, 12, 15, 81-83, 97, 101-105, 107, 108, 114-127, 129-130, 132-133, 135-136, 142, 153, 161, 166- 167, 175, 184-185, 188, 198, 200, 201, 203, 219, 222, 224, 228, 231, 234, 250, 255
Extension exercise guidelines, 81-82
External oblique, 9, 15, 56, 95, 97-101, 115, 156, 180, 192, 207-209, 212, 228

F

Facet (Joint), 74, 84, 86-91. 93, 108, 122, 127, 128, 140, 148, 152, 165, 166, 175, 198, 218, 220
Facet syndrome - *Synovitis, stiffness or laxity in the posterior facet joints, degenerated articular cartilage, and enlarged and locked facets are all possible depending on the stage of degeneration.*

Facilitated, 8, 153
Fascia, 3, 6, 8, 11, 22, 35, 38, 39, 46, 74, 83, 84, 91, 92, 94, 95, 97, 102, 103, 106, 175, 176, 205, 226
Fibrosis, 7 – *The formation of excessive fibrous tissue, as in a reparative or reactive process; as opposed to formation of fibrous tissue as a normal part of the tissue or organ.*

Fitness vs. Health, 16-17
Functional tests, 187-193

G

Gait, 26-27, 74, 97, 102, 164, 218-219

disorder can then be quickly identified through objective findings for each individual patient. The McKenzie classification of spinal pain provides reproducible means of separating patients with apparently similar presentations into definable sub-groups (syndromes) to determine appropriate treatment. As defined by the McKenzie Institute

Motor control, 10, 13, 14, 79, 177, 236
Motor patterns, 27, 47, 79
Multifidus, 9-13, 15, 62, 79, 80, 81, 95-97, 101, 103, 104, 112, 114-118, 122-130, 135, 177, 182, 184, 200, 209, 222, 227, 237, 240, 241, 243
Muscle activation patterns, 13, 28, 37, 80, 185, 240
Muscle classifications, 8-12
Muscle energy techniques- (MET)*, 35, 208, 209, 221 - Muscle energy techniques are active (requires patient utilization of force) and direct (engages the barrier) techniques that promote muscle relaxation by activating the golgi tendon reflex. It has also been proposed that temporary muscle fatigue blocks reflex-contraction thus allowing for an increase of range of motion to beyond the barrier. The purpose is to gain motion that is limited by restrictions of neuromuscular structures. There are several distinct techniques which may be called muscle energy techniques including reciprocal inhibition, and post-isometric relaxation.*

Muscles of the low back, 85
Muscle spindles, 34, 43, 46, 49, 50, 128, 289, 293
Muscle tension, 6, 8, 13, 41, 78, 79, 83, 122, 167, 207
Muscle testing, 24, 25, 27-28, 73, 75, 149, 176-177, 194, 197, 227-233

N

Non-weight bearing, 12, 140, 199, 248, 301
Nucleus, 82, 84, 86-88, 94, 151
Neuromuscular, 2, 3, 5-8, 10, 11, 13, 17, 22-26, 33-35, 37-40, 46, 47, 49, 53, 54, 56, 70, 79, 104, 145, 147, 148, 176, 177, 198, 234, 236, 239, 293
Neutral position, 81, 84, 94, 123, 130, 154, 172, 173, 200, 209
Nutation, 92, 106, 135, 136 - *The superior border of the sacrum rotates anteriorly.*

O

One leg standing, 152, 177, 302
Open chain, 10, 48, 61, 64, 76, 80, 82, 239, 248, 249 - *Exercises performed where the hand or foot is not fixed and does move. The hand/foot is free to move without contacting a surface.*

Origin, 95, 231
Osteophyte, 87, 198 – *A pathological bony outgrowth.*

P

Pain and exercise, 17
Pain and dysfunction cycle, 303
Pain patterns, 7, 92, 95, 96, 140
Pain questions, 25-26
Palpation, 21, 25, 27, 73-75, 110, 127, 128, 136, 149, 152, 168, 174-176, 183, 184, 186, 197, 212, 219, 226

Paraspinal muscles, 9, 56, 83, 95, 107, 115, 118, 120-128, 137, 139, 150, 152, 165, 213, 220, 228, - *All of the muscles along the spine vertically.*

Pelvic tilt, 42, 122, 136, 153, 156, 157, 163, 181, 184, 185, 194, 202, 205, 215-217, 223, 229, 232
Physical therapy, 22, 73, 75, 76, 122
Piriformis, 9, 12, 95-97, 101, 102, 110, 115, 120, 134-136, 138-140, 142, 149, 151, 164, 167, 169, 170, 175, 177, 190, 194, 198, 199, 202, 205, 207, 215, 222, 225, 233
Piriformis syndrome, 135-136, 138, 151 - *Pain in the low back, groin, buttocks, back of thigh and leg, foot, and in the rectum during defecation, swelling of the limb, sexual dysfunctions, tender piriformis to palpation, and pain and weakness against resisted thigh abduction at 90° hip flexion.*

Plyometrics, 55, 57, 58, 65, 121, 264, 271, 274, 275, 277 -*Exercises that promote a maximum muscular force in the shortest amount of time.*[267] *The unique quality of plyometrics is the fact that the transition phase (as well as the three other phases of power) is utilized with every exercise.*

PMAP - proper muscle activation patterns
PMAP, 13, 28, 37, 80, 185, 240
    hip abduction, 186
    hip extension, 185
    multifidus, 184
    transverse abdominis, 182-183

Posture, 1, 3, 5, 10, 13, 24-28, 46-47, 53, 56, 73, 74, 78, 84, 149, 153-164, 168, 194, 197, 198, 200-219, 243, 285, 286, 301, 302
PNF techniques – 2, 47-50, 52, 74, 76 - *Proprioceptive neuromuscular facilitation;* these techniques are mostly for the extremities

Post-rehabilitative, 2, 17, 75, 76, 78, 83, 104, 107, 197, 241 - *The program implemented after being cleared by and having worked with a licensed professional.*

occurs with aging. Often there is herniation of the nucleus pulposus of one or more intervertebral discs and/or the formation of osteophytes.

Squats, 187, 188, 194, 227, 234, 246, 247
Stabilizers
 local, 9-12, 15, 80, 237, 238, 240
 global, 9-12, 15, 59, 80, 237, 238, 244
Sub-acute, 1, 21, 22, 62, 63, 73, 76, 240, 244, 248
Symptomatic – *Having/showing signs of symptoms*
Synergistic Dominance, 3, 13, 41, 54, 108, 204 – *This occurs when a synergist compensates for a muscle that is weak or inhibited.*

T

Tensor fascia lata- *(TFL)*, 95, 96, 107, 110, 112, 132, 137-138, 140, 164, 171-174, 186, 194, 202, 204, 205, 207, 223, 225, 233
Thoracic spine exercises, 243
Tightness, 2, 4, 5, 7, 8, 25-27, 38, 39, 40, 41, 43, 75
Tissue healing times, 76
Torsion/twisting forces, 77, 88, 89, 94
Transverse abdominis- *(T.A.)*, 11, 13, 15, 80, 83, 95, 99, 102, 104-105, 179, 182-183, 188, 198
Trigger point- *(TP)*, 16 – *TP's are tender nodules in soft tissue within a palpable taut band that elicit a distinct referred pain pattern if digital pressure is applied or they are aggravated enough.*

U

Upper-crossed syndrome, 154-155, 163

V

Vertebrae, 86-89
Vibration, 93, 147

W

Warm-up, 39, 40, 42, 58, 70-72, 251, 252, 299
Weakness, 4, 7, 8, 10, 27, 28, 41-42, 46, 74, 303
Weightbearing, 10, 12, 50, 61, 78-80, 93, 102, 237-239, 241, 244-248, 250, 255

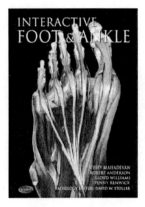 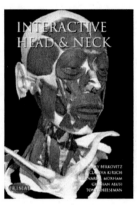 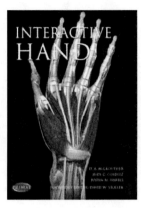 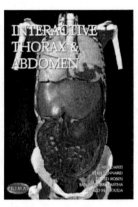
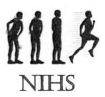